Handbook of Corticosteroids

Handbook of Corticosteroids

Edited by Bradlee Smith

STATES ACADEMIC PRESS
www.statesacademicpress.com

States Academic Press,
109 South 5th Street,
Brooklyn, NY 11249, USA

Visit us on the World Wide Web at:
www.statesacademicpress.com

ISBN: 978-1-63989-257-0

Cataloging-in-Publication Data

Handbook of corticosteroids / edited by Bradlee Smith.
p. cm.
Includes bibliographical references and index.
ISBN 978-1-63989-257-0
1. Adrenocortical hormones. 2. Steroid hormones. 3. Adrenal cortex. I. Smith, Bradlee.
QP188.A28 H36 2022
612.45--dc23

Table of Contents

Preface

The main aim of this book is to educate learners and enhance their research focus by presenting diverse topics covering this vast field. This is an advanced book which compiles significant studies by distinguished experts in the area of analysis. This book addresses successive solutions to the challenges arising in the area of application, along with it; the book provides scope for future developments.

Corticosteroids are a class of steroid hormones which are mainly produced in the adrenal cortex of the vertebrates but are also synthesized artificially. They ease redness, itching, swelling and allergic reactions. There are two main classes of corticosteroids that are involved in a wide range of physiological processes. These two classes are glucocorticoids and mineralocorticoids. Glucocorticoids have immunosuppressive, anti-inflammatory, vasoconstrictive and anti-proliferative effects, and they also affect carbohydrate and fat metabolism. Mineralocorticoids mainly regulate water and electrolyte balance by modulating ion transport. Some examples of naturally occurring steroids are aldosterone, corticosterone, cortisone and cortisol. This book presents the complex subject of corticosteroids in the most comprehensible and easy to understand language. Its objective is to give a general view of the different classes of corticosteroids. The topics covered in this book offer the readers new insights in this field.

It was a great honour to edit this book, though there were challenges, as it involved a lot of communication and networking between me and the editorial team. However, the end result was this all-inclusive book covering diverse themes in the field.

Finally, it is important to acknowledge the efforts of the contributors for their excellent chapters, through which a wide variety of issues have been addressed. I would also like to thank my colleagues for their valuable feedback during the making of this book.

Editor

1

Current Therapy in Autoimmune Bullous Diseases

Danka Svecova

Abstract

The goal of the treatment of autoimmune bullous disease is to reduce the production of pathogenic autoantibodies or increase elimination of pathogenic autoantibodies from serum of the patients. Immunosuppressive therapy reduces the production of autoantibodies. The therapy protocol is divided into three phases. The first is a control phase with the highest dose of immunosuppressive drugs suppressing activity of disease, followed with a consolidation phase, when the bulk of lesions is healed. The last phase is a maintenance phase when immunosuppressive medication is gradually tapered to the lowest level that suppresses the appearance of new lesions. In complete remission off therapy, the patient reached complete clinical remission and does not use any immunosuppressive medication. In complete remission on therapy, the patient uses a minimal immunosuppressive therapy. The first-line treatment is corticosteroids in pemphigus and pemphigoid groups. Adjuvant immunosuppressive drugs are combined with systemic corticosteroids and display a corticosteroid sparing effect. First-line immunosuppressive adjuvants comprise azathioprine, mycophenolate mofetil and mycophenolic acid. Rituximab, intravenous immunoglobulin G, immunoadsorption, cyclophosphamide, dapsone, and methotrexate are regarded as the second-line adjuvants. In dermatitis herpetiformis, a gluten free diet eliminates the clinical symptoms. Dapsone is regarded to be a valid therapeutic option in management of dermatitis herpetiformis.

Keywords: immunosuppressive therapy, corticosteroids, azathioprine, mycophenolate mofetil, cyclophosphamide, methotrexate, dapsone, rituximab, intravenous immunoglobulin G, immunoadsorption, tetracycline, gluten free diet

1. Introduction

Autoimmune bullous diseases belong to disorders that have low incidence but a high morbidity and mortality. Rupturing of blisters leads to painful erosions that cause significant loss of body fluid, electrolytes and proteins, especially in cases with extensive body surface involvement. If mucous membrane of the mouth, pharynx and esophagus are involved, the patient may not be able to tolerate adequate intake of food and medication. Erosions on the skin and mucosa can lead to secondary infections which may cause life-threatening events such as sepsis and cardiac failure. Autoimmune bullous diseases warrant the use of high dose of systemic corticosteroids and immunosuppressive drugs that may be associated with various adverse and other side effects. Moreover, considerable risk for serious systemic complications should be predicted.

Pemphigus vulgaris is a rare autoimmune bullous disease, but one of the most severe with the highest morbidity and mortality rates, and one requiring the highest doses of corticosteroids and adjuvant agents. Before the advent of systemic corticosteroids, the prognosis of pemphigus vulgaris was fatal within 2 years from diagnosis. The introduction of corticosteroids in the 1950s dramatically reduced mortality rates from around 70 to 30%. The use of adjuvant immunosuppressive agent in management of autoimmune bullous diseases in the 1960s decreases mortality rates to 10% [1]. Nowadays, it is estimated that mortality rates of pemphigus is in the range of 5–10% [2]. Among autoimmune bullous disease, the most frequent disorder is bullous pemphigoid. The mortality rate of bullous pemphigoid is age dependent and ranges in 2.43–9.5% [3]. A higher mortality is influenced by old age, widespread disease, high dose of oral corticosteroids and life-threatening comorbidities. Bullous pemphigoid has shown increasing incidence rates in recent decades, especially in Western societies. However, bullous pemphigoid rarely represents a life-threatening disease. In bullous pemphigoid, the risk factors that can evoke disease should be identified and eradicated. A provoking drug or underlying malignancy is the most frequent risk factors in bullous pemphigoid. In therapy management, many immunosuppressive drugs are contraindicated because of comorbidities or malignancy in the history.

The therapy modalities used to treat autoimmune bullous disease have different mechanisms affecting the pathophysiology of the disease. Some medications yield in suppression production of the pathogenic autoantibodies and some have anti-inflammatory activity. Immunosuppressive activity is used in the corticosteroids, azathioprine, mycophenolate mofetil, cyclophosphamide, methotrexate, and others. Medication with anti-inflammatory activity is aimed at suppressing the inflammatory process. The last group includes topical corticosteroids, dapsone and sulfonamides, as well as anti-inflammatory antibiotics. Immunoadsorption is another modality using the removal of the pathogenic autoantibodies and inflammatory mediators. A new biologic therapy is intravenous immunoglobulin G and rituximab, monoclonal antibody to transmembrane protein CD20 of B-cells. In general, immunosuppressive and anti-inflammatory medications are commonly utilized in various autoimmune bullous diseases. Dermatitis herpetiformis is one of the diseases with specific treatment regimen, namely a gluten free diet that may improve gluten reverses of underlying gluten-sensitive enteropathy and so the results in remission of the skin disease.

2. Management of autoimmune bullous diseases

Management of autoimmune bullous disease should start with initial evaluation of the disease and the patient's condition in order to evaluate the risk of complications developing from immunosuppressive therapy. The clinical diagnosis should be confirmed with the histopathology of the blister, direct immunofluorescence microscopy (DIF) of the perilesional skin, serological detection of autoantibodies by indirect immunofluorescence microscopy (IIF), enzyme-linked immunosorbent assay (ELISA), or immunoblot or immunoprecipitation.

The work-up before corticosteroid or immunosuppressive therapy should account for: a complete blood count, creatinine, urea, blood electrolytes, transaminases, gamma GT, alkaline phosphatase, total serum protein, albumin, glucose, hepatitis B, C and HIV, and chest X-ray. Optional examination predicting used medication includes analysis of thiopurine methyltransferase (TPMT) activity when azathioprine is considered; glucose-6-phosphate dehydrogenase (G6PD) serum activity, bilirubin, and reticulocytes if dapsone is recommended; and serum IgA deficiency should be ruled out prior to intravenous immunoglobulin therapy. Abdominal sonography is optional. QuantiFERONE or PPD is recommended where there is a risk of tuberculosis; a βhuman chorionic gonadotropin (βHCG) blood test is used to exclude pregnancy in women of childbearing age; osteodensitometry is recommended prior to corticosteroid therapy and periodically evaluated during the regimen; ophthalmological examination is performed prior to corticosteroid therapy and periodically repeated to exclude glaucoma and cataract.

A general examination should asses the patient's general condition including bodyweight, arterial blood pressure, and comorbidities such as cardiovascular, musculoskeletal or neoplastic, diabetes, etc.

Laboratory monitoring of pathogenic autoantibodies should be performed in autoimmune bullous diseases to predict outcome of the disease as well as to evaluate the efficacy of the employed therapy regimen.

In pemphigus patients, detection of pathogenic IgG antibodies by ELISA is positive in 90% of patients and correlates with disease activity. A quantitative evaluation of anti-Dsg3 and anti-Dsg1 IgG is evaluated using ELISA or IIF. Both methods can predict activity or curability of disorder. Determination of serum antibodies is performed on initiation of therapy, after 3 months and every 3–6 months based on disease activity and relapse [4]. Immunoblot and immunoprecipitation can also be used. In paraneoplastic pemphigus, the autoantibody to various antigens can be detected, including envoplakin, periplakin, desmocollin, desmoplakin, desmogleins, BP180 antigen, BP230 antigen, and plectin.

In patients with bullous pemphigoid, pathogenic anti-BP180 IgG autoantibodies are evaluated by ELISA or IIF. A quantitative evaluation should be monitored at days 0, 60, and 150 during treatment. A negative anti-BP180 IgG antibody at day 150 has a good predictive value of durable remission in approximately 90% [5].

In patients with dermatitis herpetiformis, pathogenic autoantibodies are IgA against tissue transglutaminase (anti-tTG) and IgA against endomysia (primate smooth muscle reticular connective tissue, EMA). Tissue transglutaminase (tTG) antigens share a 64% homology with epidermal transglutaminase, which is the target antigen in dermatitis herpetiformis. Detection by ELISA anti-tTG IgA is positive in 90% of patients with dermatitis herpetiformis. Detection of EMA IgA antibody uses IIF and is positive in 100% of patients with dermatitis herpetiformis [6]. Both markers are useful in detection of bowel damage and gluten-free diet compliance in patients with dermatitis herpetiformis and they disappear, if a gluten-free diet is strictly adherent. In general, monitoring of autoantibodies reflect patient's adherence to a gluten-free diet. Serological evaluation is sensitive to detecting major but not minor failure in diet.

Therapy protocol of pemphigus group diseases and pemphigoid diseases is divided into three phases, based on the activity of the disease. The first is the induction phase, followed by a consolidation phase and then a maintenance phase. During the induction phase, control of disease should be established usually by a high dose of immunosuppressant agent, mostly corticosteroids. Bullous disease usually responds to treatment within 2 weeks, provided the correct dose is used. In the consolidation phase, the dropped dose of medication is used until the bulk of lesions have been healed. Slow healing is an indicator that the dose of medication is inadequate and should be boosted. The maintenance phase begins once most lesions have been healed (80%). The rate of medication tapering is based on clinical improvement of the disease and the physician's experience. If new lesions (one to five) appear while medication is tapering, these can be treated with high potency topical or intralesional corticosteroid, while maintaining patients on their current dose of systemic medications. If many new lesions appear, the dose of corticosteroids should be increased in 25–50% increments until control of disease is achieved. In most patients, the healing is slow, often requiring a period of 1–3 months for complete clearance of lesions. Discontinuation of immunosuppressive therapy may be proposed if complete remission is achieved with a low dose of systemic corticosteroid (prednisolone ≤10 mg/day) for a period of 6–12 months. Remission should be supported by negative DIF data. DIF data is a sensitive method for autoantibody detection in tissue in active disease, as well as in remission. Furthermore, DIF data correlate with the immunological activity of the disease. Patients with a higher autoantibody titer and positive DIF data are likely to experience disease relapse. In pemphigus group, the titer of autoantibodies correlates with disease activity, while not so closely in the bullous pemphigoid group, but also is used in monitoring.

The aim of treatment is to suppress disease activity with the minimum dose of drug necessary to induce complete remission, with minimum dose resulting in minimum adverse events, allowing all therapies to be discontinued. Duration of different treatment regimens is not standardized, ranging from 1 to 5 years or even longer. Long-term treatment leads to a high accumulation of corticosteroids and adjuvant drugs, leading to the development of adverse events from all used medications. In general, minimizing potential adverse effects of corticosteroids could be managed by agent that reduces osteoporosis and antacids, following a diet low in sugar and salt. In methotrexate protocol, the bone marrow depression could be reduced with folic acid. It is also important to reduce risk factors such as bacterial or viral infections, sun exposure and radiation therapy, large dental procedure, and psychical stress. In dermatitis herpetiformis, the most preferred precaution is to avoid a diet failure. Physicians and patients should be aware that autoimmune bullous diseases may not require lifelong treatment. However, patients with autoimmune bullous diseases should be monitored in their clinical remission and blood analysis for autoantibody detection. Both help to evaluate the risk of disease flaring up.

3. Systemic treatment of pemphigus group

3.1. Systemic induction therapy

Systemic induction therapy should be started with systemic immunosuppressive medication in combination with topical antiseptic agents and possible topical corticosteroids. Only in exceptional cases of limited disease and minor severity, monotherapy with topical corticosteroids or with topical calcineurin inhibitors may be considered. However, patient clinical symptoms and the presence of autoantibody level should be evaluated.

Corticosteroids are the mainstay therapy in management of mild to severe disease of all subtypes of pemphigus due to their rapid effects, resulting in a significant improvement in morbidity and mortality rates. Corticosteroids are regarded as a first-line treatment for initial management of pemphigus. Prednisolone equivalent of 0.5–1.5 mg/kg/day is recommended as the initial dose in induction therapy, depending on disease severity, patient age, and comorbidities. To control pemphigus foliaceus, generally, lower doses than that of pemphigus vulgaris are required. If the control of the disease is not achieved within 2 weeks, a higher prednisolone equivalent up to 2.0 mg/kg/day is optional. In severe and recalcitrant disease, a daily dose above 100 mg should be utilized intravenously in pulse therapy mode. Doses of pulse therapy are not standardized. Methylprednisolone 10–20 mg/kg/day (250–1000 mg) is administered every day on 3 consecutive days in intervals of 3–4 weeks, subsequently for 6–8 weeks [7]. Another choice is to use dexamethasone 2–5 mg/kg (50–200 mg). The aim of pulsing is to achieve more rapid and effective disease control compared with conventional oral dosing. However, adverse effects are common and dose related. The dosing schedule is advocated according to disease severity. Patients with mild disease are treated with initial prednisolone equivalent 40–60 mg/day, and more severe cases with 60–100 mg/day. If the patient does not respond within 5–7 days, the dose should be increased in 50–100% increments until disease control is achieved. When a patient does not respond well to systemic prednisolone therapy even at higher doses, the change of prednisolone to other oral corticosteroid (e.g., betamethasone, dexamethasone or methylprednisolone) might improve patient's condition [8]. Autoantibody titers fall with clinical healing, but the decrease of autoantibody titer is slower than clinical improvement.

Systemic corticosteroids can be combined with an immunosuppressive adjuvant agent at the start of therapy, especially in individuals with increased risk of corticosteroid-related side effects (**Table 1**). However, the addition of an adjuvant agent in induction therapy was not exactly confirmed and documented. Adjuvant drugs are usually administered in combination with a systemic corticosteroid to reduce related adverse and side effects and increase the immunosuppressive efficacy of medication. Their corticosteroid-sparing effect may lead to corticosteroid-free remission. If an adjuvant agent is utilized at the induction phase of treatment combined with corticosteroid, its efficacy should be expected in within approximately 1 month, depending on the specific adjuvant drug. Some authorities believe that the time to induce remission is shorter in high dose oral prednisolone monotherapy than with low dose oral prednisolone combined with an adjuvant drug. Moreover, rapidly progressive lesions necessitate a high dose of corticosteroid for early and adequate control of the disease. However, the significantly higher dose directly correlates to increased rates of treatment-associated adverse events. Therapy-related side and adverse effects and complications should be expected in prolonged administration of more than 4 months or at prednisolone dose ≥10 mg/day [1].

In severe and refractory cases, the induction therapy can be started with second-line adjuvant agents' rituximab, intravenous immunoglobulins or by immunoadsorption.

First-line therapy	Dose initial therapy
Prednisolone	0.5–1.5 mg/kg/day
Second-line therapy (first-line adjuvant agent)	
Azathioprine	1–3 mg/kg/day
Mycophenolate mofetil	2 g/day
Mycophenolic acid	1440 mg/day
Third-line therapy (second-line adjuvant agent)	
Cyclophosphamide	500 m i.v. bolus or 2 mg/kg/day orally
Methotrexate	10–20 mg/week
Dapsone	100 mg/day or up to ≤1.5 mg/kg/day
Anti-CD20 monoclonal antibody (rituximab)	2 × 1 g i.v. (2 weeks apart) or 4 × 375 mg/m^2 (each 1 week apart)
Intravenous immunoglobulin G	2 g/kg/4 weeks i.v.
Immunoadsorption	2 cycles a 4 days, 4 weeks apart
Pemphigus herpetiformis	
Dapsone + prednisolone	100–300 mg/day + low dose of prednisolone
IgA pemphigus	
Dapsone + prednisolone	100–300 mg/day + low dose of prednisolone
Acitretin	50 mg/day

First-line therapy uses systemic corticosteroid that has rapid immunosuppressive efficacy. Second-line therapy is used in refractory disease or in contraindications to systemic corticosteroids. First-line adjuvant agents have corticosteroid-sparing effect. Second-line adjuvant agents are used in refractory disease or in contraindications to first-line adjuvant agents.

Table 1. Systemic treatment of pemphigus group.

3.2. Systemic consolidation therapy

Systemic consolidation therapy in pemphigus vulgaris starts as soon as control of disease activity is achieved and approximately 80% of lesions are healed. Tapering of the corticosteroid can start by approximately 25% of the dose at 7–14-days intervals. If tapering reached a prednisolone equivalent of 20 mg/day, slower tapering at 2- to 4-week intervals is recommended. If relapse of the disease develops in the consolidation phase, systemic corticosteroid dose should be returned to two reduction intervals before. If control of disease activity is achieved within 14 days, tapering of corticosteroid can continue. If control of disease activity is not achieved, it is recommended to return to the initial systemic corticosteroid dose [1, 7].

Immunosuppressive efficacy of systemic corticosteroid is enhanced, if combination with other immunosuppressive adjuvant is used, including azathioprine, mycophenolate mofetil, cyclophosphamide, methotrexate or dapsone. Most adjuvant immunosuppressive drugs act more slowly than corticosteroids and their efficacy manifests within several weeks. Therefore, adjuvant agents are most frequently utilized after control of disease activity is achieved.

3.3. Systemic maintenance therapy

In the systemic maintenance phase, systemic corticosteroid is gradually tapering to the lowest level that suppresses the appearance of new lesions, with the goal being to discontinue all medications eventually. If a patient is treated with two or more immunosuppressive drugs, these should be tapered one at a time. Corticosteroid tapering continues from the consolidation phase and other immunosuppressive agents should be tapered later. Tapering too rapidly increases the chance of relapse, while tapering too slowly may lead to medication-related side effects. In complete remission on therapy, the patient receives minimal therapy, i.e., less than 10 mg/day prednisolone and/or minimal adjuvant therapy for at least 2 months. Minimal adjuvant therapy is defined as half of the initial dose. The systemic corticosteroid dose is reduced by approximately 25% at 7 to 14 days and gradual conversion to an alternate day schedule once the daily dose is at 10–8 mg. The rate of medication tapering is based on the clinical outcome and physician's experience. If autoantibody does not continue to fall and new lesions (one to three) appear while medication is being tapered, new lesions could be treated with intralesional or highly potent topical corticosteroid while maintaining the patients on their current dose of systemic medications [9]. The appearance of three to five lesions in a month that do not heal spontaneously within 1 week is regarded to be a relapse of disease in the maintenance phase. The dose of medication should be returned to the dose given two reduction intervals before until control of the disease is achieved.

Remission on minimal maintenance dose, negative autoantibody level, and negative DIF data are indicating markers for discontinuation of immunosuppressive medication. It is recommended to control the DIF data, if the patient is on a minimal maintenance dose for about 6–12 months with total clinical clearance [1]. Healthy skin from the sacral area not irradiated by the sun and covered with suits is a suitable sample for DIF. In addition, discontinuation of medication can ultimately be compassed in most patients. The proportion of patients in whom discontinuation of immunosuppressive therapy can be achieved increases steadily with time, and it can be discontinued in approximately 50% of patients after 3 years and in 75% of patients after 10 years [10, 11].

Prolonged treatment lead to high cumulative doses of corticosteroids and adjuvant drugs and medication-related side and adverse effects.

3.4. Adjuvant drugs

The application of adjuvant drugs into the therapy regimen of autoimmune bullous skin disorders allows the period of high dose corticosteroids application to be shortened. Adjuvant drugs have a corticosteroid-sparing effect, following with a decrease of corticosteroid-related side and adverse effects and an increase in the immunosuppressive efficacy of the regimen. Recently, several adjuvant agents have been utilized as an initial treatment in combination with corticosteroids.

3.4.1. Azathioprine

Among adjuvant agents, azathioprine is regarded as a first-line adjuvant with corticosteroid-sparing efficacy, most frequently used to treat autoimmune bullous disease including pemphigus. Azathioprine is a purine analog with specific activity to lymphocytes and is more selective for T-cells than B-cells [12]. Azathioprine interferes with purine synthesis and metabolism, leading to delayed action of drug, as it usually takes at least 1–2 months [13].

Extensive experience with azathioprine refers to good efficacy, tolerability and safety profiles. One study compared four regimens in 120 patients with pemphigus vulgaris. The efficacy of prednisolone was enhanced, when the drug was combined with an immunosuppressive adjuvant. Among adjuvants, azathioprine showed the highest corticosteroid-sparing effect. Other compared adjuvants were mycophenolate mofetil, intravenous cyclophosphamide, and prednisolone alone. In general, azathioprine is believed to be more effective than corticosteroid alone, both in terms of mortality and morbidity rates [14]. Another review evaluated 20 clinical studies comprehending data of 826 patients with pemphigus vulgaris and pemphigus foliaceus and confirmed the very good corticosteroid-sparing effect of azathioprine better than cyclophosphamide. However, azathioprine did not increase the remission rate [15]. The next review evaluated 10 clinical studies that comprehended data of 559 participants treated with various adjuvants, including azathioprine, mycophenolate mofetil, cyclophosphamide, intravenous immunoglobulins, plasma exchange and infliximab. All adjuvants collectively decreased the risk of relapse by 29%, but all of them did not increase the remission rate [16]. The corticosteroid-sparing effect of azathioprine was also confirmed in a review study of 11 studies with 404 participants [17].

The activity of thiopurine methyltransferase (TPMT) should be evaluated before the beginning of therapy with azathioprine. Decreased activity of TPMT takes place in induction of an adverse event. In the Japanese population, an adverse event of azathioprine was associated with gene mutation of inosine triphosphate pyrophosphohydrolase (ITPA), another enzyme metabolizing azathioprine [18]. It is recommended to start therapy with a low initial dose of azathioprine 50 mg/day to detect idiosyncratic reactions. If the activity of TPMT shows normal levels, the dose can be increased to 1–3 mg/kg/day depending on the clinical outcome. If TPMT activity shows an intermediate or low level, it should be applied in a lower dose up to 0.5–1.5 mg/kg/day. Patients with insufficiency of TMPT activity are at risk and should not be treated with azathioprine because they may experience rapid bone marrow suppression after initiation of therapy. Furthermore, some patients may experience complications despite normal TPMT activity. All patients at risk of severe toxicity should undergo close monitoring of clinical and hematologic parameters, including liver enzyme levels. Likewise, an abrupt increase in liver enzymes observed soon after administration of azathioprine is a clue to deficient TPMT activity. In addition, concurrent therapy with TPMT-inhibiting drugs, such as allopurinol or sulfasalazine, can also increase the risk of myelotoxicity [19].

If the clinical outcome improves, the lowest effective dosage should be administered. If no improvement occurs within 3 months, the drug should be withdrawn and changed for another adjuvant agent. However, in patients who achieve improvement in clinical outcome, care should be taken in monitoring for myelosuppression and hepatotoxicity. It is strictly recommended to monitor the full blood count weekly over a period of 8 weeks, then at a minimum of once every 3 months. In addition, liver functions should be monitored.

Adverse drug reactions with azathioprine occur in 15–30% of patients and include leucopenia, thrombocytopenia, anemia, pancytopenia, and hepatotoxicity [13]. Long-lasting immunosuppression increases the risk of infections and only a minor increase of neoplasia, mostly lymphoma [20]. In addition, alopecia, rash or gastrointestinal disturbances (nausea, vomiting, anorexia, diarrhea, aphthous stomatitis, and pancreatitis) can be observed. In pregnancy and breastfeeding, azathioprine is contraindicated due to the risk to the child [21].

Extensive experience with azathioprine refers to good efficacy and safety profile and the drug is recommended as a first-line adjuvant agent with corticosteroid-sparing immunosuppressive in the second line of treatment in moderate to severe pemphigus vulgaris and pemphigus foliaceus, and other types of pemphigus.

3.4.2. Mycophenolate mofetil and mycophenolic acid

Mycophenolate mofetil is an esterified prodrug of mycophenolic acid. Both belong to first-line adjuvants. Mycophenolic acid is an active metabolite that selectively inhibits inosine monophosphate dehydrogenase, an enzyme involved in *de novo* synthesis of quanosine nucleotides. Mycophenolate mofetil inhibits T-cells and B-cells proliferation, and antibody production by B-cells [22]. The induction of disease remission often requires at least 8 weeks of treatment.

One study compared combined therapy of corticosteroid with mycophenolate mofetil or azathioprine. Both adjuvants demonstrated similar efficacy, sparing effect, and safety profiles [23]. Very good efficacy was demonstrated in 18 patients with pemphigus vulgaris treated with mycophenolate mofetil using a conventional dose, with 89% of them achieving complete disease control. The average time to achieve 75% clearance of lesions was 4.5 months. Three patients discontinued all immunosuppressive therapy, including mycophenolate mofetil, in an average of 3 years [24]. Another review of 11 clinical studies comprehended data of 404 patients with pemphigus vulgaris and pemphigus foliaceus and evaluated mycophenolate mofetil as more effective in achieving disease control than azathioprine [17]. Mycophenolate mofetil is regarded to be less myelosuppressive and hepatotoxic than azathioprine [20].

Adverse drug reactions include especially gastrointestinal events such as diarrhea, nausea, vomiting, following with infections, leucopenia, and anemia. Hematologic findings are dose-related and reversible. In general, mycophenolate mofetil is well-tolerated and serious adverse effects are rarely observed. The recommended dose of mycophenolate mofetil is 0.5–2 g/day or mycophenolic acid at 1440 mg/day. However, increasing the daily dose by 1 capsule (500 mg) per week is recommended until the final dose of 2 g/day to evoke better gastrointestinal tolerance. Enteric-coated mycophenolate sodium was prepared to minimize gastrointestinal side effects and improve quality-of-life and compliance to treatment [25]. Mycophenolate mofetil is contraindicated in pregnancy because of the increased risk of miscarriage and congenital malformations [21]. Mizoribine is a newly developed immunosuppressive agent affecting purine synthesis similar to mycophenolate mofetil and can be utilized in patients with autoimmune bullous diseases, including pemphigus vulgaris [26]. It is suspected that mizoribine would have lower toxicity and higher tolerability than other immunosuppressants, such as azathioprine or cyclosporine.

Mycophenolate mofetil displayed a very good safety and efficacy profile as a first-line adjuvant agent and could replace azathioprine as an antimetabolite adjuvant of choice in the second-line treatment of many autoimmune and inflammatory diseases, including moderate to severe pemphigus vulgaris and pemphigus foliaceus as well as other types of pemphigus.

3.4.3. Cyclophosphamide

Cyclophosphamide is a second-line adjuvant agent that can be utilized when first-line adjuvant agents fail to evoke remission or a corticosteroid-sparing effect. Cyclophosphamide is an alkylating agent with highly effective immunosuppressive activity. It alkylates DNA at various positions, resulting in cell cycle arrest, DNA repair, and apoptosis. Proliferating tissues with a high mitotic rate are the most susceptible to cyclophosphamide. However, its activity is not cell cycle-dependent. Both cellular and humoral immunity is suppressed [27]. The toxicity is significantly higher than that of azathioprine and therefore it is reserved for the most severe and refractory diseases.

Several studies demonstrated that oral cyclophosphamide is an effective adjuvant in the treatment of severe and refractory pemphigus vulgaris and pemphigus foliaceus in dose 2–2.5 mg/kg/day each morning followed by massive oral hydration of at least 2–3 L of fluids [28]. One retrospective study evaluated therapy in 101 patients with pemphigus vulgaris. Authors compared oral cyclophosphamide, azathioprine, and cyclosporine. Cyclophosphamide was evaluated as the drug with the best remission and relapse rates [29]. Another comparative study of 16 patients with pemphigus vulgaris showed a faster onset of activity in cyclophosphamide than azathioprine, but the evaluation of efficacy in both did not differ [30]. One prospective study of 11 patients with pemphigus compared dexamethasone-cyclophosphamide pulse therapy with oral corticosteroid (methylprednisolone)-azathioprine therapy in conventional doses and failed to find significant benefits between these two regimens, besides fewer recurrences in pulse therapy with cyclophosphamide [31]. Cyclophosphamide showed a very good corticosteroid-sparing effect [29].

Several dosing schedules have been developed to minimize cumulative dose and susceptibility to adverse events. These include monthly intravenous administration (500 mg) in conjugation with low oral dose daily between infusions (2.0 mg/kg/day). A single dose of intravenous immunoablative therapy can also be used. However, daily oral cyclophosphamide results in the highest cumulative dose. On the other hand, continuous daily exposure provides optimal immunosuppression. In severe recalcitrant pemphigus vulgaris, a combined regimen of pulsed intravenous cyclophosphamide with corticosteroid could be used. The pulse regimen consists of the intermittent administration of a high dose of corticosteroid and cyclophosphamide, usually as three daily doses of corticosteroid (dexamethasone 100 mg or methylprednisolone 500–1000 mg) and a single dose of cyclophosphamide (500 mg). Such corticosteroid-cyclophosphamide pulses can be administered once a month over a period of several months. Between these pulses, the patient receives cyclophosphamide 2 mg/kg/day.

In cyclophosphamide therapy, adverse events are frequent, including hemorrhagic cystitis and high susceptibility to infection. Mutagenic activity increases an individual's lifetime risk for transitional cell carcinoma of the bladder and hematologic malignancies. This risk is proportional to the cumulative dose of the drug. Moreover, acute myelosuppression can be developed in 6–10 days and recovered in 14–21 days after discontinuation of cyclophosphamide.

However, another adverse gastrointestinal event may develop, including mucosal ulcers, nausea, vomiting, stomach pain, and diarrhea. Potential gonadal toxicity is associated with amenorrhea, azoospermia, and infertility [19]. In addition, cardiotoxicity, hepatotoxicity, interstitial lung fibrosis, darkening of the skin and nails, alopecia, changes to hair color and texture, and lethargy may develop.

The efficacy and safety profile raised cyclophosphamide as a second-line adjuvant drug of choice in the third line of treatment in severe and refractory pemphigus vulgaris and pemphigus foliaceus.

3.4.4. Methotrexate

Methotrexate was primarily developed to treat malignancies. Recently, methotrexate has been used as an immunosuppressive and anti-inflammatory agent. Methotrexate is a folate antagonist that competitively inhibits dihydrofolate reductase, resulting in blocking of several folate-dependent enzymes integral to DNA synthesis. The synthesis of purine and pyrimidine nucleotides is involved, which in turn is necessary for synthesis of DNA and RNA. The drug affects the S-phase of the cell cycle, thus inhibiting rapidly proliferating cells, including malignant, hematopoietic, and mucosal [32]. However, methotrexate inhibits cell proliferation especially at higher doses. At lower doses, the drug has anti-inflammatory activity. The mechanism of anti-inflammatory activity is not fully understood. It could be mediated via a pathway separate from folate antagonism. The drug may evoke the inhibition of polyamines, resulting in a net increase in intracellular and extracellular adenosine. Adenosine is a purine nucleoside with potent anti-inflammatory effect on many different target cells [32, 33].

Methotrexate was the first adjuvant drug to be combined with corticosteroid in the management of autoimmune bullous diseases. A retrospective analysis of 7 clinical studies evaluated the efficacy of methotrexate in 116 patients with pemphigus vulgaris. Of those, 83% showed clinical improvement. Fourteen patients achieved total remission and were off therapy by a mean of 2.6 years after discontinuation of methotrexate and systemic corticosteroid. Nausea and infection were the most frequent side effects and one patient died due to bronchopneumonia [34].

At present, a methotrexate dose of 10–20 mg/week is used orally to treat autoimmune bullous diseases, including pemphigus vulgaris. A test dose of 2.5–5 mg is recommended at the initiation of therapy. If the drug is tolerated, the dose can be escalated to the therapeutic dose. Methotrexate has good oral bioavailability and is akin to parenteral administration. However, interindividual absorption variability exists. Therefore, in patients with an inadequate answer to oral administration, a switch to intramuscular dosing is recommended. Folic acid is used to decrease the deleterious side effects of methotrexate and can be used the next day in a dose of 1–5 mg or daily. Folic acid supplementation can prevent folate deficiency, improving tolerance and preventing anemia, neutropenia, stomatitis, and oral ulcers. Methotrexate is a corticosteroid-sparing agent with delayed, beneficial effect on oral lesions, whereas the cutaneous lesions usually respond very well and rapidly. Methotrexate may interact with nonsteroidal anti-inflammatory drugs, trimethoprim-sulfamethoxazole, sulfasalazine and phenytoin, resulting in increased time to eliminate methotrexate. These interactions may result in severe bone marrow toxicity. Adverse events involving methotrexate are usually mild and self-limiting or preventable. When an adverse event occurs, the dosage should be decreased or withdrawn. In a relatively brief time, the adverse effects may consolidate in a normal condition. The most frequent adverse effects include nausea, anorexia, vomiting, diarrhea, fatigue, and malaise. Fatigue and nausea may be minimized by taking the drug before bedtime and by folic acid supplementation. In general, adverse effects are dose-dependent and usually appear around the initiation of therapy. A serious adverse event is myelosuppression, which can develop in patients with potential risk factors like renal insufficiency, senescence, concomitant serious illness or infection, drug overdose or drug interaction. In severe cases, myelosuppression is considered a potentially fatal condition, but usually improves after dose reduction or withdrawal. Mucositis is regarded as precursor of developing pancytopenia, and should be taken seriously. Patients with significant pancytopenia (WB ≤ 3000, Hg ≤ 11, platelets ≤ 50,000) should be treated immediately with intravenous leucovorin (folinic acid), the antidote to methotrexate, that is able to bypass dihydrofolate reductase [35]. In addition, hepatotoxicity, resulting in fibrosis and cirrhosis, is a serious adverse event associated with long-term administration of methotrexate, when the cumulative dose reached 9.5–26 g [34]. Obesity, diabetes mellitus and excessive alcohol consumption are regarded as risk factors for liver toxicity. According to the Manchester protocol, serum procollagen III aminopeptide (PIIINP) assay may be used to monitor liver toxicity resulting from methotrexate toxicity [36]. If PIIINP assay is not approachable, some authors predict a liver biopsy. A liver biopsy is recommended when the total cumulative dose reaches 3.5–4.0 g [37]. Monitoring of liver function and bone marrow is recommended to be repeated regularly to avoid myelosuppression and hepatotoxicity. Methotrexate is contraindicated in pregnancy due to its teratogenic and abortifacient properties. Moreover, it causes reproductive toxicity and decreases the sperm account [38]. Mucocutaneous toxicity occurs more commonly in patients without adequate folic acid supplementation. In severe cases, it can be associated with diarrhea and myelosuppression. Mucocutaneous toxicity can start with mucositis or very painful oral ulceration. More rarely, ulceration of the skin could be an early harbinger of methotrexate toxicity.

Methotrexate is a corticosteroid sparing agent and is recommended as a second-line adjuvant in the third-line treatment of moderate to severe pemphigus vulgaris and pemphigus foliaceus. The drug is relatively inexpensive.

3.4.5. Dapsone

Dapsone is a sulfone-derived drug that primarily possesses both antimicrobial and antiprotozoal activities. Additionally, dapsone has anti-inflammatory properties like non-steroidal anti-inflammatory drugs. Dapsone suppresses neutrophilic infiltration by inhibition of neutrophil activation and recruitment through many different pathways [39].

One multicenter randomized, double blind study confirmed the glucocorticoid-sparing efficacy of dapsone in 19 patients with pemphigus vulgaris. Seventy-three percent of patients treated with dapsone achieved remission [40]. A retrospective review study analyzed 35 case series and case reports comprehending data of 427 patients with autoimmune bullous disease. Among them were 55 patients with pemphigus (32 patients with pemphigus vulgaris and 14 with pemphigus foliaceus). Dapsone was evaluated as an effective and useful corticosteroid-sparing agent in therapy of autoimmune bullous disease, including pemphigus. Adverse events were dose-dependent and reversible. The most frequent adverse event was hemolysis and concomitant anemia secondary to hemolysis [41].

The recommended dose of dapsone is 100 mg/day or up to ≤1.5 mg/kg/day. Prior to start dapsone therapy, glucose-6-phosphate dehydrogenase deficiency should be excluded, and cell blood counts, renal and liver functions must be examined. During dapsone therapy, cell blood counts including reticulocyte, leukocyte and platelet, and the level of methemoglobin, should be regularly monitored. It is recommended to start dapsone therapy with a low dose of 0.5 mg/kg/day. If the drug is tolerated, the dose can escalate slowly up to the effective dose [39]. A rapid enhancement of medication may result in a severe hemolytic anemia. Adverse events are dose-dependent and transient. However, frequent adverse effects include hemolytic anemia and methemoglobinemia which may necessitate halting treatment. A high dose of vitamin C supplementation can evoke better tolerability of dapsone, including a drop in the methemoglobin level. In addition, headache is a common adverse event. More serious complications are hepatitis, hypersensitivity syndrome and agranulocytosis. Peripheral neuropathy is a rare adverse event and may involve both motor and sensory nerves [39]. Most complications are referred in the first 3 months of treatment. Precaution should by mentioned in the second trimester of pregnancy, when dapsone should be reduced or stopped. If dapsone is not tolerated, it could be replaced with other sulfonamides, e.g., sulfapyridine (1.5 g/day) or sulfamethoxypyridazine (0.25–1.5 g/day). In addition, sulfonamides are contraindicated in breastfeeding women because they may induce hemolytic anemia in an infant.

Dapsone is recommended as a second-line adjuvant agent to treat mild to severe pemphigus vulgaris and pemphigus foliaceus, especially in the maintenance phase of their management. The drug is a corticosteroid-sparing agent recommended with either low or intermediate doses of systemic corticosteroid and may allow tapering or discontinuation of corticosteroid doses. Dapsone is regarded as a third-line therapy in pemphigus diseases.

3.4.6. Anti-CD20 monoclonal antibody (rituximab)

Rituximab is a murine/human chimeric monoclonal antibody, targeting the CD20 molecule found on the cell surface of B-cells of various maturate stages up to the preplasma cell stage. Stem cells or B-cell progenitors, plasmablasts, and plasma cells, do not express the CD20 molecule and do not respond to rituximab. Among several mechanisms involved in pathophysiology of autoimmune bullous disease, rituximab exerts B-cell cytotoxic activity mainly through antibody-dependent cell-mediated cytotoxicity, resulting in depletion of B-cells that presumably produce pathogenic antibodies. Depletion of B-cells persists in circulation for 6–12 months. However, after the rituximab treatment, the B-cell count returns to normal levels. Even so, replacement of B-cells is not associated with relapse in a considerable number of patients with autoimmune disease. These data suggest that rituximab-mediated depletion of B-cells may influence also other cells participating in immune tolerance and homeostasis. In addition, the depletion of B-cells may participate in decreasing resistance against infection. One study demonstrated a significant reduction of T regulatory cells after rituximab therapy. This event may be due to increased skin homing of these cells [42].

Primarily, rituximab was used for treating non-Hodgkin's B-cell lymphoma. The use of rituximab in pemphigus began after a marked improvement in lymphoma-associated paraneoplastic pemphigus [43]. Rituximab has a late onset of action to control acute disease and produces an initial clinical response in 69 weeks or less. It should therefore, be used as an adjuvant agent combined with systemic corticosteroids and/or another adjuvant agent. Two FDA protocols for rituximab management can be used to treat autoimmune bullous disease, including pemphigus. The lymphoma protocol utilizes four infusions of rituximab 375 mg/m^2 given in four consecutive weeks, a week apart. The rheumatoid arthritis protocol uses two infusions at a dose of 1 g, given 2 weeks apart. Even though both protocols are effective, the rheumatoid arthritis protocol could prove better because both rheumatoid arthritis and pemphigus are autoimmune diseases. One retrospective review report evaluated 42 clinical studies comprehending data of 272 patients with pemphigus vulgaris who have been treated with rituximab. Data of the review study showed that a complete remission was achieved in 66.6% of patients on the lymphoma protocol and 75% on the rheumatoid arthritis protocol within an 18-month follow-up. During this period, 11.1% of patients treated with the lymphoma protocol achieved remission and were off therapy and 33.3% on minimal immunosuppressive therapy. Meanwhile, on the rheumatoid arthritis protocol, 53.3% of patients achieved remission off therapy and 17.4% on minimal immunosuppressive therapy. A partial response was observed in 12.8% of patients on the lymphoma protocol, and in 23.9% of patients on the rheumatoid arthritis protocol. The relapse rates were 22.8% on the lymphoma protocol and 35.9% on the rheumatoid arthritis protocol. The incidence of serious infections was 3.9% on the lymphoma protocol and 15.2% on the rheumatoid arthritis protocol. The mortality rate on the lymphoma protocol was 2.2% and 1.1% on the rheumatoid arthritis protocol [44]. Remarkable differences were observed in patient's response between both protocols. At present, the reason for protocol differences cannot be detected. Rituximab has a corticosteroid-sparing effect. In the future, a modified protocol for autoimmune bullous disease should be designed and evaluated. Some patients can develop resistance and do not respond to the rituximab regimen. The resistance can be due to the autoantibody to rituximab that interferes with drug binding or the pharmacokinetics of the drug could be changed by other ways.

Intravenous administration of rituximab should be initiated with premedication before each infusion using an antipyretic, e.g., paracetamol 1000 mg orally, or antihistamine. Prior to the first infusion, prednisolone 100 mg orally is advised. Rituximab infusion should be administered over 4–5 h. One cycle of rituximab may be repeated. Pathological lesions start to heal within just a few weeks after the first rituximab infusion and maximal effect can be expected after 3–4 months. Remission rates after the first-treatment cycle reached 76%. Repeating treatment further increased the remission rates to 91% [45].

Rituximab is generally well tolerated, and serious adverse effects are rare. Infusion-related reactions include anaphylaxis, hypotension, fever, chills, headache, weakness, nausea, pruritus and rash. Infusion-related reactions could be ameliorated by premedication before each infusion, then by decelerating or temporarily stopping of infusion. In addition, deep venous thrombosis of the lower limb and pulmonary embolism are serious complications. A frequent adverse event is the infection afflicting around 30% of patients, with a larger account of bacterial than viral infections. Moreover, herpes zoster is reported in several cases. Higher rates of infection could be influenced by concomitant treatment with an immunosuppressive agent, including corticosteroids. Another serious adverse event may accompany rituximab treatment like *Pneumocystis carinii* infection causing pneumonia or septic shock, which may cause death.

In addition, rituximab is an effective drug in controlling recalcitrant disease and is recommended as the second-line adjuvant to treat severe refractory autoimmune bullous diseases, including pemphigus vulgaris, pemphigus foliaceus and pemphigus paraneoplastic. Complications such as fatal infections and other serious adverse events place the drug to the last resort treatment restricted for severe and refractory cases. Rituximab is recommended when other second-line adjuvant agents, including immunoadsorption and intravenous immunoglobulins, fail in the treatment or patients have multiple relapses. Despite the threat of serious adverse events, several reports would like to recommend rituximab as a first-line treatment accompanied with low dose of corticosteroids in patients with moderate to severe pemphigus [46]. The regimen proved effective and caused fewer adverse events than the regimen using corticosteroids alone [47]. First-line treatment with rituximab should be regarded in pemphigus patients, who are contraindicated to corticosteroid and other immunosuppressive therapy [47–49]. In near future, a new protocol for pemphigus patients should be elaborated and confirmed in clinical trials. Another study recommended rituximab combined with intravenous immunoglobulins as a first-line therapy in severe and refractory pemphigus. This regimen can evoke prolonged remission and could be used when corticosteroids and immunosuppressive adjuvants are contraindicated [50].

Research into biologic agents discovered new molecules that could be used in the management of autoimmune bullous diseases. New humanized anti-CD20 monoclonal antibodies modify or bind to different sites to the target molecules. The new molecules escalate activity and possess a higher efficacy in preclinical trials. All of them are of second or third generations of humanized anti-CD20 monoclonal antibody. Furthermore, efficacy, safety, and tolerability should be evaluated in clinical trials. Among them, veltuzumab is an anti-CD20 monoclonal antibody that is largely identical to rituximab. Its advantage is subcutaneous administration. Obinutuzumab possesses 50-fold greater binding and stronger induction of apoptosis than rituximab resulting in a rapid and profound B-cell depletion during the first infusion. Ofatumumab possesses a superior and longer-lasting cytotoxic effect than rituximab. It is used intravenously. Ocaratuzumab has a higher binding affinity and 10-fold higher cytotoxicity, which results in smaller dosage using subcutaneous administration. PRO131921 has 30-fold higher binding affinity and 10-fold higher cytotoxicity than rituximab. It is used intravenously [51]. New humanized anti-CD20 monoclonal antibodies require further clinical trials to evaluate and establish dosing, efficacy and safety, including the monitoring of potential adverse events.

According to the guidelines rituximab is recommended as a second-line adjuvant for severe and refractory pemphigus vulgaris. Rituximab can be utilized, when the failure of conventional therapy is present, e.g., severe adverse events in conventional therapy, contraindications to use a high dose of other immunosuppressive therapies and progressive and rapid uncontrolled disease. Rituximab is regarded as a third-line therapy in pemphigus diseases.

3.4.7. Intravenous immunoglobulin G

Primarily, high intravenous immunoglobulin G was used to treat primary immunodeficiencies, immune thrombocytopenic purpura, Kawasaki disease, chronic B-cell lymphocytic leukemia, pediatric AIDS and others. In recent years, intravenous immunoglobulin has been used in the treatment of autoimmune and chronic inflammatory diseases, including autoimmune bullous diseases.

Immunoglobulin preparations are a special type of biologic treatment obtained from the pooled plasma of multiple healthy donors amounting 3000–10,000. Purified, pooled plasma contains natural antibodies of the IgG subclass. Natural autoantibodies are believed to play a role in maintaining immune homeostasis. Moreover, it contains a repertoire of the all IgG antibodies from populations as a mirror of the interaction of intravenous immunoglobulin individuals with external pathogens. Plasma may contain also natural autoantibodies, which presents the risk of preparation, but a considerable number of donors assists in dilution of these molecules. In addition, pooled plasma may contain a minimal refused amount of IgA or IgM. The guidelines for processing plasma are precise and stringent to avoid especially viral and bacterial contaminations. For this reason, pooled plasma is stored for 60 days and donors are checked for seroconversation to several pathogens. Individual plasma is also examined by polymerase chain reaction (PCR) for the presence of HCV RNA, HBV DNA, HIV RNA, HAV RNA and Parvovirus B19 DNA [52]. Only plasma with no pathogens may be collected to the pool preparation. Pulled plasma is evaluated for the main biological and pharmacological properties, the degree of purity and the antibody spectrum. The half-life of intravenous immunoglobulin is approximately 3 weeks.

The mechanism of intravenous immunoglobulin assesses several activities involving in activity complex. The desired response of intravenous immunoglobulin is a rapid decline in pathogenic autoantibodies and improvement of disease. The intravenous immunoglobulin produces complement blockade and degradation, Fc-receptor blockade and induces immunomodulatory Fc receptors, inhibits B-cells, and alters T-cell function, modulates cytokine production and cellular migration [53, 54]. Anti-idiotypic antibodies of intravenous immunoglobulin bind to the pathogenic autoantibodies, helping in their rapid decline. Despite partial knowledge of the intravenous immunoglobulin activity, the objective mechanism is not fully understood as it possesses multiple modes of action related to its ability to interact with both innate and adaptive compartment of the immune system [55]. The intravenous immunoglobulin appears to have increased clearance of pathogenic IgG autoantibodies, but failed in the suppression of autoantibody production. However, intravenous immunoglobulin is an adjuvant treatment and suppression of autoantibody production is operated by corticosteroids and other immunosuppressive adjuvants.

The good efficacy and safety profile of intravenous immunoglobulin was documented in multiple reports, mostly small series. The first multicentric, randomized, placebo-controlled, double-blind trial of intravenous immunoglobulin confirmed objectively the efficacy of intravenous immunoglobulin in 61 patients with pemphigus and confirmed a decrease in the autoantibody level in treated patients. After 7 days, anti-Dsg antibody clearance was documented in 42–74.4% of patients [56]. One review study evaluated 23 clinical studies and comprehended data of 260 patients with autoimmune bullous disease treated with intravenous immunoglobulin, among them 191 patients with pemphigus. The intravenous immunoglobulin showed improvement in 245 patients and demonstrated a corticosteroid-sparing effect [57]. In addition, many studies confirmed intravenous immunoglobulin therapy to have a very good safety profile [58, 59].

Some authors offer intravenous immunoglobulin not only for severe and refractory pemphigus vulgaris but also for mild and recalcitrant cases of pemphigus foliaceus [60]. Intravenous immunoglobulin may trigger the shift from an intractable condition to remission using a yet not fully understood mechanism, possibly based on immunomodulation. In recalcitrant pemphigus, a combination of intravenous immunoglobulin and rituximab is recommended. This combination could be useful, when response fails to a high corticosteroid dose in combination with adjuvant immunosuppressive drugs. The mechanism of combined activity of both medications is not known and should be elucidated. However, rituximab affects pathogenic B-cells and blocks production of pathogenic autoantibody and intravenous immunoglobulin rapidly declines pathogenic autoantibody and influences the innate and adaptive immune system. A 10-year follow-up study reported long-lasting remission, in 10 patients with refractory pemphigus vulgaris who have been treated with rituximab combined with intravenous immunoglobulin [9]. The intravenous immunoglobulin preparations are safe and effective and can treat juvenile autoimmune bullous diseases including pemphigus [61]. Several studies reported good safe and efficacy profiles also in pregnancy [38, 62].

An intravenous immunoglobulin response is rapid and administration should be repeated after 4 weeks initially. If the clinical response is good, the interval between cycles could be increased gradually to 6 weeks. If the patient does not respond to an intravenous immunoglobulin therapy, it should be discontinued. In pemphigus vulgaris, the recommended dose is 2 g/kg divided over 3–5 consecutive days. The number of intravenous immunoglobulin cycles should be repeated depending on the severity of disease. In standard regimen, 3–5 cycles are recommended to achieve the desired response. However, severity of the disease may require further intravenous immunoglobulin cycles, without restriction. A repeated dose can be applied also in relapse of the disease. The intravenous immunoglobulin is a relatively safe and well-tolerated therapy. Premedication with an antipyretic, e.g., acetaminophen or antihistamine is recommended to avoid adverse events. Oral or intravenous corticosteroid may be useful, if patient has had a prior reaction or is of elevated risk. The intravenous immunoglobulin should be administered as a long-lasting infusion over 4–5 h.

Systemic adverse events are relatively common, occurring in 20–40% of patients [63], but are mild and most frequently treatable. Immediate adverse reactions account for 60% of all adverse events. They occur during or within 6 h of the infusion and could be avoided by long-lasting infusion. Discontinuation of drug administration may treat immediate adverse events or the treatment is symptomatic. The most frequent immediate adverse event is headache (8.9–43.8%) [63]. Others include muscles aches, fatigue, chills, and fever. Delayed adverse reactions develop within more than 6 h to 1 week after administration. Very rare events occur weeks and months after infusion [63]. A serious adverse event is acute renal failure developing in patients with renal insufficiency. Risk patients are diabetics, older individuals, or patients using concomitantly nephrotoxic agents. Sucrose-free intravenous immunoglobulin preparations are recommended to prevent acute renal failure in risk patients. In these risk patients, an intravenous immunoglobulin should be administered very slowly and at the lowest effective dose. Another serious adverse event is thromboembolism associated with a large dose administered during a fast infusion, which may cause high plasma viscosity. A low dose of intravenous immunoglobulin is imperative also to respect precaution to avoid plasma viscosity.

Thromboembolism may develop within hours, days, or weeks. Risk patients should be monitored. A very rare and serious adverse event is aseptic meningitis, which may develop within 6 h to 1 week [64]. A minimal amount of IgA intravenous immunoglobulin may evoke the production of anti-IgA antibody in patients with IgA deficiency. Subsequently, anti-IgA antibody can cause immediate anaphylactic or anaphylactoid reactions. An intravenous immunoglobulin administration may lead to mild hemolytic reactions, due to the presence of anti-A or anti-B isoagglutinins. Furthermore, mild neutropenia and hyponatremia may occur 2–4 days after infusion and resolves in less than 1 week [63].

Intravenous immunoglobulin is a second-line adjuvant agent and is utilized with corticosteroids or other immunosuppressive adjuvant in refractory pemphigus vulgaris and pemphigus foliaceus. Indication criteria for intravenous immunoglobulin use include the failure of conventional therapy, including significant adverse events in conventional therapy, contraindications to high doses of other immunosuppressive therapies and progressive and rapid uncontrolled disease. However, in exceptional cases intravenous immunoglobulin can be utilized as a first-line treatment, e.g., aseptic bone necrosis, poorly controlled diabetes, advanced osteoporosis, and cataracts. Intravenous immunoglobulin is regarded as a third-line therapy in pemphigus diseases.

3.4.8. *Immunoadsorption*

Immunoadsorption is a specific method used to selectively clear pathogenic autoantibodies from the circulation in autoantibody-mediated disease, including autoimmune bullous diseases. Immunoadsorption is most frequently used to treat severe and refractory pemphigus vulgaris. In addition, immunoadsorption also removes immune complexes and produces cytapheresis by removing inflammatory cells or platelets from the peripheral circulation. In dermatology, the last can be used to treat pyoderma gangrenosum and psoriasis [65, 66]. Rapid removal of autoantibodies is performed extracorporally by adsorber system, which contains a high-affinity IgG adsorber or low-affinity IgG adsorber. Both adsorber systems differ with respect to ligands, matrix, volume of columns, affinity to certain immunoglobulin classes, and reusability. Reusable adsorbers can be utilized several times for the same patient. The reusable adsorbers are: Immunosorba® (ligand: ligand Staphylococcal protein A), Ig-Therasorb® (ligand: polyclonal anti-human antibodies from sheep), and Globaffin® (ligand: synthetic peptide-PGAM146). Reusable adsorbers are very effective and produce approximately similar depletion rates [67]. A number of one-time adsorbers are available, including adsorber Selesorb® (ligand: dextransulfate), Prosorba® (ligand: Staphylococcal protein A ligand), adsorber IM TR350® (ligand: tryptophan) and IM PH350® (ligand: phenylalanine), and adsorber Coraffin® (ligand: combination of synthetic peptides). One-time use adsorbers achieve only a low degree of IgG decline and usually show little specificity. In the induction phase of therapy, a high-affinity adsorber is recommended. Autoantibody levels can drop by about 75% utilizing a single procedure with a reusable adsorber system. A decrease about of 95% can be reached at the end of one cycle; 3 procedures applied over 3 consecutive days. The 3-day procedure is necessary to avoid a rebound phenomenon, which can appear after the first procedure within 24 h. Autoantibodies re-diffuse from the tissue to circulation and may reach 40% of the initial autoantibody level [68]. In selected cases, the induction phase could be realized with two consecutive treatments with low-affinity adsorbers (e.g., IM TR350® and IM PH350®). This procedure is utilized in individuals with known hypersensitivity towards material used in columns or other materials. After reaching control of disease, the therapy protocol may continue with subsequent regimen depending on clinical outcome. Single immunoadsorption can be utilized in weekly intervals and later in longer intervals. Another modality is to use a 3- to-4-day procedure repeated monthly. In pemphigus patients, the level of anti-Dsg IgG autoantibody should be evaluated regularly before and after each individual procedure using ELISA or the titer in indirect immunofluorescence. For pemphigus, a new adsorber system is developing with new highly specific adsorber selectively binding anti-Dsg IgG antibodies. Recombinant full-length Dsg1 and Dsg3 ectodomains could be used as a ligand in a highly specific adsorber system [69].

In general, immunoadsorption is recommended to treat severe autoimmune disease, including pemphigus vulgaris in combination with immunosuppressive medication, which can decrease the production of pathogenic autoantibodies. A retrospective study evaluated data of 82 patients with pemphigus treated with immunoadsorption. In most patients, reusable systems were applied with corticosteroids combined with other immunosuppressive drugs, usually azathioprine, mycophenolate mofetil, or cyclophosphamide used in conventional doses. Immunoadsorption showed a sharp decline of anti-Dsg IgG autoantibodies followed by clinical improvement [70]. The recent combination of immunoadsorption with rituximab and immunosuppressive adjuvants azathioprine or mycophenolate mofetil showed complete remission in 88% of patients with autoimmune bullous diseases, including pemphigus vulgaris (6 patients). The combination regimen evokes long-lasting improvement in disease outcome. However, the relapse rate was 13% with an average follow-up of 22 months [71]. In addition, another recent protocol used immunoadsorption combined with rituximab and dexamethasone pulses in conjugation with azathioprine or mycophenolate mofetil, all medication used in conventional doses. Autoantibody levels declined by more than 50% between the first two cycles. This combined regimen demonstrated a long-lasting complete remission in 83% of patients. However, at follow up of 11–43 months a relapse occurred in 26% of patients. In general, the therapy was well tolerated. However, severe adverse events were documented in 9% of patients, including Staphylococcal sepsis and transient paraplegia of the legs [72]. Immunoadsorption combined with another immunosuppressive medication showed a corticosteroid-sparing effect.

Adverse events in immunoadsorption are rare and may occur in ≤1% of procedures [68]. Some severe adverse effects were referred, including deep venous thrombosis, perforating diverticulitis, and sepsis [72]. Other adverse effects may develop such as hypotension, bradycardia, citrate-induced paresthesia, and hypocalcemia [67]. Contraindications for immunoadsorption include known hypersensitivity towards material used in the columns, treatment with ACE inhibitors and anticoagulants, severe cardiovascular disease, hypofibrinogenemia, severe systemic infection and body weight under 15 kg.

Immunoadsorption is a second-line adjuvant treatment in autoimmune bullous disease, including pemphigus. Immunoadsorption is indicated in acute severe disease, if the first-line treatment proved ineffective or is contraindicated. It is a rapid acting mode of treatment and is recommended if a rapid response is required. It can also be used in chronic refractory disease, if the response to standard treatment is inadequate. Immunoadsorption is almost always utilized in combination with immunosuppressive agents that reduce the production of pathogenic autoantibodies. Systemic corticosteroids are used in high dose orally or intravenously in bolus and usually are combined with adjuvant immunosuppressant, e.g., azathioprine, mycophenolate mofetil or cyclophosphamide. Immunoadsorption is regarded as a third-line therapy in pemphigus diseases.

3.5. Therapy of pemphigus herpetiformis

Pemphigus herpetiformis is a very rare variant in the pemphigus group. The clinical symptoms resemble dermatitis herpetiformis, but the pathogenic autoantibody IgG is directed mostly against Dsg1 (occasionally against Dsg3 or desmocollin) [73]. In general, the prognosis is more favorable than in pemphigus vulgaris. Furthermore, some cases may progress into pemphigus vulgaris, requiring more aggressive treatment. The therapy regimen of pemphigus herpetiformis differs from that of pemphigus vulgaris. Dapsone 100–300 mg/day is utilized as a treatment of choice and can be combined with low dose of systemic corticosteroids. In some severe disease, improvement of disease could be induced with adjuvant agents that are used to treat pemphigus vulgaris. Several authors referred to the good efficacy and tolerability of adjuvant agents, including azathioprine, mycophenolate mofetil, methotrexate, and cyclophosphamides [74, 75]. In refractory disease, intravenous immunoglobulin and plasmapheresis may improve the clinical outcome [73]. One case series report of 8 patients with pemphigus herpetiformis referred to the minimal clinical improvement of two patients treated with rituximab [74].

3.5.1. Therapy of IgA pemphigus

IgA pemphigus is a very rare variant of the pemphigus group. Disease differs in clinical affliction from those in the pemphigus group, because of the pustular lesions accompanied by vesicular ones. Based on clinical and pathological symptoms, it is divided into two variants: the subcorneal pustular dermatosis type and intraepidermal neutrophilic IgA dermatosis type. Pathogenic autoantibodies IgA are most frequently directed against desmocollin-1 and desmocollin-2, -3. Occasionally, IgA autoantibodies can be directed against Dsg1 and Dsg3 [76]. Dapsone is regarded as a first-line treatment. A dose of 100–300 mg/day may improve clinical symptoms of IgA pemphigus. Dapsone can be combined with a low dose of corticosteroids. Refractory cases could utilize etretinate or acitretin (50 mg/day), which can be used alone or in combination with dapsone [77, 78]. No objective clinical study was performed to demonstrate the efficacy and tolerability of various therapy regimens in IgA pemphigus. All recommendations result from clinical experience and small series or case reports.

3.5.2. Therapy of paraneoplastic pemphigus (paraneoplastic autoimmune syndrome)

Paraneoplastic pemphigus or paraneoplastic autoimmune syndrome is a rare condition with a variety of lesions including florid oral involvement, generalized polymorphous cutaneous rash resembling various skin disorders and pulmonary involvement. Moreover, it is associated with malignant neoplasm, most frequently hematoblastosis like non-Hodgkin's lymphoma, chronic lymphocytic leukemia or thymoma. However, paraneoplastic pemphigus may occasionally accompany benign neoplasia like Castleman's disease or monoclonal gammopathy. Therapy of paraneoplastic pemphigus is almost always very difficult and suboptimal. The mainstay of therapy is to treat underlying neoplasm. Early detection and complete resection of neoplasm are of paramount importance. Subsequently, the removal of neoplasm reduces the production of autoantibodies released from the tumor. Perioperative intravenous immunoglobulins administration in an obvious dose (2 g/kg/cycle) is recommended to block autoantibody release from the tumor during surgery [79]. In the case of benign neoplasm, surgical removal ameliorates the condition and may induce remission of paraneoplastic pemphigus with contemporary decrease of autoantibodies within 6–8 weeks [80]. In malignant neoplasm, the prognosis is poor and depends on the behavior of malignant tumor and development of severe respiratory failure. The mortality rate is high and ranges from 75 to 90% [80]. The disease may progress despite surgery and chemotherapy. The prognosis of paraneoplastic pemphigus is obviously unfavorable with rapid fatal outcome. Treatment of clinical symptoms of paraneoplastic pemphigus can be started with systemic corticosteroid, prednisone 0.5–1.0 mg/kg. Adjuvant agents with corticosteroid-sparing effect including azathioprine, mycophenolate mofetil, and cyclophosphamide in conventional doses could be used, but they have mostly potentially tumorigenic properties and their utilization in this condition is limited. However, patients are often resistant to all conventional therapies and therefore a new therapy regimen should be sought. The preferred treatment in paraneoplastic pemphigus is rituximab, which could probably reduce the risk of tumorigenicity. Several studies referred to the efficacy of rituximab, and some of them about rituximab combined with intravenous immunoglobulin. In several cases, rituximab was combined with chemotherapy depending on underlying malignancy [81]. Separaliter administration of intravenous immunoglobulin may also ameliorate the clinical outcome of paraneoplastic pemphigus and has a corticosteroid-sparing effect [59]. Reports about treatment efficacy and tolerability in paraneoplastic pemphigus embrace only small series or case reports. In addition, the therapy protocol embraces aggressive immunosuppressive agents and adverse events are the rule, including serious infections; among them sepsis is the most frequent cause of death. Respiratory failure, if evident, is a fatal complication. Other fatal complications may result from underlying neoplasm.

4. Therapy of bullous pemphigoid group

Bullous pemphigoid is the most frequent autoimmune blistering disorder and may last several years in the absence of treatment followed by total remission. The tendency to relapse is obligate and can be evoked with/without any risk factors. In general, the course of bullous pemphigoid is less severe and requires less aggressive treatment than pemphigus vulgaris (**Table 2**). However, a very severe course of bullous pemphigoid is not excluded. Relapse of disease starts with pruritus, consequently followed by skin eruption and occasionally also oral mucosa involvement. Advanced age in patients supports a large list of comorbidities, including cardiovascular, neurological, neoplastic, metabolic and respiratory comorbidities. The concomitant treatment regimen of comorbidities can hardly influence the choice of treatment regimen in patients with bullous pemphigoid.

First-line therapy	Dose initial therapy
Topical corticosteroid	High potency corticosteroid up 30–40 g/day
Prednisolone	0.5–0.75 mg/kg/day
Second-line therapy (first-line adjuvant agent)	
Tetracyclines	Oxytetracycline 2 g/day, doxycycline 200 mg/day
Azathioprine	1–3 mg/kg/day
Mycophenolate mofetil	2 g/day
Mycophenolic acid	1440 mg/day
Dapsone	100 mg/day or up to ≤1.5 mg/kg/day
Methotrexate	10–20 mg/week
Cyclophosphamide	500 m i.v. bolus or 2 mg/kg/day orally
Third-line therapy (second-line adjuvant agent)	
Anti-CD20 monoclonal antibody (rituximab)	2 × 1 g i.v. (2 weeks apart) or 4 × 375 mg/m^2 (each 1 week apart)
Intravenous immunoglobulin G	2 g/kg/4 weeks i.v.
Immunoadsorption	2 cycles a 4 days, 4 weeks apart
Linear IgA dermatosis	
Prednisolone	0.25–0.5 mg/kg/day
Dapsone	100 mg/day
Epidermolysis bullosa acquisita	
Prednisolone	1–1.5 mg/kg/day
Dapsone	25–100 mg/day
Colchicine	0.6–1.2 mg/day
Dermatitis herpetiformis	
Gluten-free diet	
Dapsone	50–150 mg/day

In mild bullous pemphigoid, a topical high potency corticosteroid may control disease. Systemic corticosteroids are used in severe disease; compared with pemphigus in lower doses. Tetracycline has an anti-inflammatory efficacy and can replace corticosteroids in mild bullous pemphigoid. Second-line therapy is used in refractory disease with precaution to comorbidities. The third-line adjuvant agents most frequently are used in severe mucous membrane pemphigoid or epidermolysis bullosa acquisita. Antihistamines are used to eliminate pruritus.

Table 2. The treatment of pemphigoid group.

4.1. Topical and systemic corticosteroids

Bullous pemphigoid can occur as localized or limited disease with mild activity. Potent topical corticosteroids, e.g., clobetasol propionate 0.05% cream or ointment is often successful to achieve remission. A dose up to 30–40 g/day can be administered twice daily to the blisters and erosions and perilesional normal skin. Initial treatment should be tapered 15 days after disease control. The tapering regimen embraces the application of corticosteroid cream or ointment every 2 days in the second month, then twice per week in the third month, and then once per week in the fourth month [82]. In relapse, topical corticosteroid therapy is increased to the previous level. High-potency topical corticosteroids are also recommended to support healing of more severe disease. Application can cover the whole body, sparing the face. However, administration of high potency corticosteroid to a large body area results in systemic absorption. Despite this, topical application of corticosteroids decreases adverse events of systemic corticosteroids. Topical corticosteroids are recommended in mild disease, especially when localized. However, topical corticosteroids can also be utilized in severe disease as they can decrease the dose of systemic corticosteroids. A large comparative study of 312 patients with bullous pemphigoid demonstrated that mild regimen of topical corticosteroid (10–30 g/day) induced co-equal clinical improvement as that of standard regimen (40 g/day). In addition, a mild regimen of topical corticosteroid allowed a 70% reduction in the cumulative doses of topical potent corticosteroid [83]. Application of topical corticosteroids requires nursing care and should be accompanied by antiseptic bath, bullae count, and bandaging.

Systemic corticosteroids are a mainstay of therapy and are used in lower doses than in pemphigus. Severe bullous pemphigoid is treated with prednisolone 0.5–0.75 mg/kg/day as an initial treatment. Prednisolone dose ≤0.5 mg/kg/day seems to be ineffective. Initial therapy starts with prednisolone 0.5 mg/kg/day and can be increased to 0.75 mg/kg/day only if control of disease is not achieved within 1–3 weeks [84]. The major goal in bullous pemphigoid is reducing the patient's cumulative dose of systemic corticosteroid. During the consolidation phase, the dose of corticosteroid is tapered 15 days after disease control. However, earlier tapering is possible, if the outcome of diseases is favorable. In the maintenance phase, the lowest dose of corticosteroid (prednisolone 0.1 mg/kg/day) should be achieved within 4–6 months after initiation of treatment [82, 85]. If the patient is in remission on maintenance dose for 3–6 months, treatment may be stopped. Total treatment from initiation phase through consolidation phase up to maintenance phase, is usually 9–12 months [82]. In the case of relapse, the previous dose of corticosteroid is recommended.

Topical and systemic corticosteroids are the first-line treatment recommended for mild to severe bullous pemphigoid.

4.2. Adjuvant therapy

In bullous pemphigoid, immunosuppressive adjuvant therapy is used with high precautions and respect to comorbidities. Adjuvants are used when systemic corticosteroids are limited or contraindicated, e.g., in diabetes, severe osteoporosis or cardiovascular disease. However, adjuvant agents have a corticosteroid-sparing effect and their use in the elderly is limited because of adverse events, which are more frequent in this population. Associated treatment of comorbidities can interact with adjuvant drugs and facilitated the involvement of adverse events.

4.2.1. Tetracycline

Tetracycline is recommended as a first adjuvant agent with anti-inflammatory activity confirmed by reduction of collagenolytic activity [86]. Several small series documented good efficacy and safety profiles of tetracycline and nicotinamide to treat mild to severe bullous pemphigoid [86, 87]. The therapy regimen is almost always combined with topical high potency corticosteroids. One randomized controlled study compared doxycycline (200 mg/day) and prednisolone

(0.5 mg/kg/day) for initial therapy in 256 patients with bullous pemphigoid. Therapy with doxycycline was evaluated as a useful alternative to prednisolone [88]. The recommended regimen is oxytetracycline 2 g/day and doxycycline 200 mg/day, both orally. Tetracycline can be used alone or in combination with nicotinamide up to 2 g/day orally. Nicotinamide, the amide derivate of vitamin B has been referred to having several types of anti-inflammatory activity, including inhibition of proinflammatory cytokines [87]. The combination of both may result in ameliorating of anti-inflammatory activity of bullous pemphigoid. The presence of circulating autoantibody after clearance of skin lesions is probably based on anti-inflammatory properties and not on decline of autoantibody production against the basement membrane zone. Tetracycline is regarded as a second-line therapy in pemphigoid diseases.

4.2.2. First-line adjuvant agents: azathioprine, mycophenolate mofetil, methotrexate, and dapsone

First-line adjuvant agents can be used in the same dose as in pemphigus vulgaris and include azathioprine, mycophenolate mofetil, methotrexate, and dapsone [22, 89, 90]. However, a daily dose in the lower range is most frequently effective and better tolerated in elderly patients. A retrospective review evaluated 35 case reports and case series and comprehended data of 170 patients with bullous pemphigoid treated with dapsone alone or combined with corticosteroids. Clinical remission was achieved in 81% of patients. Adverse events were developed in 37% of patients and in 5% of patients required discontinuation of dapsone. The most frequent adverse event was hemolysis and concomitant anemia, both were dose-dependent and reversible [41]. A small series study compared the efficacy and safety of azathioprine and dapsone in 15 patients with bullous pemphigoid. Both drugs were effective and showed an acceptable safety profile [91]. Another small series study compared the corticosteroid-sparing effect of azathioprine and dapsone in 8 patients with bullous pemphigoid. The corticosteroid-sparing effect was moderately higher in dapsone [92]. A retrospective review evaluated 6 studies comprehending data of 79 patients with bullous pemphigoid treated with methotrexate. Clinical improvement was achieved in 94% of patients [34]. Another small series study evaluated 16 patients with bullous pemphigoid treated with methotrexate combined with prednisone. Eight of 16 patients achieved remission off therapy after 25.3 months and during the 5.5 years of follow-up [93]. A retrospective study evaluated data of 70 patients with bullous pemphigoid treated with low-dose methotrexate (5–15 mg/week) combined with short-term high potent topical corticosteroid (clobetasol propionate). The regimen demonstrated very good efficacy and induced clinical improvement in all patients in a mean time interval of 21.9 days. Long-term disease control was achieved in 76% of patients [94]. Cyclophosphamide is a very effective immunosuppressant, but also toxic agent, and so its use in bullous pemphigoid is limited and not generally recommended.

4.2.3. Second-line adjuvant agents: intravenous immunoglobulin G, rituximab, immunoadsorption

Second-line adjuvant agents are used in severe or refractory bullous pemphigoid nonresponsive to corticosteroids or adjuvants of the first line. They must be used with extreme precaution in respect of adverse events. Second-line adjuvant medications are the same as in pemphigus and are utilized by standard rule. However, the number of patients treated with this modality is much lower compared with pemphigus. The efficacy and safety of second-line adjuvants were referred to in several small series and case reports [89, 90]. One review study evaluated 7 clinical studies and comprehended data of 69 patients with bullous pemphigoid treated with intravenous immunoglobulin. All of the patients showed clinical remission within 14–27 months of post-intravenous immunoglobulin follow-up. In 10 patients, the titer of both anti-BP180 IgG and anti-BP230 IgG autoantibodies showed a gradual decline and non-detectable titer after 11 months and 10 months, respectively. No serious adverse event was documented in all patients treated with intravenous immunoglobulin [57]. Another review study summarized 16 patients with bullous pemphigoid treated with rituximab; among them 14 patients were treated according to the lymphoma protocol and 2 patients according to the rheumatoid arthritis protocol. Complete clinical remission was achieved in 69% of patients and 6% of patients did not show any response. The mortality rate was 19%. Two patients died from sepsis and one from cardiac event [95]. The combination of intravenous immunoglobulin and rituximab showed good efficacy and no serious adverse events in 12 patients with severe and refractory bullous pemphigoid, who did not respond to previous conventional immunosuppressive therapy. Complete clinical improvement was achieved in a mean of 4.6 months and previous immunosuppressive therapy was discontinued. Clinical improvement was correlated with rapid decline of anti-BP180 IgG and anti-BP230 IgG autoantibodies and thereafter remained undetected. The therapy regimen was well tolerated without adverse events, including infections. Ten patients remained in remission in the follow-up at 73.8 months [96]. This regimen could be recommended, if conventional therapy fails. Patients with bullous pemphigoid and elevated level of IgE and eosinophilia who do not respond to conventional therapy regimen could be treated with omalizumab, monoclonal antibody that binds to and declines IgE. It is expected that the anti-BP180 IgE autoantibody could be pathogenic in some individuals [97].

Immunoadsorption can be used in severe refractory autoimmune bullous diseases has shown utilization in bullous pemphigoid not responsive to conventional treatment. Only small case series, or several patients were included into a group of pemphigus patients treated with immunoadsorption. Respectable patients for this regimen are those with markedly elevated levels of pathogenic autoantibodies. Clinical improvement is associated with rapid decline of anti-BP180 IgG and anti-BP230 IgG autoantibodies [67, 68, 70, 98]. Depending on the disease outcome, immunoadsorption can be used in several cycles. Adverse events do not differ from those in pemphigus patients and the incidence is low. One case series study documented good efficacy and safety of immunoadsorption combined with rituximab in various severe and refractory autoimmune bullous diseases, including bullous pemphigoid (3 patients), mucous membrane pemphigoid (3 patients), and epidermolysis bullosa acquisita (1 patients). Concomitant medication with systemic corticosteroids and other immunosuppressive drugs was administered. The clinical improvement was compounded with persistent decrease in both anti-BP180 IgG and anti-BP230 IgG autoantibodies. Complete remission was achieved in all patients and, in one patient, all immunosuppressive therapy was interrupted. Combined therapy proved rapid with long-lasting response, and was well tolerated and produced a corticosteroid-sparing effect [71]. Immunoadsorption is a second-line adjuvant treatment in autoimmune bullous disease including bullous pemphigoid, mucous membrane pemphigoid and epidermolysis bullosa acquisita. These second-line adjuvant agents are regarded as a third-line therapy in pemphigoid diseases.

4.3. Therapy of pemphigoid gestationis

Treatment of pemphigoid gestationis is influenced by pregnancy and should be secure to the fetus. In general, treatment is based on clinical experience. Disorder is almost always self-limiting, but can be associated with post-partum relapse. The goal of the therapy is to reduce pruritus and block the production of autoantibodies. Topical high-potency corticosteroids are the first-line therapy. Usually, topical corticosteroids are combined with systemic antihistamine which is respectable in pregnancy, e.g., chlorpheniramine or cetirizine. If the topical corticosteroid is ineffective, a systemic corticosteroid at a low-mild dose is recommended, e.g., prednisolone up to 0.25 mg/kg/day, as an initial dose with subsequent reduction based on clinical outcome [90, 99]. Severe cases require a high dose of 0.5–1 mg/kg/day of prednisolone [100]. Small and moderate doses of systemic corticosteroid do not affect pregnancy and the fetus, whereas placental enzyme inactivates 88% of prednisolone [101]. The initial dose should continue for 1–2 weeks after disease control is reached, then gradually tapered to an adequate maintenance dose. Alternate day therapy is preferred [102]. Discontinuation of prednisolone therapy depends on the clinical outcome and can be realized after or before delivery. In addition, prednisolone is excreted in breast milk in small amount. A dose up to 40 mg/day is regarded as safe [101]. Severe disease can be treated with intravenous immunoglobulin in a conventional dose. The safety profiles of intravenous immunoglobulin in pregnant women were confirmed by several clinical studies in pregnant women with pemphigus [38, 62]. Another choice of treating severe disease and unresponsive disease to conventional treatment is immunoadsorption [70]. One case report referred to a pregnant patient with severe pemphigoid gestationis who was successfully treated with immunoadsorption followed by systemic corticosteroids. After three procedures, disease control was achieved and pathogenic autoantibodies declined by 89% [103]. Immunoadsorption was evaluated as an effective and safe treatment modality in pemphigoid gestationis.

4.3.1. Therapy of linear IgA dermatosis

IgA dermatosis is a rare diagnosis that can affect adults, especially women of fertile age and children. Treatment should be started with topical high-potency corticosteroids. If topical therapy is ineffective, a systemic corticosteroid should be started, e.g., prednisolone in a dose of 0.25–0.5 mg/kg/day. In severe cases, when corticosteroids do not achieve disease control, prednisolone should be combined with dapsone 1 mg/kg/day. It is recommended to initiate the treatment with dapsone 0.5 mg/kg/day to avoid adverse effects, e.g., hemolytic anemia. According to the clinical outcome, initial therapy can be enhanced up to a conventional dose of 100 mg/day or up to ≤1.5 mg/kg/day. In children, dapsone 0.5–2 mg/kg/day is utilized [89]. Another treatment option is tetracycline (2 g/day) combined with nicotinamide (1.5–2 g/day) [104]. A gluten-free diet is ineffective.

4.3.2. Therapy of mucous membrane pemphigoid (cicatricial pemphigoid)

Treatment of mucous membrane pemphigoid is usually very difficult because of the sequela that may result in blindness and esophageal stricture despite utilization of immunosuppressive medications. The therapy regimen is based on whether ocular mucosa is afflicted or not.

Mucous membrane pemphigoid without ocular involvement requires systemic corticosteroids, e.g., prednisolone over 1 mg/kg/day combined with first-line adjuvant agents like dapsone, azathioprine or mycophenolate mofetil [105]. All immunosuppressive agents are used in conventional doses. The preferred medication in mild disease is dapsone being effective in 30–70% of patients. Response to dapsone can be expected within 2–12 weeks [89]. Mucous membrane pemphigoid with ocular involvement has more severe outcome of disease. In mild-to-moderate ocular mucous membrane pemphigoid, dapsone is recommended at a dose of 50 mg/day up to a maximum dose of 200 mg/day. Another choice, especially if dapsone cannot be used, is to utilize sulfapyridine (500 mg/day or two times daily), or sulfasalazine (1–4 g/day). The anti-inflammatory activity of the last three medications is used in the therapy regimen [106]. A retrospective study of 23 patients with mucous membrane pemphigoid with ocular involvement referred to the good efficacy of mycophenolate mofetil. Control of conjunctival inflammation was achieved in 69.6% of patients within 6 months and in 82.6% of patients within 12 months of therapy [107]. In patients with ocular involvement, another choice is a low dose methotrexate. A retrospective clinical study of 17 patients with mucous membrane pemphigoid demonstrated an improvement in ocular inflammation in 72% of afflicted eyes and improvement of visual acuity in 85% of eyes [108]. Progressive disease in ocular involvement requires a more aggressive therapy regimen. Systemic corticosteroid (prednisolone 1 mg/kg/day) with second-line adjuvant agent, like cyclophosphamide (1–2 mg/kg/d), is recommended. A retrospective study of 94 patients documented the good efficacy of cyclophosphamide combined with prednisolone, resulting in total remission of conjunctival inflammation in 82.9% of patients within 1 year [109]. Recently, new strategies have been employed to treat a severe refractory disease. Small series documented the good efficacy and tolerability of intravenous immunoglobulin. Ten patients with progressive ocular involvement in mucous membrane pemphigoid who were unresponsive to conventional immunosuppressive therapy reported good efficacy and tolerability of intravenous immunoglobulin after receiving 4–12 cycles. Clinical improvement and stabilization of ocular disease was achieved in all patients [110]. Another choice is rituximab. One retrospective study documented the efficacy of rituximab to 61 eyes of 32 patients with ocular involvement in mucous membrane pemphigoid. Twenty-six patients achieved clinical remission with an absence of progressive ocular scarring and ocular inflammation within ≥2 months (average remission of 24.5 months). The therapy regimen of rituximab was used as a monotherapy (6 patients) or in combination (6 patients), rituximab combined with intravenous immunoglobulin (14 patients) and rituximab combined with intravenous immunoglobulin and other immunosuppressive adjuvant (6 patients). The progression of ocular involvement was controlled and no cicatrization developed in the follow-up. Adverse effects were mild and transient [111].

4.3.3. Therapy of epidermolysis bullosa acquisita

It is very difficult to treat epidermolysis bullosa acquisita, especially the classic mechanobullous form associated with high skin fragility at trauma-prone areas. This form is associated with dystrophic changes, digital contracture and esophageal stricture. Inflammatory epidermolysis bullosa acquisita resembles other autoimmune bullous diseases with responses to anti-inflammatory and immunosuppressive medications. The main stay therapy is systemic corticosteroids, prednisolone 1–1.5 mg/kg/day. Adjuvant agents with corticosteroid-sparing effect used to treat other autoimmune bullous disease are also effective in the management of epidermolysis bullosa acquisita. Such adjuvants include azathioprine (1–2 mg/kg/day), mycophenolate mofetil (1–2 g/day), methotrexate (7.5 mg/week), and cyclophosphamide (500 mg /day in mode of pulse therapy). In small series, anti-inflammatory drugs including dapsone (25–100 mg/day) and colchicine (0.6–1.2 mg/day) induced remission [112]. Colchicine can be used as a single or combined with systemic corticosteroid or dapsone. Adverse events of colchicine include diarrhea, and renal or hepatic toxicity [113]. One retrospective study of 30 patients with epidermolysis bullosa acquisita referred to the time remission of combined methylprednisolone with mycophenolate mofetil or cyclophosphamide or azathioprine. One year after initiation therapy, complete remission was achieved in 33.3% of patients and partial remission in 32.8% [114]. In severe and refractory cases unresponsive to conventional therapy regimen, intravenous immunoglobulin, rituximab, plasmapheresis, and immunoadsorption could be utilized in conventional doses for autoimmune bullous diseases. All of the therapy modalities were used and documented only in small series of patients with epidermolysis bullosa acquisita, almost always with good efficacy and total or partial remission. In all regimens, a good safety profile was documented. Adverse events did not differ from adverse events in other autoimmune bullous disease [115]. Rituximab combined with intravenous immunoglobulin was referred in 5 patients with refractory epidermolysis bullosa acquisita. Patients received a high number of intravenous immunoglobulin (10–26) and 1–2 cycles of rituximab and achieved adequate improvement of disease, while being well tolerated [116]. The education of patients in the management of topical therapy and preventive measures against common trauma are obligatory.

5. Therapy of dermatitis herpetiformis

The mainstay therapy in dermatitis herpetiformis is a gluten-free diet that ameliorates both skin disease and gluten sensitive enteropathy. Precise maintenance of a gluten-free diet of 2 years cleans the skin disease and heals enteropathy. Adherence to a gluten-free diet should be provided for the whole life. After many years, IgA-antibody deposits disappear from the dermo-epidermal junction in both bowel and skin [6]. The reintroduction of gluten to the diet evokes the recurrence of gluten sensitive enteropathy and cutaneous rash within 12 weeks, frequently sooner. Good adherence to a gluten-free diet within 5–10 years induces improvement of enteropathy and is regarded to have a protective property against lymphoma, which might be associated with dermatitis herpetiformis [117]. Patients on a gluten-free diet must exclude cereals containing gluten and its toxic fractions, including wheat, rye, and barley. Based on some authors, oats can be incorporated into a gluten-free diet, whereas the majority of patients with dermatitis herpetiformis and gluten-sensitive enteropathy can tolerate moderate amounts of pure oats [118, 119]. Furthermore, oats increase the nutrition value of a gluten-free diet. Some studies reported that pure oats do not induce systemic or mucosal antibody response in patients with coeliac disease [119, 120]. However, oats can be contaminated with prolamines from other cereals and pure oats are difficult to prepare. This issue requires further investigation and new agricultural processing and manufacture of oats. Long-term administration of a gluten-free diet could permit the discontinuation of systemic medication, meaning self-sustaining treatment in dermatitis herpetiformis.

The mainstay medication in dermatitis herpetiformis is dapsone at a dose of 50–150 mg/day. Dapsone usually has a rapid and dramatic effect in suppressing skin symptoms within a few days, but does not have a curable effect on the underlying enteropathy. The effectiveness of dapsone has not been confirmed by clinical studies. Multiple and long-lasting empirical utilization of dapsone in practice confirmed its efficacy and safety in dermatitis herpetiformis.

Another choice to treat dermatitis herpetiformis is sulfonamides, when dapsone fails to control the disease or is not tolerated. Three sulfonamides may be an alternative to dapsone: sulfapyridine (1.5 g/day), sulfamethoxypyridazine (0.25–1.5 g/day), and sulfasalazine (1–2 g/day) [6]. Several case reports referred to an alternative treatment using sulfasalazine, which is commonly utilized in the long-term management of inflammatory bowel disease and as a second-line agent in rheumatoid arthritis and psoriatic arthritis [121]. All three sulfonamides may cause the same adverse events, including hypersensitivity reactions and bone marrow toxicity, resulting in agranulocytosis, aplastic anemia, and methemoglobinemia. More common and not severe adverse effects are nausea, anorexia, and vomiting. Gastro-enteric events could be avoided with administration of an enteric-coated form of medication.

Systemic corticosteroids are not recommended for treating dermatitis herpetiformis, because they are not effective. On the other hand, topical corticosteroids, especially of high potency (e.g., clobetasol propionate) may reduce itching. Another choice to ameliorate pruritus is third-generation antihistamine with specific activity on eosinophil activity.

6. Local therapy in autoimmune bullous diseases

In autoimmune bullous disease, the local therapy is important to prevent infection, to control reepithelization of denuded areas, and to ameliorate pain. Management of bullae depends on their size. Small bullae stay intact and large bullae should be punctured, but the covering should stay at the site of previous bullae. The released roof of blister built up a protective covering that shield the denuded area from secondary infection as well as loss of serum contents. In extensive disease, bathing with antiseptic agent should be applied, e.g., potassium permanganate (1:10,000), chlorhexidine or other commercial agent. Denuded areas should be covered with antiseptic or antibiotic agent in the form of lotions, sprays or cream. A potent topical corticosteroid, e.g., 0.05% clobetasone propionate cream, is preferably used in bullous pemphigoid and can be the self-sustaining therapy in mild bullous pemphigoid [82]. The advantage of topical corticosteroids is their local anti-inflammatory and immunosuppressive activity, which may be helpful in dropping of the systemic corticosteroid. Topical corticosteroids are also successfully utilized to treat minor forms of pemphigus or in the maintenance phase of therapy management [122]. One clinical study demonstrated the good efficacy of clometasone propionate 0.05% cream applied to afflicted areas on skin and mucosa in 7 patients with pemphigus vulgaris and pemphigus foliaceus. Topical corticosteroid was used as self-sustaining therapy. Another topical corticosteroid, betamethasone valerate 0.1% cream, was applied to the face. The creams were used twice daily for at least 15 days, up to remission. Moreover, when clinical improvement was achieved, topical creams were applied in tapering mode to the area of previous lesions. In 4 patients, relapses occurred when topical treatment was discontinued, but were successfully controlled by reapplication of topical corticosteroid. In 3 patients, topical therapy failed, and a systemic corticosteroid was utilized and combined with other adjuvant agents (dapsone or methotrexate). Topical treatment did not influence anti-Dsg IgG autoantibody titer. No serious side effect was noticed [123]. Topical corticosteroids seem to have only postponed activity in autoimmune bullous disease, because they do not influence the production of pathogenic autoantibody and utilize only anti-inflammatory activity. However, topical corticosteroids may help bypass the period before the systemic immunosuppressive drug should be used to control disease. In addition, minor disease can be controlled by self-sustained topical corticosteroid. Moreover, the monitoring of pathogenic autoantibody may indicate a relative threat of relapse and utilization of systemic medication. In mild disease, a combination of topical corticosteroid with systemic immunosuppressive agent may induce improvement of clinical outcome. In addition, topical corticosteroids may support the systemic agent and advocate healing through their local anti-inflammatory activity. A topical corticosteroid agent can be combined with antibiotic, e.g., gentamycin having dual activity, anti-inflammatory, and antibacterial.

The therapeutic challenge is the pathologic lesions in mucosa, especially in the oral cavity. The response to conventional therapy in oral mucosa occurs in a special environment resulting in delayed healing compared with skin lesions. Topical administration in mucosa should be modified because the saliva dilutes and shortens the therapeutic activity of medication. Therefore, corticosteroid should be implicated into an adhesive paste, which allows longer persistence and activity of the medication. Fluocinonide 0.05%, clobetasol 0.05%, and halobetasol 0.05% ointments compounded 1:1 with Orabase have shown good efficacy in oral management in 12 patients with oral pemphigus vulgaris. The only adverse effect was candida infection in the oral cavity, which afflicted most of the patients [124].

Another option in topical management of the oral cavity is triamcinolone acetonide, a high potency corticosteroid administered perilesional or intralesional to treat recalcitrant and remnant lesions. One clinical study compared perilesional or intralesional triamcinolone acetonide application and topical cream of 0.1% in 35 patients with recalcitrant oropharyngeal pemphigus vulgaris. Perilesional or intralesional triamcinolone displayed a better clinical outcome than topical application and induced complete clinical remission, while reducing the total amount of corticosteroids [125]. A perilesional or intralesional corticosteroid is recommended only in the maintenance phase of therapy, when 4–6 oropharyngeal sites are involved and do not respond to conventional immunosuppressive therapy. In addition, immediate use can be recommended to treat new lesions appearing in the maintenance phase. This regimen is not recommended upon relapse of disease, because the first step is to enhance systemic immunosuppressive medication. Good and meticulous personal oral hygiene and periodic professional oral hygiene sessions are advisable. Topical antiseptic mouthwash solution containing anesthetic agent is useful. However, afflicted mucosa especially that of the oral cavity, shows a refractory clinical outcome and slow response to systemic therapy. Perilesional or intralesional triamcinolone acetonide may improve vegetative tissue formation, especially in intertriginous location in pemphigus vegetans [126].

The topical immunomodulatory agents, calcineurin inhibitors, are new choice in local management of autoimmune bullous disease that promote healing and may enhance reepithelization. A double-blind, placebo-controlled clinical study referred to the good efficacy and safety profile of pimecrolimus 1% cream for cutaneous lesions in 11 patients with pemphigus vulgaris [127]. Another new topical agent, epidermal growth factor (10 μg in cream) was evaluated in a double-blind, randomized, controlled clinical trial and showed accelerating efficacy and a good safety profile in 20 patients with cutaneous lesions of pemphigus vulgaris [128]. Nicotinamide gel 4%, an adjunctive topical gel, was referred as an effective new treatment modality for cutaneous lesions of pemphigus vulgaris in 8 patients in a double-blind, placebo-controlled study [129]. All new topical medications should be confirmed in large clinical studies and eventually in practice.

Author details

Danka Svecova

Address all correspondence to: danka.svecova@fmed.uniba.sk

Faculty of Medicine, Comenius University in Bratislava, Bratislava, Slovakia

References

[1] Bystryn JC, Steinman NM. The adjuvant therapy of pemphigus. An update. Archives of Dermatology. 1996;**16**:203-212 PMID: 8629830

[2] Chams-Davatchi C, Valikhani M, Daneshpazhooh M, Esmaili N, Balighi K, Hallaji Z, Barzegari M, Akhiani M, Ghodsi Z, Mortazavi H, Naraghi Z. Pemphigus: Analysis of 1209 cases. International Journal of Dermatology. 2005;**44**:470-476. DOI: 10.1111/j.1365-4632.2004.02501.x

[3] Lee JH, Kim SC. Mortality of patients with bullous pemphigoid in Korea. Journal of the American Academy of Dermatology. 2014;**71**:676-683. DOI: 10.1016/j.jaad.2014.05006

[4] Hertl M, Jedlickova H, Karpati S, Martinovic B, Uzun S, Yayli S, Mimouni D, Borradori L, Feliciani C, Ioannides D, Joly P, Kowalewski C, Zambruno G, Zillikens D, Jonkman MF. Pemphigus. S2 Guideline for diagnosis and treatment-guided by the European Dermatology Forum (EDF) in cooperation with the European Academy of Dermatology and Venereology (EADV). Journal of the European Academy of Dermatology and Venereology. 2015;**29**:405-414. DOI: 10.1111/jdv.12772

[5] Bernad P, Reguiai Z, Tancréde-Bohin E, Cordel N, Platin P, Pauwels C, Vaillant L, Grande F, Richard-Lallemand MA, Sassolas B, Roujeau JC, Lok C, Picard-Dahan C, Chosidow O, Vitry F, Joly P. Risk factors for relapse in patients with bullous pemphigoid in clinical remission: A multicenter, prospective, cohort study. Archives of Dermatology. 2009;**145**:537-542. DOI: 10.1001/archdermatol.2009.53

[6] Caproni M, Antiga E, Melani L, Fabbri P. Guidelines for the diagnosis and treatment of dermatitis herpetiformis. Journal of the European Academy of Dermatology and Venereology. 2009;**23**:633-638. DOI: 10.1111/j.1468-3083.2009.03188.x

[7] Eming R, Sticherling M, Hofmann SC, Hunzelmann N, Kern JS, Kramer H, Pfeifer C, Schuster V, Zillikens D, Goebeler M, Hertl M, Nast A, Orzechowski HD, Sárdy M, Schmidt E, Sitaru C, Sporbeck B, Worm M. S2k guidelines for the treatment of pemphigus vulgaris/foliaceus and bullous pemphigoid. Journal der Deutschen Dermatologischen Gesellschaft. 2015;**13**:833-844. DOI: 10.1111/ddg.12606

[8] Ratnam KV, Phay KL, Tan CK. Pemphigus therapy with oral prednisolone regimens. A 5-years study. International Journal of Dermatology. 1990;**29**:363-367 PMID: 2361795

[9] Bystryn JC, Rudolph JL. Pemphigus. Lancet. 2005;**366**:61-73. DOI: 10.1016/S0140-6736(05)66829-8

[10] Herbst A, Bystryn JC. Patterns of remission in pemphigus vulgaris. Journal of the American Academy of Dermatology. 2000;**42**:422-427 PMID: 10688711

[11] Almugairen N, Hospital V, Bedane C, Duvert-Lehembre S, Picard D, Tronquony AF, Houivet E, Díncan M, Joly P. Assessment of the rate of long-term complete remission off therapy in patients with pemphigus treated with different regimens including medium- and high-dose corticosteroids. Journal of the American Academy of Dermatology. 2013;**69**:583-588. DOI: 10.1016/j.jaad.2013.05.016

[12] Patel AA, Swerlich RA, McCall CO. Azathioprine in dermatology: The past, the present, and the future. Journal of the American Academy of Dermatology. 2006;**55**:369-389. DOI: 10.1016/j.jaad.2005.07.059

[13] Meyer V, Beissert S. Azathioprine in the treatment of autoimmune blistering disease. Immunology and Allergy Clinics of North America. 2012;**32**:295-307. DOI: 10.1016/j.iac.2012.04.009

[14] Chams-Davatchi C, Esmaili N, Daneshpazhooh M, Valikhani M, Balighi K, Hallaji Z, Barzegari M, Akhyani M, Ghodsi SZ, Seifari H, Nazemi MJ, Mortazavi H, Mirshams-Shahshahani M. Randomized controlled open-label trial of four treatment regimens for pemphigus vulgaris. Journal of the American Academy of Dermatology. 2007;**57**:622-628. DOI: 10.1016/j.jaad.2007.05.024

[15] Atzmony L, Hodak E, Gdalevich M, Rosenbaum O, Minouni D. Treatment of pemphigus vulgaris and pemphigus foliaceus: A review and meta-analysis. American Journal of Clinical Dermatology. 2014;**15**:503-515. DOI: 10.1007/s40257-014-0101-9

[16] Atzmony L, Hodak E, Leshem YA, Rosenbaum O, Gdalevich M, Anhalt GJ, Mimouni D. The role of adjuvant therapy in pemphigus: A systemic review and meta-analysis. Journal of the American Academy of Dermatology. 2015;**73**:264-271. DOI: 10.1016/j.jaad.2015.04.038

[17] Martin LK, Werth VP, Villaneuva EV, Murrell DF. A systematic review of randomized controlled trials for pemphigus vulgaris and pemphigus foliaceus. Journal of the American Academy of Dermatology. 2011;**64**:903-908. DOI: 10.1016/j.jaas.2010.04.039

[18] Uchiyama K, Nakamura M, Kubota T, Yamane T, Fujise K, Tajiri H. Thiopurine S-methyltransferase and inosine triphosphate pyrophosphohydralase genes in Japanese patients with inflammatory bowel disease in whom adverse drug reactions were induced by azathioprine/6-mercaptopurine treatment. Journal of Gastroenterology. 2009;**44**:197-203. DOI: 10.1007/s00535-008-2307-1

[19] Schiavo AL, Puca RV, Ruocco V, Ruocco E. Adjuvant drugs in autoimmune bullous diseases, efficacy versus safety: Facts and controversies. Clinics in Dermatology. 2010;**28**:337-343. DOI: 10.1016/j.clindermatol.2009.06.018

[20] Meurer M. Immunosuppressive therapy for autoimmune bullous diseases. Clinics in Dermatology. 2012;**30**:78-83. DOI: 10.1016/j.clindermatol.2011.03.013

[21] Garritsen FM, van den Broek MP, van Zuilen AD, Fidder HH, de Bruin-Weller MS, Spuls PI. Pregnancy and fetal outcomes after paternal exposure to azathioprine, methotrexate or mycophenolic acid: A critically appraised topic. The British Journal of Dermatology. 2017;**176**:866-877. DOI: 10.1111/bjd.15320

[22] Eskin-Schwartz M, David M, Mimouni D. Mycophenolate mofetil for management of immune bullous diseases. Dermatologic Clinics. 2011;**29**:555-559. DOI: 10.1016/j.det.2011.06.012

[23] Beissert S, Werfel T, Frieling U, Böhm M, Sticherling M, Stadler R, Zillikens D, Rzany B, Hunzelmann N, Meuer M, Gollnick H, Ruzicka T, Pillekamp H, Junghans V, Luger TA. A comparison of oral methyleprednisolone plus azathioprine or mycophenolate mofetil for treatment of pemphigus. Archives of Dermatology. 2006;**142**:1447-1454. DOI: 10.1001/archderm.142.11.1447

[24] Strowd LC, Taylor SL, Jorizzo JL, Namazi MR. Therapeutic ladder for pemphigus vulgaris: Emphasis on achieving complete remission. Journal of the American Academy of Dermatology. 2011;**64**:490-494. DOI: 10.1016/j.jaad.2010.02.052

[25] Doukaki S, Platamone A, Alaimo R, Bongiorno MR. Mycophenolate mofetil and enteric-coated mycophenolate sodium in the treatment of pemphigus vulgaris and pemphigus foliaceus. Journal of Dermatological Treatment. 2015;**26**:67-72. DOI: 10.3109/09546634.2014.880395

[26] Hashimoto T, Kawakami T, Koga H, Ohyama B, Hamada T, Dainichi T, Nakama T, Yasumoto S, Tsuruta D, Ishii N. Therapeutic effects of mizoribine on pemphigus vulgaris and pemphigus foliaceus. Dermatologic Therapy. 2012;**25**:382-385. DOI: 10.1111/dth.12386

[27] Ahlmann M, Hempel G. The effect of cyclophosphamide on the immune system: Implications for clinical cancer therapy. Cancer Chemotherapy and Pharmacology. 2016;**78**:661-671. DOI: 10.1007/s00280-016-3152-1

[28] Cummins DL, Mimouni D, Anhalt GJ, Nousari CH. Oral cyclophosphamide for treatment of pemphigus vulgaris and foliaceus. Journal of the American Academy of Dermatology. 2003;**49**:276-280. DOI: 10.1067/S0190-9622(03)00859-4

[29] Olszewska M, Kolacinska-Strasz Z, Sulei J, Labecka H, Cwikla J, Natorska U, Blaszczyk M. Efficacy and safety of cyclophosphamide, azathioprine, and cyclosporine (ciclosporin) as adjuvant drugs in pemphigus vulgaris. American Journal of Clinical Dermatology. 2007;**8**:85-92 PMID: 17428113

[30] Sardana K, Agarwal P, Bansal S, Uppal B, Garg VK. A comparative effectiveness research of azathioprine and cyclophosphamide on the clinical and serological response in pemphigus vulgaris. Indian Journal of Dermatology. 2016;**61**:418-426. DOI: 10.4103/0019-5154.185710

[31] Rose E, Wever S, Zilliken D, Linse R, Haustein UF, Bröcker EB. Intravenous dexamethasone-cyclophosphamide pulse therapy in comparison with oral methylprednisolone-azathioprine therapy in patients with pemphigus: Results of a multicentric prospectively randomized study. Journal der Deutschen Dermatologischen Gesellschaft. 2005;**3**:200-206 PMID: 16372814

[32] Chan ES, Cronstein BN. Methotrexate-how does it really work? Nature Reviews Rheumatology. 2010;**6**:175-178. DOI: 1630.1038/nrrheum.2010.5

[33] Shen S, O'Brien T, Yap LM, Prince HM, McCormack CJ. The use of methotrexate in dermatology: A review. The Australasian Journal of Dermatology. 2012;**53**:1-18. DOI: 10.1111/j.1440-0960.2011.00839.x

[34] Gürcan HM, Ahmed R. Analysis of current data on the use of methotrexate in the treatment of pemphigus and pemphigoid. The British Journal of Dermatology. 2009;**161**:723-731. DOI: 10.1111/j.1365-2133.2009.09246.x

[35] Bangert CA, Costner MI. Methotrexate in dermatology. Dermatologic Therapy. 2007;**20**:216-228. DOI: 10.1111/j.1529-8019.2007.00135.x

[36] Chalmers RJ, Kirby B, Smith A, Burrows P, Little R, Horan M, Hextall JM, Smith CH, Klaber M, Rogers S. Replacement of routine liver biopsy by procollagen III aminopeptide for monitoring patients with psoriasis receiving long-term methotrexate: A multicenter audit and health economic analysis. The British Journal of Dermatology. 2005;**152**:444-450. DOI: 10.1111/j.1365-2133.2005.06422.x

[37] Kalb RE, Strober B, Weinstein G, Lebwohl M. Methotrexate and psoriasis: 2009 National Psoriasis Foundation Consensus Conference. Journal of the American Academy of Dermatology. 2009;**60**:824-837. DOI: 10.1016/j.jaad.2008.11.906

[38] Tavakolpour S, Mirasafaei HS, Delshad S. Management of pemphigus disease in pregnancy. American Journal of Reproductive Immunology. 2017;**77**:e1261. DOI: 10.1111/aji.12601

[39] Piette EW, Werth VP. Dapsone in the management of the autoimmune bullous diseases. Dermatologic Clinics. 2011;**29**:561-564. DOI: 10.1016/j.det.2011.06.018

[40] Werth VP, Fivenson D, Pandya AG, Chen D, Rico MJ, Albrecht J, Jacobus D. Multicenter randomized, double-blind, placebo-controlled, clinical trial of dapsone as a glucocorticoid-sparing agent in maintenance-phase pemphigus vulgaris. Archives of Dermatology. 2008;**144**:25-32. DOI: 10.1001/archDerm.144.1.25

[41] Gürcan HM, Ahmed AR. Efficacy of dapsone in the treatment of pemphigus and pemphigoid: Analysis of current data. American Journal of Clinical Dermatology. 2009;**10**:383-396. DOI: 10.2165/11310740-000000000-00000

[42] El-Zawahry B, Bassiouny D, Hegazy R, Gawdat H, Shalaby S, Khoshied M, Saleh MA. Rituximab treatment in pemphigus vulgaris: Effect on circulating T regs. Archives of Dermatological Research. 2017;Jun 19. DOI: 10.1007/s00403-017-1754-z

[43] Borradori L, Lombardi T, Samson J, Girardet C, Saurat JH, Hügli A. Anti-CD20 monoclonal antibody rituximab for refractory erosive stomatitis secondary to $CD20^+$ follicular lymphoma-associated paraneoplastic pemphigus. Archives of Dermatology. 2001;**137**:269-272 PMID: 11255323

[44] Zakka LR, Shetty SS, Ahmed R. Rituximab in the treatment of pemphigus vulgaris. Dermatologic Therapy. 2012;**2**:17. DOI: 10.1007/s13555-012-0017-3

[45] Leshem YA, Hodak E, David M, Anhalt GJ, Mimouni D. Successful treatment of pemphigus with biweekly 1-g infusions of rituximab: A retrospective study of 47 patients. Journal of the American Academy of Dermatology. 2013;**68**:404-411. DOI: 10.1016/j.jaad.2012.08.010

[46] Joly P, Maho-Vaillant M, Prost-Squarcioni C, Hebert V, Houivet E, Calbo S, Caillot F, Golinski ML, Labeille B. Picard-Dahan C et French study group on autoimmune bullous diseases. First-line rituximab combined with short-term prednisone versus prednisone alone for the treatment of pemphigus (Ritux 3): A prospective, multicenter, parallel-group, open-label randomized trial. Lancet. 2017;**389**:2031-2040. DOI: 10.1016/S0140-6736(17)30070-3

[47] Cho YT, Lee FY, Chu CY, Wang LF. First-line combination therapy with rituximab and corticosteroids is effective and safe for pemphigus. Acta Dermato-Venereologica. 2014;**94**:472-473. DOI: 10.2340/00015555-1746

[48] Ingen-Housz-Oro S, Valeyrie-Allanore L, Cosnes A, Ortonne N, Hüe S, Paul M, Wolkenstein P, Chosidow O. First-line treatment of pemphigus vulgaris with a combination of rituximab and high-potency topical corticosteroids. JAMA Dermatology. 2015;**151**:200-203. DOI: 10.1001/jamadermatol.2014.2421

[49] Kasperkiewicz M, Ellebrecht CT, Takahashi H, Yamagami J, Zillikens D, Payne AS, Amagai M: Pemphigus. Nature Reviews Disease Primers. 2017;**3**:17026. DOI:10.1038/nrdp.2017.26

[50] Ahmed AR, Nguyen T, Kaveri S, Spigelman ZS. First line treatment of pemphigus vulgaris with a novel protocol in patients with contraindications to systemic corticosteroids and immunosuppressive agents: Preliminary retrospective study with a seven year follow-up. International Immunopharmacology. 2016;**34**:25-31. DOI: 10.1016/j.intimp.2016.02.013

[51] Huang A, Madan RK, Levitt J. Future therapies for pemphigus vulgaris: Rituximab and beyond. Journal of the American Academy of Dermatology. 2016;**74**:746-753. DOI: 10.1016/j.jaad.2015.11.008

[52] Enk A. European Dermatology Forum Giudeline Subcomittee. Guidelines on the use of high-dose intravenous immunoglobulin in dermatology. European Journal of Dermatology. 2009;**19**:90-98. DOI: 10.1684/ejd.2008.0580

[53] Nagelkerke SO, Kuijpers TW. Immunomodulation by IVIG and the role of Fc-gamma receptors: Classic mechanisms of action after all? Frontiers in Immunology. 2015;**5**:674. DOI: 10.3389/fimmu.2014.00674

[54] Czernik A, Toosi S, Bystryn JC, Grando S. Intravenous immunoglobulin in the treatment of autoimmune bullous dermatoses: An update. Autoimmunity. 2012;**45**:111-118. DOI: 10.3109/08916934.2011.606452

[55] Tha-In T, Bayry J, Metselaar HJ, Kaveri SV, Kwekkeboom J. Modulation of the cellular immune system by intravenous immunoglobulin. Trends in Immunology. 2008;**29**:608-615. DOI: 10.1016/j.it.2008.08.004

[56] Amagai M, Ikeda S, Shimizu H, Iizuka H, Hanada K, Aiba S, Kaneko F, Izaki K, Tamaki K, Ikezawa Z, Takigawa M, Seishima M, Tanaka T, Miyachi Y, Katayama I, Horiguchi Y, Miyagawa S, Furukawa F, Iwatsuki K, Hide M, Tokura Y, Furue M, Hashimoto T, Ihn H, Fujiwara S, Nishikawa T, Ogawa H, Kitajima Y, Hashimoto KA. Randomized double-blind trial of intravenous immunoglobulin for pemphigus. Journal of the American Academy of Dermatology. 2009;**60**:595-603. DOI: 10.1016/j.jaad.2008.09.052

[57] Gürcan HM, Jeph S, Ahmed AR. Intravenous immunoglobulin therapy in autoimmune mucocutaneous blistering diseases: A review of the evidence for its efficacy and safety. American Journal of Clinical Dermatology. 2010;**11**:315-326. DOI: 10.2165/11533290-000000000-00000

[58] Svecova D. IVIG therapy in pemphigus vulgaris has corticosteroid-sparing and immunomodulatory effects. The Australasian Journal of Dermatology. 2016;**57**:141-144. DOI: 10.1111/ajd.12422

[59] Seidling V, Hoffmann JH, Enk AH, Hadaschik EN. Analysis of high-dose intravenous immunoglobulin therapy in 16 patients with refractory autoimmune blistering skin disease: High efficacy and no serious adverse events. Acta Dermato-Venereologica. 2013;**93**:346-349. DOI: 10.2340/00015555-1471

[60] Kawakami T, Koga H, Saruta H, Ueda A, Inoue Y, Soma Z, Ishii N, Hashimoto T. Four mild but refractory cases of pemphigus foliaceus successfully treated with intravenous immunoglobulin. The Journal of Dermatology. 2013;**40**:869-873. DOI: 10.1111/1346-8138.12280

[61] Gürcan HM, Mabrouk D, Ahmed AR. Management of pemphigus in pediatric patients. Minerva Pediatrica. 2011;**63**:279-291 PMID: 21909064

[62] Ahmed AR, Gürcan HM. Use of intravenous immunoglobulin therapy during pregnancy in patients with pemphigus vulgaris. Journal of the European Academy of Dermatology and Venereology. 2011;**25**:1073-1079. DOI: 10.1111/j.1468-3083.2010.03925.x

[63] Stiehm ER. Adverse effects of human immunoglobulin therapy. Transfusion Medicine Reviews. 2013;**27**:171-178. DOI: 10.1016/j.tmrv.2013.05.004

[64] Bharath V, Eckert K, Kang M, Chin-Yee IH, Hsia CC. Incidence and natural history of intravenous immunoglobulin-induced aseptic meningitis: A retrospective review at a single tertiary care center. Transfusion. 2015;**55**:2597-2605. DOI: 10.1111/trf.13200

[65] Watanabe Y, Yamada H. Leukocyte adsorption apheresis for the treatment of pyoderma gangrenosum. The Journal of Dermatology. 2008;**35**:792-794. DOI: 10.1111/j.1346-8138.2008.00572.x

[66] Liumbruno GM, Centoni PE, Molfettini P, Ceretelli S, Ceccarini M, Bachini L, Pomponi A, Bagnoni G, Vitolo M, Eberle O, Biondi A, Sodini ML. Lymphocytapheresis in the treatment of psoriasis vulgaris. Journal of Clincal Aheresis. 2006;**21**:158-164. DOI: 10.1002/jca.20079

[67] Zillinkens D, Derfler K, Eming R, Fierlbeck G, Goebeler M, Hertl M, Hofmann SC, Karlhofer F, Kautz O, Nitschke M, Opitz A, Quist S, Rose C, Schanz S, Smidt E, Shimanovich I, Sticherling M. Recommendations for the use of immunoapheresis in the treatment of autoimmune bullous diseases. Journal der Deutschen Dermatologischen Gesellschaft. 2007;**5**:881-887. DOI: 10.1111/j.1610-0387.2007.06342.x

[68] Schmidt E, Zillikens D. Immunoadsorption in dermatology. Archives of Dermatological Research. 2010;**302**:241-253. DOI: 10.1007/s00403-009-1024-9

[69] Langenhan J, Dworschak J, Saschenbrecker S, Komorowski L, Schlumberger W, Stöcker W, Westermann J, Recke A, Zillikens D, Schmidt E, Probst C. Specific immunoadsorption of pathogenic autoantibodies in pemphigus requires the entire ectodomains of desmogleins. Experimental Dermatology. 2014;**23**:253-259. DOI: 10.1111/exd.12355

[70] Meyersburg D, Schmidt E, Kasperkiewicz M, Zillikens D. Immunoadsorption in dermatology. Therapeutic Apheresis and Dialysis. 2012;**16**:311-320. DOI: 10.1111/j.1744-9987.2012.01075.x

[71] Kolesnik M, Becker E, Reinhold D, Ambach A, Heim MU, Gollnick H, Bonnekoh B. Treatment of severe autoimmune blistering skin diseases with combination of protein a immunoadsorption and rituximab: A protocol without initial dose or pulse steroid medication. Journal of the European Academy of Dermatology and Venereology. 2014;**28**:771-780. DOI: 10.1111/jdv.12175

[72] Kasperkiewicz M, Shimanovich I, Meier M, Schumacher N, Westermann L, Kramer J, Zillikens D, Schmidt E. Treatment of severe pemphigus with a combination of immunoadsorption, rituximab, pulsed dexamethasone and azathioprine/mycophenolate mofetil: A pilot study of 23 patients. The British Journal of Dermatology. 2012;**166**:154-160. DOI: 10.1111/j.1365-2133.2011.10585.x

[73] Kasperkiewicz M, Kowalewski C, Jablonska S. Pemphigus herpetiformis: From first description until now. Journal of the American Academy of Dermatology. 2014;**70**:780-787. DOI: 10.1016/j.jaad.2013.11.043

[74] Laws PM, Heelan K, Al-Mohammedi F, Walsh S, Shear NH. Pemphigus herpetiformis: A case series and review of the literature. International Journal of Dermatology. 2015;**54**:1014-1022. DOI: 10.1111/ijd.12582

[75] Duarte IB, Bastazini I, Barreto JA, Carvalho CV, Nunes AJ. Pemphigus herpetiformis in childhood. Pediatric Dermatology. 2010;**27**:488-491. DOI: 10.1111/j.1525-1470.2010.01256.x

[76] Hashimoto T, Teye K, Ishi N. Clinical and immunological studies of 49 cases of various types of intercellular IgA dermatosis and 13 cases of classical subcorneal pustular dermatosis examined at Kurume University. The British Journal of Dermatology. 2017;**176**:168-175. DOI: 10.1111/bjd.14780

[77] Tsuruta D, Ishii N, Hamada T, Ohyama B, Fukuda S, Koga H, Imamura K, Kobayashi H, Karashima T, Nakama T, Dainichi T, Hashimoto T. IgA pemphigus. Clinics in Dermatology. 2011;**29**:437-442. DOI: 10.1016/j.clindermatol.2011.01.014

[78] Monshi B, Richter L, Hashimoto T, Groiß E, Haensch N, Rappersberger K. IgA pemphigus of the subcorneal pustular dermatosis type. Successful therapy with a combination of dapsone and acitretin. Der Hautarzt. 2012;**63**:482-486. DOI: 10.1007/s00105-011-2270-2

[79] Yong AA, Tey HL. Paraneoplastic pemphigus. The Australasian Journal of Dermatology. 2013;**54**:241-250. DOI: 10.1111/j.1440-0960.2012.00921.x

[80] Wieczorek M, Czernik A. Paraneoplastic pemphigus: A short review. Clinical, Cosmetic and Investigational Dermatology. 2016;**9**:291-295. DOI: 10.2147/CCID.S100802

[81] Czernik A, Camilleri M, Pittelkow MR, Grando SA. Paraneoplastic autoimmune multiorgan syndrome: 20 years after. International Journal of Dermatology. 2011;**50**:905-914. DOI: 10.1111/j.1365-4632.2011.04868.x

[82] Feliciani C, Joly P, Jonkman MF, Zambruno G, Zillikens D, Ioannides D, Kowalewski C, Jedlickova H, Kárpáti S, Marinovic B, Mimouni D, Uzun S, Yayli S, Hertl M, Borradori L. Management of bullous pemphigoid: The European Dermatology Forum consensus in collaboration with the European Academy of Dermatology and Venereology. The British Journal of Dermatology. 2015;**172**:867-877. DOI: 10.1111/bjd.13717

[83] Joly P, Roujeau JC, Benichou J, Delaporte E, D'Incan M, Dreno B, Bedane C, Sparsa A, Gorin I, Picard C, Tancrede-Bohin E, Sassolas B, Lok C, Guillaume JC, Doutre MS, Richard MA, Caux F, Prost C, Plantin P, Chosidow O, Pauwels C, Maillard H, Saiag P, Descamps V, Chevrant-Breton J, Dereure O, Hellot MF, Esteve E, Bernard P. A comparison of two regimens of topical corticosteroids in the treatment of patients with bullous pemphigoid: A multicenter randomized study. The Journal of Investigative Dermatology. 2009;**129**:1681-1687. DOI: 10.1038/jid.2008.412

[84] Culton DA, Diaz LA. Treatment of subepidermal immunobullous diseases. Clinics in Dermatology. 2012;**30**:95-102. DOI: 10.1016/jclindermatol.2011.03.015

[85] Bagci IS, Horváth ON, Ruzicka T, Sárdy M. Bullous pemphigoid. Autoimmunity Reviews. 2017;**16**:445-455. DOI: 10.1016/j.autrev.2017.03.010

[86] Henehan M, Montuno M, De Benedetto A. Doxycycline as an anti-inflammatory agent: Updates in dermatology. Journal of the European Academy cf Dermatology and Venereology. 2017;**31**:1800-1808. DOI: 10.1111/jdv.14345

[87] Siohara J, Yoshida K, Hasegawa J, Uhara H, Takata M, Saida T, Ohyama B, Hashimoto T. Tetracycline and niacinamide control bullous pemphigoid but not pemphigus foliaceus when these conditions coexist. The Journal of Dermatology. 2010;**37**:657-661. DOI: 10.1111/j.1346-8138.2010.00920.x

[88] Chalmers JR, Wojnarowska F, Kirtschig G, Nunn AJ, Bratton DJ, Mason J, Foster KA, Whitham D, Williams HC. A randomized controlled trial to compare the safety and effectiveness of doxycycline (200 mg daily) with oral prednisolone (0.5 mg kg^{-1} daily) for initial treatment of bullous pemphigoid: A protocol for the bullous pemphigoid steroids and tetracyclines (blister) trail. The British Journal of Dermatology. 2015;**173**:227-234. DOI: 10.1111/bjd.13729

[89] de Vega IF, Iranzo-Fernández P, Mascaró-Galy JM. Bullous pemphigoid: Clinical practice guidelines. Actas Dermo-Sifiliográficas. 2014;**105**:328-346. DOI: 10.1016/j.ad.2012.10.022

[90] Schmidt E, Zillikens D. The diagnosis and treatment of autoimmune blistering skin diseases. Deutsches Ärzteblatt International. 2011;**108**:399-405. DOI: 10.3238/arztebl. 2011.0405

[91] Tirado-Sanchez A, Diaz-Molina V, Ponce-Olivera RM. Efficacy and safety of azathioprine and dapsone as an adjuvant in the treatment of bullous pemphigoid. Allergologia et Immunopathologia. 2012;**40**:152-155. DOI: 10.1016/j.aller.2010.12.009

[92] Sticherling M, Franke A, Aberer E, Gläser R, Hertl M, Pfeiffer C, Rzany B, Schneider S, Shimanovich I, Werfel T, Wilczek A, Zillikens D, Schmidt E. An open, multicenter, randomized clinical study in patients with bullous pemphigoid comparing methylprednisolone and azathioprine with methylprednisolone and dapsone. The British Journal of Dermatology. 2017;**117**:1299-1305. DOI: 10.1111/bjd.15649

[93] Kwarta SG, Jorizzo JL. Bullous pemphigoid: A case series with emphasis on long-term remission off therapy. Journal of Dermatological Treatment. 2013;**24**:327-331. DOI: 10.3109/09546634.2012.660519

[94] Du-Thanh A, Merlet S, Maillard H, Bernard P, Joly P, Esteve E, Richard MA, Pauwels C, Ingen-Housz-Oro S, Guillot B, Dereure O. Combined treatment with low-dose methotrexate and initial short-term superpotent topical steroids in bullous pemphigoid: An open, multicetre, retrospective study. The British Journal of Dermatology. 2011;**165**:1337-1343. DOI: 10.1111/j.1365-2133.2011.10531.x

[95] Shetty S, Ahmed AR. Treatment of bullous pemphigoid with rituximab: Critical analysis of the current literature. Journal of Drugs in Dermatology. 2013;**12**:672-677 23839185

[96] Ahmed AR, Shetty S, Kaveri S, Spigelman ZS. Treatment of recalcitrant bullous pemphigoid (BP) with a novel protocol: A retrospective study with a 6-year follow-up.

Journal of the American Academy of Dermatology. 2016;**74**:700-708.e3. DOI: 10.1016/j.jaad.2015.11.030

[97] London VA, Kim GH, Fairley JA, Woodley DT. Successful treatment of bullous pemphigoid with omalizumab. Archives of Dermatology. 2012;**148**:1241-1243. DOI: 10.1001/archdermatol.2012.1604

[98] Herrero-Gonzalez JE, Sitaru C, Klinker E, Bröcker EB, Zillikens D. Successful adjuvant treatment of severe bullous pemphigoid by tryptophan immunoadsorption. Clinical and Experimental Dermatology. 2005;**30**:519-522. DOI: 10.1111/j.1365-2230.2005.01853.x

[99] Chi CC, Wang SH, Charles-Holmes R, Ambros-Rudolph C, Powell J, Jenkins R, Black M, Wojnarowska F. Pemphigoid gestationis: Early onset and blister formation are associated with adverse pregnancy outcomes. The British Journal of Dermatology. 2009;**160**:1222-1228. DOI: 10.1111/j.1365-2133.2009.09086.x

[100] Lipozencic J, Ljubojevic S, Bukvic-Mokos Z. Pemphigoid gestationis. Clinics in Dermatology. 2012;**30**:51-55. DOI: 10.1016/j.clindermatol.2011.03.009

[101] Semkova K, Black M. Pemphigoid gestationis: Current insights into pathogenesis and treatment. European Journal of Obstetrics, Gynecology, and Reproductive Biology. 2009; **145**:138-144. DOI: 10.1016/j.ejogrb.2009.05.012

[102] Jackson S, Gilchrist H, Nesbitt LT. Update on the dermatologic use of systemic glucocorticosteroids. Dermatologic Therapy. 2007;**20**:187-205. DOI: 10.1111/j.1529-8019.2007.00133.x

[103] Marker M, Derfler K, Monshi B, Rappersberger K. Successful immunoapheresis of bullous autoimmune diseases: Pemphigus vulgaris and pemphigoid gestationis. Journal der Deutschen Dermatologischen Gesellschaft. 2011;**9**:27-31. DOI: 10.1111/j.1610-0387.2010.07500.x

[104] Shan XF, Zhang FR, Tian HQ, Wang N, Zhou SJ, Wang GJ. A case of linear IgA dermatosis successfully treated with tetracycline and niacinamide. International Journal of Dermatology. 2016;**55**:e216-e217. DOI: 10.1111/ijd.12524

[105] Chan LS. Ocular and oral mucous membrane pemphigoid (cicatricial pemphigoid). Clinics in Dermatology. 2012;**30**:34-37. DOI: 10.1016/j.clindermatol.2011.03.007

[106] Sobolewska B, Deuter C, Zierhut M. Current medical treatment of ocular mucous membrane pemphigoid. The Ocular Surface. 2013;**11**:256-266. DOI: 10.1016/j.jtos.2013.02.003

[107] Nottage JM, Hammersmith KM, Murchison AP, Felipe AF, Penne R, Raber I. Treatment of mucous membrane pemphigoid with mycophenolate mofetil. Cornea. 2013;**32**:810-815. DOI: 10.1097/ICO.0b013e31826af7b8

[108] McCluskey P, Chang JH, Singh R, Wakefield D. Methotrexate therapy for ocular cicatricial pemphigoid. Ophthalmology. 2004;**111**:796-801. DOI: 10.1016/j.ophtha.2003.07.010

[109] Thorne JE, Woreta FA, Jabs DA, Anhlat GJ. Treatment of ocular mucous membrane pemphigoid with immunosuppressive drug therapy. Ophthalmology. 2008;**115**:2146-2152.e1. DOI: 10.1016/j.ophtha.2008.08.002

[110] Foster CS, Ahmed AR. Intravenous immunoglobulin therapy for ocular cicatricial pemphigoid: A preliminary study. Ophthalmology. 1999;**106**:2136-2143. DOI: 10.1016/S0161-6420(99)90496-7

[111] You C, Lamba N, Lasave AF, Ma L, Diaz MH, Foster CS. Rituximab in the treatment of ocular cicatricial pemphigoid: A retrospective cohort study. Graefe's Archive for Clinical and Experimental Ophthalmology. 2017;**255**:1221-1228. DOI: 10.1007/s00417-017-3603-3

[112] Kim JH, Kim SC. Epidermolysis bullosa acquisita. Journal of the European Academy of Dermatology and Venereology. 2013;**27**:1204-1213. DOI: 10.1111/jdv.12096

[113] Arora KP, Sachdeva B, Singh N, Battacharya SN. Remission of recalcitrant epidermolysis bullosa acquisita (EBA) with colchicine monotherapy. The Journal of Dermatology. 2005;**32**:114-119 PMID: 15906541

[114] Hoon J, Kim YH, Kim SC. Epidermolysis bullosa acquisita: A retrospective clinical analysis of 30 cases. Acta Dermato-Venereologica. 2011;**91**:307-312. DOI: 10.2340/0001 5555-1065

[115] Gürcan HM, Ahmed AR. Current concept in the treatment of epidermolysis bullosa acquisita. Expert Opinion on Pharmacotherapy. 2011;**12**:1259-1268. DOI: 10.1517/1465 6566.2011.549127

[116] Oktem A, Akay BN, Boyvat A, Kundakci N, Erdem C, Bostanci S, Sanli H, Kocyigit P. Long-term results of rituximab-intravenous immunoglobulin combination therapy in patients with epidermolysis bullosa acquisita resistant to conventional therapy. The Journal of Dermatological Treatment. 2017;**28**:50-54. DOI: 10.1080/09546634.2016.1179711

[117] Cardones AR, Hall RP. Management of dermatitis herpetiformis. Dermatologic Clinics. 2011;**29**:631-635. DOI: 10.1016/j.det.2011.06.015

[118] Pulido OM, Gillespie Z, Zarkadas M, Dubois S, Vavasour E, Rashid M, Switzer C, Godefroy SB. Introduction of oats in the diet of individuals with celiac disease. Advances in Food and Nutrition Research. 2009;**57**:235-285. DOI: 10.1016/S1043-4526(09)57006-4

[119] Fric P, Gabrovska D, Nevoral J. Celiac disease, gluten-free diet, and oats. Nutrition Reviews. 2001;**69**:107-115. DOI: 10.1111/j.1753-4887.2010.00368.x

[120] Koskinen O, Villanen M, Korponay-Szabo I, Lindfors K, Mäki M, Kaukinen K. Oats do not induce systemic or mucosal autoantibody response in children with coeliac disease. Journal of Pediatric Gastroenterology and Nutrition. 2009;**48**:559-565. DOI: 10.1097/MPG.0b013e3181668635

[121] Willsteed E, Lee M, Wong LC, Cooper A. Sulfasalazine and dermatitis herpetiformis. The Australasian Journal of Dermatology. 2005;**46**:101-103. DOI: 10.1111/j.1440-0960.2005.00152.x

[122] Ujiie H, Aoyagi S, Horie K, Shimizu H. Cutaneous-type pemphigus vulgaris successfully treated with topical corticosteroids. The Journal of Dermatology. 2016;**43**:840-841. DOI: 10.1111/1346-8138.13271

[123] Dumas V, Roujeau JC, Wolkenstein P, Revuz J, Cosnes A. The treatment of mild pemphigus vulgaris and pemphigus foliaceus with topical corticosteroid. British Journal of Dermatology. 1999;**140**:1127-1129 PMID: 10354082

[124] Robinson JC, Lozada-Nur F, Frieden I. Oral pemphigus vulgaris. Oral Surgery, Oral Medicine, Oral Pathology, Oral Radiology, and Endodontics. 1997;**84**:349-355 PMID: 9347496

[125] Mignogna MD, Fortuna G, Leuci S, Adamo D, Dell'Aversana Orabona G, Ruoppo E. Adjuvant triamcinolone acetonide injections in oro-pharyngeal pemphigus vulgaris. Journal of the European Academy of Dermatology and Venereology. 2010;**24**:1157-1165. DOI: 10.1111/j.1468-3083.2010.03610.x

[126] Ruocco V, Ruocco E, Caccavale S, Gambardella A, Lo Schiavo A. Pemphigus vegetans of the folds (intertriginous areas). Clinics in Dermatology. 2015;**33**:471-476. DOI: 10.1016/j.clindermatol.2015.04.011

[127] Iraji F, Asilian A, Siadat AH. Pimecrolimus 1% cream in the treatment of cutaneous lesions of pemphigus vulgaris: A double-blind, placebo-controlled clinical trial. Journal of Drugs in Dermatology. 2010;**9**:684-686 PMID: 20645531

[128] Tabrizi MN, Chams-Davatchi C, Esmaeeli N, Noormohammadpoor P, Safar F, Etemadzadeh H, Ettehadi HA, Gorouhi F. Accelerating effects of epidermal growth factor on skin lesions of pemphigus vulgaris: A double-blind, randomized, controlled trial. Journal of the European Academy of Dermatology and Venereology. 2007;**21**:79-84. DOI: 10.1111/j.1468-3083.2006.01873.x

[129] Iraji F, Banan L. The efficacy of nicotinamide gel 4% as an adjuvant therapy in the treatment of cutaneous erosions of pemphigus vulgaris. Dermatologic Therapy. 2010;**23**:308-311. DOI: 10.1111/j.1529-8019.2010.01329.x

2

Action Mechanisms and Pathophysiological Characteristics of Cortisol in Horses

Katiuska Satué Ambrojo,
María Marcilla Corzano and
Juan Carlos Gardon Poggi

Abstract

Cortisol (CORT), also known as stress hormone, plays a vital role in physiological processes such as electrolyte and fluid balance, cardiovascular homeostasis, carbohydrate, protein and lipid metabolism, immune and inflammatory responses, and sexual development and reproduction. Cortisol levels are influenced by various physiological factors such as race, age, circadian rhythm, seasonality, exercise and pregnancy. Also, some stressful conditions including isolation or transport, among others, modify levels of this hormone in the body. Excesses or deficiencies of cortisol cause important clinical problems such as Cushing's and Addison's syndromes, which contribute substantially to morbidity in equine medicine. Thus, in this review, we will develop the mechanisms of synthesis and regulation, as well as the physiological factors involved and the most important diseases related to the alteration of cortisol secretion in horses and foals.

Keywords: cortisol, horse, pathophysiology, regulatory mechanisms

1. Introduction

1.1. Synthesis of cortisol, regulatory mechanisms and participation in physiological functions in the horse

The glucocorticoid activity of adrenocortical cortex secretion comes from cortisol (CORT) almost entirely. The adrenal synthesis of CORT is regulated by the hypothalamic-pituitary-adrenal axis (HPA) and plays an important role in the integral endocrine response to stress. The HPA axis is activated when various physiological, pathophysiological or environmental stress factors drive the signals of peripheral components and the central nervous system, which are interpreted and integrated into the hypothalamus. The activation of the hypothalamic paraventricular nuclei promotes the release of the corticotropin-releasing hormone (CRH) in the hypothalamus-hypophysis support system. CRH acts on the anterior pituitary gland to activate type 1 CRH receptors on the surface of corticotrophic cells and thereby induces the release of adrenocorticotropic hormone (ACTH) into systemic circulation [1]. These hormones are important for the health of the body and help control both physical and mental stress [1, 2]. Thus, chronic responses to stress are mediated by glucocorticoids.

The hormone ACTH binds to the melanocortin 2 (MC2R) receptors located in adrenocortical cells and stimulates the adrenal glands to synthesize and secrete mainly CORT and to a lesser extent also aldosterone. MC2R is a transmembrane receptor coupled to the G protein that acts through adenylate cyclase to increase the levels of cyclic AMP. Cyclic AMP activates a variety of critical enzymes for the synthesis of CORT [1, 3]. Currently, the expression of this subtype of melanocortin receptor in the equine adrenal cortex has not been characterized, but it is presumed to be similar to that described in humans.

The critical enzymes necessary for the synthesis of CORT are expressed in cells of the fasciculated area of the adrenal cortex. These enzymes include 3-β-hydroxysteroid dehydrogenase (3-β-HSD), 17-α-hydroxylase, 21-α-hydroxylase and 11-β-hydroxylase [4]. The last enzyme catalyzes the final step in the synthesis of CORT from the precursor molecule of 11-deoxycortisol, and is present only in glucocorticoid-producing cells.

CORT is not stored in adrenocortical cells, but is secreted into the systemic circulation immediately after synthesis is induced by ACTH [5]. CORT is lipophilic and, therefore, is transported in plasma predominantly bound to plasma proteins, including cortisol-binding globulin (CBG) and albumin [6].

In most adult mammals, including horses, approximately 90% of circulating CORT is bound to CBG [6]. Nicolaides et al. [7] reported that, since CORT receptors are located in the cytoplasm of steroid-sensitive cells, only the free and free portion of circulating CORT is available to enter the cells by diffusion through the plasma membrane and bind to these intracellular glucocorticoid receptors (GR).

The binding of CORT to the cytoplasmic GR causes conformational changes that allow the dissociation of heat shock regulatory proteins (HSP), allowing the GR-CORT complex to dimerize, localize in the nucleus, bind to the DNA in glucocorticoid-response elements (GRE) and regulate transcription of genes that respond to glucocorticoids [8]. However, the equine GR isoforms and their respective activities are not well characterized [9, 10]. In addition, CORT itself acts through negative feedback mechanisms at the HPA axis to regulate this activity [11].

In healthy horses, approximately 90% of plasma CORT is bound to CBG and albumin [10, 12]. It is the remaining 10% of unbound, free CORT that is considered biologically active, and is available to bind cytoplasmic steroid receptors to mediate the majority of CORT's systemic effects [5].

In the organism, there are many cell types sensitive to glucocorticoids. In this way, the CORT has different effects, necessary for the responses to stress to both health and illness. CORT also regulates vital functions such as blood glucose, maintenance of normal vascular tone and blood pressure [13]. Likewise, CORT increases the absorption of electrolytes by direct action on the renal tubules and indirectly, through the secretion of atrial natriuretic peptide (ANP) at the cardiac level. CORT is a lipolytic agent that induces hyperglycemia and leads to fat mobilization and protein catabolism (amino acids mobilization) to support higher energy requirements and a high demand for protein biosynthesis in compromised situations [14]. Proteins with few critical functions are degraded into amino acids for mobilization into circulation before proteins with essential functions such as brain neurotransmitters and muscle contractile proteins.

CORT stimulates the production of erythrocytes and platelets. Another effect of CORT is the reversal and low regulation of inflammatory responses resulting from a stressful event [15]. The production of CORT increases in response to stress and is a physiological adaptation that promotes survival [16]. A stress response mediated by CORT is to ensure that adequate nutrients are delivered to the brain and other areas of the body that could be compromised by a stressful event or injury. Glucocorticoids are powerful inhibitors of the immune system, which limits the secretion of cytokines by macrophages and the production of antibodies. In fact, it has been demonstrated that different stressful situations such as resistance exercise, fatigue, lack of food or water and extreme temperatures induce the release of glucocorticoids and immunosuppression [17].

1.2. Reference values for cortisol levels

The CORT levels in the circulation reflect the activity of the HPA axis. Therefore, excretion in saliva and feces allows non-invasive sampling of CORT metabolites [18, 19]. Plasma CORT binds mainly to transporter proteins, while salivary CORT is not bound, that is, it is found as free CORT [20]. CORT levels in saliva and plasma reflect acute changes in release [21]. Fecal CORT as a circulating CORT index has a delay of 24 hours until excretion. Therefore, the collection protocols should uniformly sample the total fecal mass due to the unequal distribution of the hormone [22]. Compared to plasma levels, the salivary CORT is clearly lower. In saliva, only free CORT is produced, that is, unbound, whereas in the plasma both free CORT and CBG are measured [23].

Fureix et al. [24] and Pawluski et al. [25] described that there is a positive correlation between nocturnal plasma CORT levels and concentrations of fecal CORT metabolites in horses. Salivary CORT can be used to measure acute stress responses and identify stress triggers. Fecal cortisol can be used to compare levels of general stress with long-term conditions [25]. While the determination of CORT metabolites in saliva allows the detection of small and transient changes in the release of CORT, the levels of fecal CORT metabolites increase only in response to marked or prolonged release of this hormone [18]. However, contradictory results have been reported when comparing salivary and blood samples. This discrepancy is related to the limited sensitivity and specificity of saliva samples and the role of corticosteroid-binding globulins in CORT plasma levels. However, Pawluski et al. [25] reported correlations between plasma and fecal CORT levels.

CORT is susceptible to be modified by the manipulation of stressful and painful stimuli, circadian rhythm, exercise, transport, hypoglycemia and stress [26–29]. Therefore, establishing a reference interval for the basal CORT is difficult. Plasma levels ranging from 12.32 ± 2.0 to 68.1 ± 22.8 ng/ml have been reported in healthy adult horses at rest [11, 28, 30–32].

2. Physiological factor that modifies cortisol levels in horses

2.1. Breed

Although it is unknown whether breed is a modifier of CORT, Söder et al. [33] reported significantly lower CORT levels in Icelandic horses compared to Standardbred horses. However, these variations were not only attributed to the genetic configuration. They were also related to the level of training and management conditions between both equine breeds.

2.2. Age

Plasma CORT levels usually change with the age of the horse. In comparison to foals born at term, premature foals have lower serum CORT concentrations before 2 hours after birth. These low basal concentrations of CORT and also of ACTH imply that foals may have either altered adrenocortical sensitivity to ACTH, the ability to synthesize limited CORT, or both [34].

It has been established that the adrenocortical function may not be fully mature at birth, even in term foals. At 12–24 hours of age, mean baseline concentrations of CORT are lower in healthy foals compared to levels reported in healthy adult horses despite the fact that in foals there are higher concurrent concentrations of ACTH [35–37].

In neonatal foals, the CORT concentration increases during the first week of life, up to about half that in adult horses in response to a comparable dose of ACTH [38, 39]. During the first year of life, great changes occur in CORT in response to the stress of weaning and growth [25].

The advance of age is associated with a loss of adrenal sensitivity to dexamethasone and greater sensitivity to CRH and ACTH. Older horses are also more prone to diseases such as Cushing's syndrome which alters the episodic and circadian rhythm of CORT [35, 40]. Cushing's disease in adult equines originates more frequently in an adenoma of the pars intermedia of the pituitary gland [41]. This adenoma stimulates the production of ACTH and thus more CORT is secreted by the adrenal glands. Hart et al. [42], indicated an increase in free CORT and nearly twice as much in the stool with this endocrine disease. However, the total CORT observed was not affected in sick animals compared to horses and healthy ponies of the same age. Likewise, it was demonstrated that the increase in CORT in feces could be related to the decrease in the capacity of CORT binding in plasma and that this fact could be a component of these endocrine disorders in horses. However, other investigations in this species disagree [32, 43, 44].

2.3. Circadian and ultradian rhythms

Horses that live in undisturbed natural habitats and trained horses, which have adapted to their environment, show a normal oscillation in CORT blood concentrations. These concentrations are generally higher in the morning and decrease throughout the day [45, 46]. These same authors have reported maximum levels between 6:00 and 10:00 am and minimum between 6:00 and 9:00 pm. Rendle et al. [47, 48], identified a circadian rhythm in horses and ponies with the highest ACTH plasma values at 8:00 am that subsequently decrease throughout the day. The circadian rhythm can be affected by various factors such as exercise, mating, training, stress, sleep patterns and individual activities [49]. The response of CORT to these factors is immediate, proportional and quickly exceeds the normal plasma concentration [12].

Ultradian rhythms with average periods ranging from 105 to 128 and from 24 to 31 minutes overlap the circadian rhythm [50]. In contrast, the loss of the circadian rhythm of CORT occurs in animals suffering from chronic stress, disease and old age [20]. For example, in horses with Cushing's disease, the circadian rhythm is lost and the CORT is constantly high [41]. For this reason, no ultradian [47] or circadian [26, 51] rhythms have been found in horses and ponies affected by intermediate pituitary dysfunction. Also, alterations of the circadian rhythm in CORT can be observed during situations of chronic stress in many species such as pigs and humans with different types of psychological disorders such as certain types of depression, chronic fatigue syndrome and post-traumatic stress disorder [52, 53].

2.4. Seasonality

CORT levels show a marked seasonality, detecting maximum values between the months of May and September [35, 54, 55]. This seasonal pattern could reflect the physiological adaptations to the lower availability of nutrients during the winter and increase the food reserves for the period of greatest reproductive activity [35, 55]. However, the seasonal patterns of CORT and ACTH are not correlated, since the peak of ACTH occurs during the fall [35, 37, 55]. This asynchrony in the HPA axis could be the result of alterations in adrenal sensitivity, changes in the metabolism of CORT or seasonal variations in the bioactivity of ACTH. In fact, Donaldson et al. [35] have described a loss of sensitivity of the HPA axis to dexamethasone during the autumnal period. On the contrary, Haritou et al. [26] showed in horses that the plasma CORT levels did not change during the year and were different only in the summer when they obtained higher values along 24 hours.

2.5. Transport

It has been shown that transport [54, 56–60], loading of horses in a trailer [61] and social stress [12] increase the synthesis of CORT. The transport of horses at short and medium distances leads to a greater release of CORT [18]. In fact, CORT levels correlate positively with transport duration [56]. In addition, the secretion of CORT depends on the transport conditions [21] and the new environment.

At the same time, this raises the possibility that both psychological and physical stress may have a negative effect on embryo recovery rates of competition mares. Tischner et al. [62], measured stress responses to transport in mares at different stages of the estrous cycle and gestation. These authors reported that "the most intense stress reaction (to transport), measured by the maximum increase in noradrenaline, adrenaline and CORT, was shown in the mares in the right and during the winter anestrus". This suggests that competition mares subjected to embryo transfer procedures could be particularly susceptible to stress if transported in the interval between insemination and uterine lavage. There are also negative effect of heat on the recovery rates of equine embryos [63]. It is possible that the combined effect of stress and heat in mares that are "bad travelers" are other factors that could limit the rates of embryo recovery in sport mares. However, the concentrations of salivary CORT and fecal glucocorticoids were not modified during transport of horses in New York [60].

2.6. Environmental factors

The variations of the CORT levels during short periods of time depend on the adaptation of the horse to its environment [45]. In addition, there is evidence in some countries of seasonal dynamics and variations between annual periods in the same geographical region [64, 65]. Therefore, environmental factors, weather or the presence of insects, cause transient changes in the diurnal pattern of cortisol release [66].

2.7. Feeding

Today's horse management practices often include restricted access to forage and feeding large quantities of concentrates in a limited number of meals throughout the day [67]. Higher concentrations of CORT were observed in serum 30 minutes before the morning food was administered compared to 30 minutes after the feed intake. A significant postprandial increase in endogenous ACTH has also been documented. This suggests that the animal's feeding status can also be a co-founder for both endogenous and dynamic ACTH tests [51].

In a study conducted on adult horses with overweight, Glunk et al. [68] determined if limit feeding combined with a slow-feed hay net could affect morphometric measurements and patterns of postprandial hormones and metabolites. The results of the study conducted during 28 days, showed that the glucose and insulin values increased, while the levels of CORT and leptin decreased. In conclusion, it could be said that when overweight adult horses are fed, the use of a slow feeding hay network together with a diet with limit of feeding seems to be an effective method to reduce body weight and maintain more homeostatic levels of postprandial metabolites and hormones.

However, it has been shown that CORT levels increase before feeding. This elevation could be due to the anticipation of receiving the morning meal after a period of several hours without grain or hay or without acclimating to the daily feeding routine. This finding may have important implications in the way a horse is handled. At times when it is important to take into account the negative impact of stress, such as times of illness or reproduction. At times like during the reproductive season, stress can affect both the immune system and reproduction. Therefore, care must be taken to avoid other circumstances that intensify the stress already experienced half an hour before feeding [69].

2.8. Exercise

CORT is frequently used to assess stress levels induced by exercise [70, 71]. Different studies have been carried out in relation to stress in horses such as the load stress in tow [61], participation in equestrian dressage competition [72–74], competition of resistance [75] jumping [76], tourist driving and education [77]. It has been shown that moderate exercise in horse increases CORT by up to 29% compared to baseline levels through the stress response. Also, the plasma concentration of CORT was more than double the normal value 60 minutes after exercise [78]. In stress-induced exercise, a marked increase in CORT levels was attributed to exercise duration and not to intensity [79]. In addition, the secretion of CORT depends on the animal's experience in competitions [80], different head and neck positions [81] and the horse character [82].

The hormonal response during exercise is also influenced by hemodilution or hemoconcentration actions related to the displacement of plasma fluids inside and outside the vascular beds. A greater secretion of CORT can be expected during and after exercise on horses during resistance competitions. This greater secretion occurs mainly in the case of mares or horses that cover longer distances or that take place at high temperatures. Janczarek et al. [83] suggested that a high level of CORT can adversely affect the heart rate of horses, but at the same time stimulates the body to combat dehydration. The permissive action of this substance enables the animal to react favorably to situations of stress and exhaustion, since the main metabolic effects of CORT are the increase in hepatic gluconeogenesis, the mobility of free fatty acids and lipolysis [79]. During exercise, CORT is also useful in suppressing insulin release and maximizing blood glucose utilization [14, 80, 84]. Thus, the availability of energy resources necessary during physical exercise is favored. On the other hand, it has been shown that high concentrations of CORT after exercise episodes can alter the anabolic responses of testosterone and growth hormone (GH) [79]. On the contrary, Zuluaga and Martínez [44] showed no significant differences in horse performance.

2.9. Sexual excitation and reproductive state

Although sexual arousal [85, 86] and mating [87] increase CORT levels in stallions, in sexually experienced and well-trained animals, ejaculation and semen collection is perceived as no more than a modest temporary stressor [88].

In the mare, the physiological status significantly alters CORT concentrations. Based on previous studies conducted in intact and ovariectomized mares, in which it was determined that the administration of synthetic analogue of ACTH (tetracosactide) stimulates the synthesis of CORT [89, 90], Satué et al. [91] described that in the natural estral cycle, the increase in ACTH secretion stimulates the synthesis of CORT at the time of ovulation in Spanish Purebred mares. However, Ginther et al. [92] found increased levels of CORT during the luteal phase, followed by a decrease during the periovulatory period at the time of follicular deviation. This decrease in CORT may be necessary for correct follicular development and LH release. This dynamic during the corpus luteum period could partially confirm the results of the investigations carried out by Satué et al. [93, 94] during the same period of the cycle. In fact, although the relationship between CORT and progesterone is not very close, the correlations obtained between both parameters ($r = 0.47$) may suggest a certain stimulation of CORT in the synthesis of luteal progesterone in Spanish Purebred mares.

Generically, non-pregnant mares show CORT concentrations 20% higher than pregnant ones [93, 94]. These differences in the adrenocortical response between non-pregnant and pregnant mares could be interpreted in terms of variations in the metabolism of this glucocorticoid. In fact, with respect to non-pregnant mares, fetal CORT levels induce a negative feedback mechanism of maternal levels during pregnancy [82].

In mares of different breeds, as in Spanish Purebred mares, Quarter Horse, Standardbred, Thoroughbred and arabians [32, 54, 95, 96] CORT levels increase during the first half of gestation. The gestational period is associated with a state of insulin resistance, due to the anti-insulin effects of CORT, GH, lactogen and placental GH [97, 98]. The purpose is to increase blood glucose to improve placental transfer and meet fetal demands [99]. In fact, mares under restriction regimes and food presage a higher incidence of abortions. These facts do not correlate with alterations in CORT levels but rather with the metabolic changes associated with the lower glucose bioavailability and the increase of free fatty acids that could stimulate the synthesis of prostaglandins and arachidonic acid [100].

On the contrary, the elevation of the CBG [101], the decrease in production and the increase in the volume of distribution, the increase in fetal metabolism and the antiglucocorticoid effects of progesterone, could reduce CORT during the last gestation period, describing an inverse correlation between both steroid hormones [32].

At the end of pregnancy, the maternal CORT rises substantially before delivery due to the increased activity of fetal adrenal and the maturational changes necessary for the correct adaptation of the fetus to extrauterine life [102]. Furthermore, CORT release during and after foaling is most likely part of the endocrine pathways regulating parturition and not a labor-associated stress response [103].

In addition, different patterns are established in the CORT cyclicity between pregnant and empty mares, establishing differences that can be between 400 and 700% between them. Compared to the usual circadian pattern characterized by the morning increase of CORT in physiologically normal mares [37, 45], CORT levels decrease in the morning [45] and increase at night [36] in ovariectomized mares. Pregnancy is considered an additional factor that modifies the diurnal and annual pattern of CORT [89, 90], and can even mask cyclicality during the second half of pregnancy in the mare [32]. These changes in the acrofase are related to the action of the gestation and lactation hormones, exerting a different influence on the secretion and use of CORT in the mare. Thus, in a pregnant and lactating mare, the increase in CORT is related to the need for glucocorticoids during the period of fetal development and intensive lactation.

2.10. Fertility

In women it has been described that CORT inhibits the release of pituitary gonadotropins and makes the gonads become resistant to sex steroids through inactivity of the receptor [104]. Along with these suppressive effects on the gonads, CORT has shown in the mare that they have inhibitory effects on steroid hormone receptors [105]. In addition, overexposure of the fetus to excess glucocorticoids could be implicated in the restriction of fetal growth [106].

In pregnant women, abnormally high levels of CORT contributed to miscarriage by altering normal reproductive function at both the tissue and hormonal levels [107]. Likewise, in a study carried out on sheep, it was determined that high levels of CORT lead to the premature activation of growth regulation mechanisms in the fetus that have deleterious prenatal and postnatal consequences [108]. It has also been determined in sheep that high levels of CORT suppress insulin-like growth factors found in the liver, skeletal muscles and adrenal glands in fetuses [109]. It has been shown that CORT in sheep is also able to reduce the activity of the gonadotropin-releasing hormone (GnRH) receptor through the improvement of negative feedback mechanisms in estradiol [110]. In adult sows it was determined that the chronic administration of cortisol delays ovulation through the deterioration of the LH peak during the estrous cycle [111]. However, research in horses has not yet established a threshold in the systemic circulation of CORT before it presents harmful effects in pregnancy.

It has been shown that hormones are important factors that contribute to the differentiation of the conceptus in the uterus. Hormones indirectly affect fetal growth, either through genetic programming or fetoplacental growth and maturation. During pregnancy, hormones are produced at maternal and fetal levels with direct effects on their outcome. Glucocorticoids have programming action in the uterus and affect the development of the tissues and organs of the fetus [108]. Kapoor et al. [112], determined that excessive exposure of the human fetus to glucocorticoids can reprogram the fetal HPA and thus permanently change the HPA activity of the offspring. Fetal exposure to glucocorticoids can occur simply by initiating the mother's response to stress. It has also shown that high concentrations of glucocorticoids impair fetal growth and are a major determinant of intrauterine growth restriction [108]. Challis et al. [113] reported that fetal HPA is responsible for the maturation of the organ systems essential for postnatal survival.

Endocrine changes initiated by elevated CORT levels may be transient, although some alterations persist after glucocorticoid concentrations return to baseline [108]. Changes initiated by chronic exposure to glucocorticoids include underdevelopment of fetal HPA and placental hormone deficiency. The critical window of fetal HPA maturation is specific to the species [112]. Fowden et al. [114] reported that the activation of fetal HPA is an essential process for delivery in the mare. Pregnancy in equines is unique since fetal CORT levels increase rapidly very close to the term. This, in turn, increases the synthesis of uteroplacental prostaglandins and initiates myometrial contractions.

In addition, transrectal ultrasound examination in non-lactating mares induces a significant increase in salivary CORT. This reflects an activation of the HPA axis and a shift toward a sympathetic domain. On the contrary, transvaginal follicular punctures guided by ultrasound did not modify the salivary levels of CORT [115]. Also, the diagnosis of transabdominal gestation does not induce an activation of the HPA axis. This finding affirms what was previously described by Schönbom et al. [116], who indicated that controls of advanced pregnancies can be easily performed by transabdominal ultrasound.

2.11. Other factors

Other factors such as painful stimulation, water or food deprivation, contraction restriction or immobilizers [117], stabling and isolation [28, 73], weaning [118] or social stress [12] have also been linked to elevation in CORT levels. Leal et al. [119] showed that horses stabled in the urban environment were in a state of stress. Likewise, report stated that the confinement type (partial full-time), type bed (big place with chips, as small without bedding) as well as the type of work (patrol or sports) did not change the ability of the horses to cope with these housing conditions.

3. Cortisol related with equine clinic

Adrenocortical dysfunction may manifest as either abnormal increases or decreases in activity. Increased adrenocortical activity (hyperadrenocorticism) may occur in horses with PPDI, but primary hyperadrenocorticism is rare in horses. Other pathological inflammatory conditions also are related with alterations with CORT levels [1].

3.1. Hyperadrenocorticism

Cushing's disease or Pituitary Pars Intermedia Dysfunction (PPID) is the most common in horses and you put over 15 years of age with a prevalence of 15–20%. As reported by McGowan et al. [74], all breeds and types of horses may be affected by the PPID, although Morgan horses and ponies seem to be at greater risk. The corticoadrenal hyperplasia that accompanies equine Cushing's disease is relatively rare and occurs in approximately 20% of affected horses [1, 120]. In fact, there is only one well-described case of functional adrenocortical adenoma in horses. This animal showed different clinical signs such as voracious appetite, loss of muscle mass, bulging supraorbital fat, delayed coat shedding, hyperhidrosis and lethargy [41, 121].

In horses with PPID, the pars intermedia of the pituitary gland enlarge over time due exclusively to hyperplasia or adenoma formation on melanotrope cell population. This pathology produces an excessive and autonomous secretion of peptides derived from proopiomelanocortin (POMC), which include ACTH, α-melanocyte-stimulating hormone (α-MSH), β-endorphin and the intermediate peptide similar to corticotropin [120].

The increase of the hormone ACTH leads to secondary hyperadrenocorticism and the increase of CORT due to hypothalamic innervation lapses. In turn, hypothalamic dopamine exerts an inhibitory control on the production and secretion of POMC peptides by melanotropes located in the pars intermedia. In horses, abnormal pars intermedia tissue contains significantly reduced amounts of dopamine. Thus, about 10% of the tissue of the pars intermedia is normal, which means a specific loss of hypothalamic dopaminergic innervation. This loss of dopaminergic innervation is due to an oxidant-induced injury in the hypothalamic tissue. Therefore, a risk factor for affected horses could be the reduction of antioxidant defense mechanisms in neural tissue. In addition, insoluble aggregates of the neural protein α-synuclein have been found in dopaminergic nerve endings in horses affected by PPID [120].

Horses with PPID present lethargy, marked hypertrichosis together with recurrent laminitis, muscle wasting, pendulous abdomen. Also it was described additional problems such as polydipsia, polyuria, recurrent infections and abnormal sweating patterns that probably represented end-stage disease. In recent years the early recognition of the disease has been an important achievement. The clinical picture is often more subtle and the symptoms include decreased performance, loss of the superior line, slight changes in attitude, lamellar changes in the hoof in the absence of pain and mild delayed coat shedding in spring time and/or regional hypertrichosis [74, 122].

3.2. Hypoadrenocorticism

Addison's disease or hypoadrenocorticism consists of permanent adrenocortical insufficiency and, in general, is rare in the horse. This syndrome is also called relative adrenal insufficiency (RAI) or critical illness related to corticosteroid failure (CIRCI). This disease can contribute substantially to the morbidity and mortality associated with the primary disease [1].

The CORT insufficiency can be transient or permanent could be a consequence of the deterioration of the HPA axis in one or several levels [5]. The permanent dysfunction of the HPA axis results in the destruction of one or more glandular components of the shaft. Despite being rare in human and veterinary medicine, adrenocortical destruction mediated by immunity (Addison's disease) is the most common manifestation of permanent HPA axis hypofunction. Patients with

Addison's disease cannot develop an appropriate CORT response to stress. Therefore, these patients are frequently present with hemodynamic instability and collapse. Aldosterone deficiency, which is added to CORT deficiency, is a typical characteristic of Addison's disease. In affected individuals, it produces fluid and electrolyte disorders that contribute to hypovolemia, hypotension and cardiovascular collapse [1, 5].

Bacterial components such as endotoxin (a lipopolysaccharide component of Gram negative bacterial cell walls) and host pro-inflammatory cytokines participate in initiating and maintaining the HPA axis response to sepsis. These factors can directly stimulate HPA axis activity at the multiple levels, ultimately resulting in stimulation of CORT synthesis and secretion [123].

In the presence of overwhelming bacterial infection or excessive host inflammatory response, HPA axis function can also be suppressed at one or more levels. For example, in patients who died from septic shock, nitric oxide-mediated induction in the death of hypothalamic neurons of cardioregulatory centers, which may be involved in HPA axis dysfunction, has been described. The bacterial endotoxin directly decreases gene expression of the pituitary CRH receptor in both rats and cattle [124]. In addition, tumor necrosis factor-α (TNF-α) can directly affect the release of pituitary ACTH and adrenal CORT synthesis [123]. Several reduced levels of high density lipoprotein (HDL) in plasma have been demonstrated in critically ill individuals. Therefore, the availability of cholesterol for the synthesis of corticosteroids may be limited during sepsis, since decreased levels of HDL are related to attenuate CORT responses to ACTH stimulation [123].

While irreversible HPA axis hypofunction due to component destruction is uncommon, recent evidence suggests that transient HPA axis dysfunction (RAI/CIRCI) can occur in a substantial number of critically ill patients with a variety of conditions. It has also been suggested that RAI/CIRCI can occur in septic neonatal foals. Couëtil and Hoffman [125] described a clinical case in a neonate foal with septicemia, a transient dysfunction of the HPA axis. This dysfunction is evidenced by a low basal CORT concentration and an altered CORT response to a high dose ACTH stimulation test. In addition, two independent studies that measured basal concentrations of ACTH and CORT in healthy and septic neonatal foals found a significant increase in the proportion of ACTH:CORT in foals with septicemia that did not survive [126, 127]. These high concentrations of ACTH and low CORT concentrations suggest that HPA axis dysfunction can occur in septic foals at term.

In two studies conducted by Hart et al. [39] and Wong et al. [128], the HPA axis function has been characterized in hospitalized foals that use stimulation tests with ACTH. None of the studies identified a significant difference in CORT peak responses between groups of healthy and diseased foals of similar age. These results were in response to a low-dose ACTH stimulation test (0.1 μg/kg) [128] or in response to a paired low-dose ACTH stimulation test (10 μg)/high dose (100 μg) [39]. However, when the criteria for human diagnosis for RAI/CIRCI [123] were adapted and applied to a group of hospitalized foals, approximately 50% fulfilled these criteria [39]. In addition, the greater severity of the disease and the worse prognosis were correlated with the decrease in CORT responses to stimulation with ACTH. Specifically, foals that did not survive had lower CORT responses to low-dose ACTH stimulation compared to survivors [128]. Likewise, foals that met the RAI/CIRCI criteria had a significantly higher incidence of shock, multiple organ dysfunction syndrome and non-survival compared to foals with an adequate CORT response to ACTH [39]. These studies provide evidence that RAI/CIRCI occurs in critically ill and septic neonatal foals with frequency and impact comparable to humans with septicemia.

In adult horses, insufficiency of the adrenal cortex is not well described. Transient adrenal insufficiency is characterized by low basal levels of ACTH and CORT and altered responses of this hormone to the stimulation test with ACTH. This situation has been described in a horse after the abrupt cessation of long-term anabolic steroid supplementation [129]. A syndrome of adrenal exhaustion that produces lethargy, anorexia and poor performance is also described anecdotally in racehorses. This syndrome has been attributed to adrenal insufficiency associated with prolonged steroid administration or chronic stress [120].

Before the ACTH stimulation test, horses with adrenal insufficiency have reduced CORT concentrations and do not respond or respond minimally. However, measurement of ACTH levels may be important in determining other causes of hypoadrenocorticism. It is suggested that the exogenous administration of glucocorticoids decreases the concentrations of ACTH (secondary hypoadrenocorticism). Likewise, adrenal insufficiency (primary adrenocorticism) results in a higher concentration of ACTH due to the decrease in endogenous glucocorticoid concentrations due to the lack of negative feedback [1].

In mares with abnormal behavior related to estrus, a diminished response of CORT to ACTH has been described [36]. However, the clinical importance of this behavior is unknown. In horses treated with chronic glucocorticoids or anabolic steroid supplements, the potential for iatrogenic adrenal insufficiency associated with the suppression of the HPA axis by exogenous steroids should be considered. In the same way, care must be taken to avoid abrupt cessation of this type of treatment.

In horses as in many other animal species, the adrenal gland is extremely vulnerable to the ischemic injury associated with endotoxic or hypovolemic shock. It is a common finding in the necropsy of adult horses with acute gastrointestinal disease and other diseases associated with endotoxic shock, adrenocortical hemorrhage and necrosis similar to Waterhouse-Friedrichsen syndrome in humans [123]. In theory, although this has not been documented to date, in surviving horses, this damage to the adrenals could contribute to long-term adrenocortical insufficiency. Furthermore, to the knowledge of the authors, classic hypoadrenocorticism or Addison's disease has not been described in horses. This disease is responsible for the adrenocortical destruction mediated by immune mechanisms and manifested by deficiency of glucocorticoids and mineralocorticoids.

In general, horses with adrenal insufficiency have a history of depression, anorexia, exercise intolerance, weight loss, bad hair or lameness. Therefore, it is necessary to obtain a complete history, including, among other things, the performance, the previous illnesses, the administration of medications and those conditions that may cause stress. Endogenous and exogenous glucocorticoids suppress the HPA axis. This produces atrophy of the fasciculate area of the adrenal gland due to the decrease in ACTH concentrations. Although there may be electrolyte disturbances in some cases of adrenal insufficiency, the glomerulosa zone is minimally affected. The clinical signs of these alterations include depression, anorexia, scanty hair, abdominal deformity and lameness. The biochemical analysis may be normal or there may be hyponatremia, hypochloremia, hyperkalemia and hypoglycemia. Severe damage from sepsis, hemorrhage, venous thrombosis and cortical necrosis may lead to atrophy and dysfunction of the adrenal gland. Therefore, hypoadrenocorticism can occur in critically ill horses with septicemia, colic, enterocolitis, endotoxemia, disseminates intravascular coagulation [10].

3.3. Other conditions

In a study conducted by Martos et al. [130], the existing CORT concentrations were compared in four groups of animals that had the following pathologies: (1) postoperative hernia, anorexia, diarrhea, castration, chronic inflammation, babesiosis, laminitis, proximal enteritis, Horner syndrome, umbilical hernia and control group (17.55–37.56 ng/ml); (2) displacement of the major colon, idiopathic ileus and obstruction of the small intestine (49.40–53.02 ng/ml); (3) impaction of the large intestine [68, 91] and (4) acute inflammation (151.08 ng/ml). The group of animals with postoperative hernia, anorexia, diarrhea, castration, chronic inflammations, babesiosis and chronic anemia had lower CORT levels compared with control group. However, animals that present significant colonic displacement, idiopathic ileus, strangulated small bowel obstruction, impaction of the large intestine, acute inflammation and obstruction of the large intestine represented with visceral pain, functional gastrointestinal disorders, hypovolemic shock, dehydration, acidic-base anomalies and the electrolyte showed acute response to stress. Recently, Ayala et al. [28] reported elevated CORT levels in horses with laminitis, acute abdominal syndrome, castration, surgery and acute and chronic diseases than control group. The major changes in the activity of the HPA axis occurred mainly in acute diseases, laminitis and abdominal syndrome.

Elevated concentrations of CORT in serum have been associated with the presentation of colic and the severity of the disease. Therefore, CORT levels can provide additional information about decision making and prognosis and thus predict the survival of horses with colic [53, 131]. Leal et al. [119] described a significant association between abnormal circadian rhythm and the incidence of colic in horses. The results show that horses with <30% circadian rhythm are more prone to colic episodes. In addition, pain and plasma CORT in clinical and surgical colic provide a physiological validation of pain scores as a marker of underlying stress in horses [132, 133].

Finally, Keating et al. [134] showed that stress management and CORT levels have an ability to influence and manage fecal egg count levels without having to use a deworming agent. Further studies may be done regarding the factors that influence CORT and determine which potential factors, if any, can be controlled. Combined with management practices that are already known to lower the levels of eggs in the feces, it has the potential to be another method that could alleviate and curb cyathostome infestation without ever having to resort to a deworming agent.

4. Conclusion

The activation of the HPA axis in stressful situations triggers behavioral and physiological changes that improve the body's adaptability and increase its chances of survival. Unlike chronic stress, acute stress subjected to various stressful conditions including isolation, transport or exercise increase significantly plasma, saliva or feces concentrations of this hormone. Diverse physiological factors such as age, circadian and ultradian rhythms, season, feeding or reproductive state influencing cortisol levels, so it will have to take it into account when interpreting this parameter. Clinical elevation of cortisol is related with Cushing's syndrome in older horses. Deficiencies of cortisol are related to serious pathologies such as sepsis or endotoxemia in foals or adult horses.

Abbreviations

3-β-HSD	3-β-Hydroxysteroid dehydrogenase
ACTH	Adrenocorticotropic hormone
CBG	Cortisol-binding globulin
CIRCI	Critical illness related to corticosteroid failure
CORT	Cortisol
CRH	Corticotropin-releasing hormone
GH	Growth hormone
GnRH	Gonadotropin-releasing hormone
HDL	High density lipoprotein
HPA axis	Hypothalamic-pituitary-adrenal axis
HSP	Heat shock regulatory proteins
POMC	Proopiomelanocortin
PPID	Pituitary pars intermedia dysfunction
RAI	Relative adrenal insufficiency
α-MSH	α-Melanocyte-stimulating hormone

Author details

Katiuska Satué Ambrojo[1]*, María Marcilla Corzano[1] and Juan Carlos Gardon Poggi[2]

*Address all correspondence to: ksatue@uchceu.es

1 Department of Animal Medicine and Surgery, School of Veterinary Medicine, University CEU-Cardenal Herrera, Valencia, Spain

2 Department of Animal Medicine and Surgery, Faculty of Veterinary and Experimental Sciences, Catholic University of Valencia "San Vicente Mártir", Valencia, Spain

References

[1] Toribio R. Endocrine diseases. The Veterinary Clinics of North America. Equine Practice 2011;**27**(1):1-58. ISBN: 978-1-4557-0518-4

[2] Hall JE. Guyton and Hall Textbook of Medical Physiology. 12th ed. Philadelphia, PA: Saunders Elsevier; 2011. 931-934 pp. ISBN: 978-1-4160-4574-8

[3] Clark A, King P. The ACTH receptor and its mutations. In: Gaillard R, editor. The ACTH Axis: Pathogenesis, Diagnosis, and Treatment. Boston: Kluwer Academic Publishers; 2003. pp. 171-190. DOI: 10.1007/978-1-4615-0501-3

[4] Arlt W, Stewart PM. Adrenal corticosteroid biosynthesis, metabolism, and action. Endocrinology and Metabolism Clinics of North America. 2005;**34**:293-313. DOI: 10.1016/j.ecl.2005.01.002

[5] Stewart P. The adrenal cortex. In: Kronenberg H, Melmed S, Polonsky K, Larsen P, editors. Williams Textbook of Endocrinology. 11th ed. Philadelphia: Saunders Elsevier; 2008. pp. 445-503. ISBN: 9781437721812

[6] Lewis JG, Bagley CJ, Elder PA, Bachmann AW, Torpy DJ. Plasma free cortisol fraction reflects levels of functioning corticosteroid-binding globulin. Clinica Chimica Acta. 2005;**359**(1-2): 189-194. DOI: 10.1016/j.cccn.2005.03.044

[7] Nicolaides N, Galata Z, Kino T, Chrousos G, Charmandari E. The human glucocorticoid receptor: Molecular basis of biologic function. Steroids. 2010;**75**:1-12. DOI: 10.1016/j.steroids.2009.09.002

[8] Gravanis A, Margioris A. Pharmacology of glucocorticoids: An overview. In: Margioris A, Chrousos G, editors. Contemporary Endocrinology: Adrenal Disorders. Totowa, NJ: Humana Press; 2001. 59-70 pp. ISBN: ISBN-10: 1617370290

[9] Hoffman CJ, McKenzie HC, Furr MO, Desrochers A. Glucocorticoid receptor density and binding affinity in healthy horses and horses with systemic inflammatory response syndrome. Journal of Veterinary Internal Medicine. 2015;**29**(2):626-635. DOI: 10.1111/jvim.12558

[10] Hart K, Barton M, Ferguson D, Berghaus R, Slovis NM, Heusner GL. Serum free cortisol fraction in healthy and septic neonatal foals. Journal of Veterinary Internal Medicine. 2011;**25**:345-355. DOI: 10.1111/j.1939-1676.2010.0667.x

[11] Walker AJ, Avenatti RC, Arent SM, McKeever KH. Effectiveness of a superoxide dismutase supplement derived from melon extract as a recovery aid for horses following strenuous exercise. Comparative Exercise Physiology. 2015;**11**(4):213-221. DOI: https://doi.org/10.3920/CEP150023

[12] Alexander S, Irvine C. The effect of social stress on adrenal axis activity in horses: The importance of monitoring corticosteroid-binding globulin capacity. The Journal of Endocrinology. 1998;**157**:425-432. DOI: 10.1677/joe.0.1570425

[13] Buckbinder L, Robienson RP. The glucocorticoid receptor: Molecular mechanism and new therapeutic opportunities. Current Drug Targets. Inflammation and Allergy. 2002;**1**(2):127-136. DOI: 10.2174/1568010023344751

[14] de Graaf-Roelfsema E, van Ginneken ME, van Breda E, Wijnberg ID, Keizer HA, van der Kolk JH. The effect of long-term exercise on glucose metabolism and peripheral insulin sensitivity in Standardbred horses. Equine Veterinary Journal. Supplement. 2006;**36**:221-225. DOI: 10.1111/j.2042-3306.2006.tb05543.x

[15] Sun X, Mammen JM, Tian X. Sepsis induces the transcription of the glucocorticoid receptor in skeletal muscle cells. Clinical Science (London, England). 2003;**105**(3):383-391. DOI: 10.1042/CS20030087

[16] Sapolsky RM, Romero LM, Munck AU. How do glucocorticoids influence stress responses? Integrating permissive, ·suppressive, stimulatory, and preparative actions. Endocrine Reviews. 2000;**21**(1):55-89. DOI: 10.1210/edrv.21.1.0389

[17] Leclere M. Corticosteroids and immune suppressive therapies in horses. The Veterinary Clinics of North America. Equine Practice. 2017;**33**(1):17-27. DOI: 10.1016/j.cveq.2016.11.008

[18] Schmidt A, Möstl E, Wehnert C, Aurich J, Müller J, Aurich C. Cortisol release and heart rate variability in horses during road transport. Hormones Behavior. 2010;**57**:209-215. DOI: 10.1016/j.yhbeh.2009.11.003

[19] Palme R. Monitoring stress hormone metabolites as a useful, non-invasive tool for welfare assessment in farm animals. Animal Welfare. 2012;**21**:331-337. DOI: 10.7120/09627286.21.3.331

[20] Mostl E, Palme R. Hormones as indicators of stress. Domestic Animal Endocrinology. 2002;**23**:67-74. DOI: 10.1016/S0739-7240(02)00146-7

[21] Schmidt A, Aurich C, Neuhauser S, Aurich J, Möstl E. Comparison of cortisol levels in blood plasma, saliva and faeces of horses submitted to different stressors or treated with ACTH. In: Proceedings, 5th International Symposium Equitation Science, Sydney. Australia: International Society for Equitation Science; July 2009. p. 53

[22] Merl S, Scherzer S, Palme R, Möstl E. Pain causes increased concentrations of glucocorticoid metabolites in horse faeces. Journal of Equine Veterinary Science. 2000;**20**:586-590. DOI: http://dx.doi.org/10.1016/S0737-0806(00)70267-X

[23] Bae YJ, Kratzsch J. Corticosteroid-binding globulin: Modulating mechanisms of bioavailability of cortisol and its clinical implications. Best Practice & Research. Clinical Endocrinology & Metabolism. 2015;**29**(5):761-772. DOI: 10.1016/j.beem.2015.09.001

[24] Fureix C, Benhajali H, Henry S, Bruchet A, Prunier M, Ezzaouia M, Coste C, Hausberger M, Palme R, Jego P. Plasma cortisol and faecal cortisol metabolites concentrations in stereotypic and non-stereotypic horses: Do stereotypic horses cope better with poor environmental conditions? BMC Veterinary Research. 2013;**9**:3. DOI: 10.1186/1746-6148-9-3

[25] Pawluski J, Jego P, Henry S, Bruchet A, Palme R, Coste C, Hausberger M. Low plasma cortisol and fecal cortisol metabolite measures as indicators of compromised welfare in domestic horses (*Equus caballus*). PLoS One. Sep 8, 2017;**12**(9):e0182257. DOI: 10.1371/journal.pone.0182257

[26] Haritou SJ, Zylstra R, Ralli C, Turner S, Tortonese DJ. Seasonal changes in circadian peripheral plasma concentrations of melatonin, serotonin, dopamine and cortisol in aged horses with Cushing's disease under natural photoperiod. Journal of Neuroendocrinology. 2008;**20**(8):988-996. DOI: 10.1111/j.1365-2826.2008.01751.x

[27] Peeters M, Sulon J, Beckers JF, Ledoux D, Vandenheede M. Comparison between blood serum and salivary cortisol concentrations in horses using an adrenocorticotropic hormone challenge. Equine Veterinary Journal. 2011;**43**(4):487-493. DOI: 10.1111/j.2042-3306.2010.00294.x

[28] Ayala I, Martos NF, Silvan G, Gutierrez-Panizo C, Clavel JG, Illera JC. Cortisol, adrenocorticotropic hormone, serotonin, adrenaline and noradrenaline serum concentrations in relation to disease and stress in the horse. Research in Veterinary Science. 2012;**93**:103-107. DOI: 10.1016/j.rvsc.2011.05.013

[29] Fazio E, Medica P, Cravana A, Ferlazzo A. Pituitary-adrenocortical adjustments to transport stress in horses with previous different handling and transport conditions. Veterinary World. 2016;**9**(8):856-861. DOI: 10.14202/vetworld.2016.856-861

[30] Reijerkerk EP, Visser EK, van Reenen CG, van der Kolk JH. Effects of various doses of ovine corticotrophin-releasing hormone on plasma and saliva cortisol concentrations in horses. American Journal of Veterinary Research. 2009;**70**(3):361-364. DOI: 10.2460/ajvr.70.3.361

[31] Haffner J, Fecteau K, Eiler H, Tserendorj T, Hoffman R, Oliver J. Blood steroid concentrations in domestic Mongolian horses. Journal of Veterinary Diagnostic Investigation. 2010;**22**:537-543. DOI: 10.1177/104063871002200407

[32] Satué K, Domingo R, Redondo JI. Relationship between progesterone, oestrone sulphate and cortisol and the components of renin angiotensin aldosterone system in Spanish purebred broodmares during pregnancy. Theriogenology. 2011;**76**(8):1404-1415. DOI: 10.1016/j.theriogenology.2011.06.009

[33] Söder J, Bröjer J, Nostel KEA. Interday variation and effect of transportation on indirect blood pressure measurements, plasma endothelin-1 and serum cortisol in Standardbred and Icelandic horses. Acta Veterinaria Scandinavica. 2012;**54**(1):37. DOI: 10.1186/1751-0147-54-37

[34] Rossdale PD, Ousey JC, Silver M, Fowden A. Studies on equine prematurity 6: Guidelines for assessment of foal maturity. Equine Veterinary Journal. 1984;**16**:300-302. DOI: 10.1111/j.2042-3306.1984.tb01931.x

[35] Donaldson MT, McDonnell SBJ, Lamb SV, McFarlane D, Beech J. Variation in plasma ACTH concentration and dexamethasone suppression test results with season, age and sex in healthy ponies and horses. Journal of Veterinary Internal Medicine. 2005;**19**:217-222. DOI: 10.1111/j.1939-1676.2005.tb02685.x

[36] Hedberg Y, Dalin A, Forsberg M, Lundeheim N, Hoffmann B, Ludwig C, Kindahl H. Effect of ACTH (tetracosactide) on steroid hormone levels in the mare. Part A: effect in intact normal mares and mares with possible estrous related behavioral abnormalities. Animal Reproduction Science. 2007;**100**:73-91. DOI: 10.1016/j.anireprosci.2006.06.008

[37] Place NJ, McGowan CM, Lamb SV, Schanbacher BJ, McGowan T, Walsh DM. Seasonal variation in serum concentrations of selected metabolic hormones in horses. Journal of Veterinary Internal Medicine. 2010;**24**(3):650-654. DOI: 10.1111/j.1939-1676.2010.0500.x

[38] Bousquet-Mélou A, Formentini E, Picard-Hagen N, Delage L, Laroute V, Toutain PL. The adrenocorticotropin stimulation test: Contribution of a physiologically based model developed in horse for its interpretation in different pathophysiological situations encountered in man. Endocrinology. 2006;**147**(9):4281-4291. DOI: https://doi.org/10.1210/en.2005-1161

[39] Hart K, Slovis N, Barton M. Hypothalamic-pituitary-adrenal axis dysfunction in hospitalized neonatal foals. Journal of Veterinary Internal Medicine. 2009;**23**:901-912. DOI: 10.1111/j.1939-1676.2009.0323.x

[40] Liburt NR, McKeever KH, Malinowski K, Smarsh DN, Geor RJ. Response of the hypothalamic-pituitary-adrenal axis to stimulation tests before and after exercise training in old and young Standardbred mares. Journal of Animal Science. 2013 Nov;**91**(11):5208-5219. DOI: 10.2527/jas.2013-6329

[41] van der Kolk JH. Equine Cushing's disease. Equine Veterinary Education. 1997;**9**(4):209-214. DOI: 10.1111/j.2042-3292.1997.tb01308.x

[42] Hart KA, Wochele DM, Norton NA, McFarlane D, Wooldridge AA, Frank N. Effect of age, season, body condition, and endocrine status on serum free cortisol fraction and insulin concentration in horses. Journal of Veterinary Internal Medicine. 2016;**30**:653-663. DOI: 10.1111/jvim.13839

[43] Aurich J, Wulf M, Ille N, Erber R, von Lewinski M, Palme R, Aurich C. Effects of season, age, sex, and housing on salivary cortisol concentrations in horses. Domestic Animal Endocrinology. 2015;**52**:11-16. DOI: 10.1016/j.domaniend.2015.01.003

[44] Zuluaga A, Martínez JR. Serum cortisol concentration in the Colombian creole horse. Rough Cut Capacity Planning. 2017;**30**(3):231-238. DOI: 10.17533/udea.rccp.v30n3a06

[45] Irvine CH, Alexander SL. Factors affecting the circadian rhythm in plasma cortisol concentrations in the horse. Domestic Animal Endocrinology. 1994;**11**(2):227-238. DOI: https://doi.org/10.1016/0739-7240(94)90030-2

[46] Giannetto C, Fazio F, Vazzana I, Panzera M, Piccione G. Comparison of cortisol and rectal temperature circadian rhythms in horses: The role of light/dark cycle and constant darkness. Biological Rhythm Research 2012;**43**(6):681-687. DOI: http://dx.doi.org/10.1080/09291016.2011.632231.

[47] Rendle DI, Litchfield E, Heller J, Hughes KJ. Investigation of rhythms of secretion and repeatability of plasma adrenocorticotropic hormone concentrations in healthy horses and horses with pituitary pars intermedia dysfunction. Equine Veterinary Journal. 2014;**46**(1):113-117. DOI: 10.1111/evj.12114

[48] Rendle DI, Litchfield E, Gough S, Cowling A, Hughes KJ. The effects of sample handling and *n*-phenylmaleimide on concentration of adrenocorticotrophic hormone in equine plasma. Equine Veterinary Journal. 2015;**47**(5):587-591. DOI: 10.1111/evj.12319

[49] Pell SM, McGreevy PD. A study of cortisol and beta-endorphin levels in stereotypic and normal thoroughbreds. Applied Animal Behaviour Science 1999;**64**:81-90. DOI: http://dx.doi.org/10.1016/S0168-1591(99)00029-5

[50] Evans JW, Winget CM, Pollak EJ: Rhythmic cortisol secretion in the equine: Analysis and physiological mechanisms. Journal of Interdisciplinary Cycle Research. 1977;**8**(2):111-121. DOI: http://dx.doi.org/10.1080/09291017709359550.

[51] Diez de Castro E, Lopez I, Cortes B, Pineda C, Garfia B, Aguilera-Tejero E. Influence of feeding status, time of the day, and season on baseline adrenocorticotropic hormone and the response to thyrotropin releasing hormone-stimulation test in healthy horses. Domestic Animal Endocrinology. 2014;**48**:77-83. DOI: 10.1016/j.domaniend.2014.02.004

[52] de Jong IC, Prelle IT, van de Burgwal JA, Lambooij E, Korte SM, Blokhuis HJ, Koolhaas JM. Effects of environmental enrichment on behavioral responses to novelty, learning, and memory, and the circadian rhythm in cortisol in growing pigs. Physiology & Behavior. 2000;**68**:571-578. DOI: 10.1016/S0031-9384(99)00212-7

[53] Hinchcliff KW, Rush BR, Farris JW. Evaluation of plasma catecholamine and serum cortisol concentrations in horses with colic. Journal of the American Veterinary Medical Association. 2005;**227**:276-280. DOI: https://doi.org/10.2460/javma.2005.227.276

[54] Fazio E, Medica P, Aronica V, Grasso L, Ferlazzo A. Circulating β-endorphin, adrenocorticotrophic hormone and cortisol levels of stallions before and after short road transport: Stress effect of different distances. Acta Veterinaria Scandinavica. 2008;**50**(1):6. DOI: 10.1186/1751-0147-50-6

[55] Cordero M, Brorsen BW, McFarlane D. Circadian and circannual rhythms of cortisol, ACTH, and α-melanocyte-stimulating hormone in healthy horses. Domestic Animal Endocrinology. 2012;**43**(4):317-324. DOI: 10.1016/j.domaniend.2012.05.005

[56] Fazio E, Ferlazzo A: Evaluation of stress during transport. Veterinary Research Communications. 2003;**27**(Suppl. I):519-524. DOI: 10.1023/B:VERC.0000014211.87613.d9

[57] Stull CL, Spier SJ, Aldridge BM, Blanchard M, Stott JL. Immunological response to long-term transport stress in mature horses and effects of adaptogenic dietary supplementation as an immunomodulator. Equine Veterinary Journal. 2004;**36**:583-589. DOI: 10.2746/0425164044864589

[58] Stull CL, Morrow J, Aldridge BA, Stott JL, McGlone JJ. Immunophysiological responses of horses to 12-hour rest during 24 hours of road transport. The Veterinary Record. 2008; **162**:609-614. DOI: 10.1136/vr.162.19.609

[59] Deichsel K, Pasing S, Erber R, Ille N, Palme R, Aurich J, Aurich C. Increased cortisol release and transport stress do not influence semen quality and testosterone release in pony stallions. Theriogenology 2015;**84**(1):70-75. DOI: http://dx.doi.org/10.1016/j.theriogenology.2015.02.015

[60] Mercer-Bowyer S, Kersey DC, Bertone JJ. Use of fecal glucocorticoid and salivary cortisol concentrations as a measure of well-being of New York City carriage horses. Journal of the American Veterinary Medical Association. Feb 1, 2017;**250**(3):316-321. DOI: 10.2460/javma.250.3.316

[61] Shanahan S. Trailer loading stress in horses: Behavioral and physiological effects of nonaversive training (TTEAM). Journal of Applied Animal Welfare Science 2003;**6**:263-274. DOI: http://dx.doi.org/10.1207/s15327604jaws0604_1

[62] Tischner Jr M, Niezgoda J, Tischner M. Intensity of stress reaction in the mare during transportation at different stages of ovarian activity and pregnancy. Animal Reproduction Science. 2006;**94**:234-237. DOI: 10.1016/j.anireprosci.2006.04.043

[63] Mortensen CJ, Choi YH, Hinrichs K, Ing NH, Kraemer DC, Vogelsang SG, Vogelsang MM. Embryo recovery from exercised mares. Animal Reproduction Science. 2009;**110**:237-244. DOI: 10.1016/j.anireprosci.2008.01.015

[64] Schreiber CM, Stewart AJ, Behrend EN, Wright J, Kemppainen R, Busch KA. Seasonal variation in diagnostic tests for pituitary pars intermedia dysfunction in normal aged geldings. Journal of Veterinary Internal Medicine. 2008;**22**:734. DOI: 10.2460/javma.241.2.241

[65] Borer-Weir KE, Menzies-Gow NJ, Bailey SR, Harris PA, Elliott J. Seasonal and annual inïuence on insulin and cortisol results from overnight dexamethasone suppression tests in normal ponies and ponies predisposed to laminitis. Equine Veterinary Journal. 2013;**45**:688-693. DOI: 10.2527/jas.2011-4236

[66] Bohák Z, Szabó F, Beckers JF, Melo de Sousa N, Kutasi O, Nagy K, Szenci O. Monitoring the circadian rhythm of serum and salivary cortisol concentrations in the horse. Domestic Animal Endocrinology. 2013;**45**(1):38-42. DOI: 10.1016/j.domaniend.2013.04.001

[67] Saul JL, Nyhart AB, Reddish JM, Alman M, Cole K. Effect of feeding practice on glucose, insulin, and cortisol responses in quarter horse mares. Journal of Equine Veterinary Science 2011;**31**(5-6):299-300. DOI: http://dx.doi.org/10.1016/j.jevs.2011.03.127

[68] Glunk EC, Hathaway MR, Grev AM, Lamprecht ED, Maher MC, Martinson KL. The effect of a limit-fed diet and slow-feed hay nets on morphometric measurements and post-prandial metabolite and hormone patterns in adult horses. Journal of Animal Science. 2015;**93**(8):4144-4152. DOI: 10.2527/jas.2015-9150

[69] Widmann C. Effect of diet on cortisol concentrations in response to feeding stress in horses [thesis]. Columbus, OH: The Ohio State University; 2010

[70] Malinowski K, Shock EJ, Rochelle P, Kearns CF, Guirnalda PD, McKeever KH. Plasma beta-endorphin, cortisol and immune responses to acute exercise are altered by age and exercise training in horses. Equine Veterinary Journal. 2006;**36**:267-273. DOI: 10.1111/j.2042-3306.2006.tb05551.x

[71] Ferlazzo A, Medica P, Cravana C, Fazio E. Endocrine changes after experimental show-jumping Comparative Exercise Physiology 2009;**6**:59-66. DOI: http://dx.doi.org/10.1016/j.jevs.2014.03.001.

[72] Moons C, Heleski CR, Leece CM, Zanella AJ. Conflicting results in the association between plasma and salivary cortisol level in foals. In: Proceedings of the Dorothy Russel Havemeyer Foundation Workshop "Horse Behavior and Welfare"; Holar College, Iceland. 2002. pp. 59-63

[73] Harewood EI, McGowan CM. Behavioral and physiological responses to stabling in naive horses. Journal of Equine Veterinary Science 2005;**4**:164-170. DOI: http://dx.doi.org/10.1016/j.jevs.2005.03.008

[74] McGowan TW, Pinchbeck GP, McGowan CM. Prevalence, risk factors and clinical signs predictive for equine pituitary pars intermedia dysfunction in aged horses. Equine Veterinary Journal. 2013;**45**(1):74-79. DOI: 10.1111/j.2042-3306.2012.00578.x

[75] Larsson L, Pilborg PH, Jonansen M, Christophersen MT, Holte A, Roepstorff L, Olsen LH, Harrison AP. Physiological parameters of endurance horses pre compared basal values post-race, correlated with performance: A two race study from Scandinavia. International Scholarly Research Notices Veterinary Science. 2013; 12 pages. Article ID 684353. DOI: 10.1155/2013/684353

[76] Peeters MM, Coline CC, Becker JF, Vandenheede M. Rider and horse salivary cortisol levels during competition and impact on performance. Journal of Equine Veterinary Science. 2013;**33**:155-160. DOI: http://dx.doi.org/10.1016/j.jevs.2012.05.073

[77] Kang OD, Lee WS. Changes in salivary cortisol concentration in horses during different types of exercise. Asian-Australasian Journal of Animal Sciences. 2016;**29**(5):747-752. DOI: 10.5713/ajas.16.0009

[78] Gordon ME, McKeever K, Betros CL, Manso Filho HC. Exercise-induced alterations in plasma concentrations of ghrelin, adiponectin, leptin, glucose, insulin, and cortisol in horses. Veterinary Journal 2007;**173**(1):91-100. DOI: 10.1016/j.tvjl.2005.11.004

[79] Hyyppä S. Endocrinal responses in exercising horses. Livestock Production Science 2005; **92**:113-121. DOI: http://dx.doi.org/10.1016/j.livprodsci.2004.11.014

[80] McKeever KH. Exercise physiology of the older horse. Veterinary Clinics of North America, Equine Practice. 2002;**18**:469-490. DOI: https://doi.org/10.1053/S1534-7516(03)00068-4

[81] Smiet E, Van Dierendonck MC, Sleutjens J, Menheere PP, van Breda E, de Boer D, Back W, Wijnberg ID, van der Kolk JH. Effect of different head and neck positions on behaviour, heart rate variability and cortisol levels in lunged Royal Dutch Sport horses. Veterinary Journal. 2014;**202**(1):26-32. DOI: 10.1016/j.tvjl.2014.07.005

[82] Fazio E, Medica P, Galvano E, Cravaca G, Ferlazzo A. Changes in the cortisol and some biochemical patterns of pregnant and barren jennies (*Equus asinus*). Veterinarski Arhiv. 2011;**81**:563-574. DOI: 2-s2.0-80054894275

[83] Janczarek I, Bereznowski A, Strzelec K. The influence of selected factors and sport results of endurance horses on their saliva cortisol concentration. Polish Journal of Veterinary Science. 2013;**16**(3):533-541. DOI: 10.2478/pjvs-2013-0074

[84] Munk R, Jensen RB, Palme R, Munksgaard L, Christensen JW. An exploratory study of competition scores and salivary cortisol concentrations in Warmblood horses. Domestic Animal Endocrinology. 2017;**61**:108-116. DOI: 10.1016/j.domaniend.2017.06.007

[85] Veronesi MC, Tosi U, Villani M, Govoni N, Faustini M, Kindahl H, Madej A, Carluccio A. Oxytocin, vasopressin, prostaglandin F(2alpha), luteinizing hormone, testosterone, estrone sulfate, and cortisol plasma concentrations after sexual stimulation in stallions. Theriogenology. Mar 1, 2010;**73**(4):460-467. DOI: 10.1016/j.theriogenology.2009.09.028

[86] Schmidt K, Deichsel K, de Oliveira RA, Aurich J, Ille N, Aurich C. Effects of environmental temperature and season on hair coat characteristics, physiologic and reproductive parameters in Shetland pony stallions. Theriogenology. 2017;**15**(97):170-178. DOI: 10.1016/j.theriogenology.2017.04.035

[87] Villani M, Cairoli F, Kindahl H, Galeati G, Faustini M, Carluccio A, Veronesi MC. Effects of mating on plasma concentrations of testosterone, cortisol, oestrone sulphate and 15-keto-dihydro-PGF2alpha in stallions. Reproduction in Domestic Animals. 2006;**41**(6):544-548. DOI: 10.1111/j.1439-0531.2006.00711.x

[88] Pasing S, von Lewinski M, Wulf M, Erber R, Aurich C. Influence of semen collection on salivary cortisol release, heart rate, and heart rate variability in stallions. Theriogenology. 2013;**80**(3):256-261. DOI: 10.1016/j.theriogenology.2013.04.003

[89] Hedberg Y, Dalin AM, Forsberg M, Lundeheim N, Hoffmann B, Ludwig C, Kindahl H. Effect of ACTH (tetracosactide) on steroid hormone levels in the mare. Part A: effect in intact normal mares and mares with possible estrous related behavioral abnormalities. Animal Reproduction Science. 2007;**100**(1-2):73-91. DOI: 10.1016/j.anireprosci.2006.06.008

[90] Hedberg Y, Dalin AM, Forsberg M, Lundeheim N, Sandh G, Hoffmann B, Ludwig C, Kindahl H. Effect of ACTH (tetracosactide) on steroid hormone levels in the mare. Part B: Effect in ovariectomized mares (including estrous behavior). Animal Reproduction Science. 2007;**100**(1-2):92-106. DOI: 10.1016/j.anireprosci.2006.06.007

[91] Satué K, Gardon JC, Marcilla M. Adrenocorticotrophic hormone, aldosterone and cortisol concentrations during estrous cycle in healthy Spanish Purebred mares. Reproduction in Domestic Animals. 2016;**51**(2):138. DOI: 10.1111/rda.12801

[92] Ginther OJ, Gastal EL, Gastal MO, Beg MA. Effect of prostaglandin F2alpha on ovarian, adrenal, and pituitary hormones and on luteal blood flow in mares. Domestic Animal Endocrinology. 2007;**32**(4):315-328. DOI: 10.1016/j.domaniend.2006.04.006

[93] Satué K, Montesinos P, Gardon JC. Association between aldosterone and cortisol levels during ovulatory period in Spanish Purebred mares. Reproduction, Fertility, and Development. 2014;**26**:146. DOI: https://doi.org/10.1071/RDv26n1Ab65

[94] Satué K, Montesinos P, Gardon JC. Relationship between cortisol and progesterone in cyclic Spanish Purebred mares during the luteal phase of estrous cycle. Reproduction in Domestic Animals. 2014;**49**(4):101. DOI: 10.1111/rda.12801

[95] Harvey JW, Pate MG, Kivipelto J, Asquith RL. Clinical biochemistry of pregnant and nursing mares. Veterinary Clinical Pathology. 2005;**34**(3):248-254. DOI: 10.1111/j.1939-165X.2005.tb00049.x

[96] Marcilla M, Muñoz A, Satué K. Longitudinal changes in serum catecholamines, dopamine, serotonin, ACTH and cortisol in pregnant Spanish mares. Research in Veterinary Science. 2017;**21**;115:29-33. DOI 10.1016/j.rvsc.2017.01.020

[97] Hoffman RM, Boston RC, Stefanovski D, Kronfeld DS, Harris PA. Obesity and diet affect glucose dynamics and insulin sensitivity in thoroughbred geldings. Journal of Animal Science. 2003;**81**:2333-2342. DOI: 10.2527/2003.8192333x

[98] George LA, Staniar WB, Cubitt TA, Treiber KH, Harris PA, Geor RJ. Evaluation of the effects of pregnancy on insulin sensitivity, insulin secretion, and glucose dynamics in thoroughbred mares. American Journal of Veterinary Research. 2011;**72**(5):666-674. DOI: 10.2460/ajvr.72.5.666

[99] Fowden AL, Giussani DA, Forhead AJ. Endocrine and metabolic programming during intrauterine development. Early Human Development. 2005;**81**:723-734. DOI: 10.1016/j.earlhum-dev.2005.06.00

[100] Hedberg Y, Dalin AM, Ohagen P, Holm KR, Kindahl H. Effect of oestrous cycle stage on the response of mares in a novel object test and isolation test. Reproduction in Domestic Animals. 2005;**40**:480-488. DOI: 10.1111/j.1439-0531.2005.00611.x

[101] Jung C, Ho JT, Torpy DJ, Rogers A, Doogue M, Lewis JG, Czajko RJ, Inder WJ. A longitudinal study of plasma and urinary cortisol in pregnancy and postpartum. The Journal of Clinical Endocrinology and Metabolism. 2011;**96**(5):1533-1540. DOI: 10.1210/jc.2010-2395

[102] Nagel C, Erber R, Bergmaier C, Wulf M, Aurich J, Möstl E, Aurich C. Cortisol and progestin release, heart rate and heart rate variability in the pregnant and postpartum mare, fetus, and newborn foal. Theriogenology. 2012;**78**:759-767. DOI: 10.1016/j.theriogenology.2012.03.023

[103] Nagel C, Erber R, Ille N, von Lewinski M, Aurich J, Möstl E, Aurich C. Parturition in horses is dominated by parasympathetic activity of the autonomous nervous system. Theriogenology 2014;**82**(1):160-168. DOI: 10.1016/j.theriogenology.2014.03.015

[104] Tsigos C, Chrousos GP. Hypothalamic-pituitary-adrenal axis, neuroendocrine factors and stress. Journal of Psychosomatic Research. 2002;**53**:865-871. DOI: 10.1016/S0022-3999(02)00429-4U

[105] Berghold P, Möstl E, Aurich C. Effects of reproductive status and management on cortisol secretion and fertility of oestrous horse mares. Health Advance. 2007;**102**(3-4):276-285. DOI: http://dx.doi.org/10.1016/j.anireprosci.2006.11.009

[106] Wyrwoll CS, Holmes MC. Prenatal excess glucocorticoid exposure and adult affective disorders: A role for serotonergic and catecholamine pathways. Neuroendocrinology. 2012;**95**(1):47-55. DOI: 10.1159/000331345

[107] Nepomnashy PA, Welch KB, McConnell DS, Low BS, Strassmann BI, England BG. Cortisol levels and very early pregnancy loss in humans. Proceedings of the National Academy of Sciences of the United States of America. Mar 7, 2006;**103**(10):3938-3942. DOI: 10.1073/pnas.0511183103

[108] Fowden AL, Forhead AJ. Endocrine regulation of fetoplacental growth. Hormone Research. 2009;**72**:257-265. DOI: 10.1159/000245927

[109] Fowden AL. The insulin-like growth factors and feto-placental growth. Placenta. 2003;**24**:803-812. DOI: http://dx.doi.org/10.1016/S0143-4004(03)00080-8

[110] Oakley AE, Breen KM, Clarke IJ, Karsch FJ, Wagenmaker ER, Tilbrook AJ. Cortisol reduces gonadotropin-releasing hormone pulse frequency in follicular phase ewes: Influence of ovarian steroids. Endocrinology. 2009;**150**(1):341-349. DOI: 10.1210/en.2008-0587

[111] Einarsson S, Brandt Y, Rodriguez-Martinez H, Madej A. Conference lecture: Influence of stress on estrus, gametes and early embryo development in the sow. Theriogenology. 2008;**70**:1197-1120. DOI: 10.1016/j.theriogenology.2008.06.015

[112] Kapoor A, Petropoulos S, Matthews SG. Fetal programming of hypothalamic-pituitary-adrenal (HPA) axis function and behavior by synthetic glucocorticoids. Brain Research Reviews. 2008;**57**:586-595. DOI: 10.1016/j.brainresrev.2007.06.013

[113] Challis JR, Sloboda D, Matthews SG, Holloway A, Alfaidy N, Patel FA, Whittle W, Fraser M, Moss TJ, Newnham J. The fetal placental hypothalamic-pituitary-adrenal (HPA) axis, parturition and post natal health. Molecular and Cellular Endocrinology. Dec 20, 2001;**185**(1-2): 135-144. DOI: https://doi.org/10.1016/S0303-7207(01)00624-4

[114] Fowden AL, Forhead AJ, Ousey JC. The endocrinology of equine parturition. Experimental and Clinical Endocrinology & Diabetes. 2008;**116**(7):393-403. DOI: 10.1055/s-2008-1042409

[115] Diego R, Douet C, Reigner F, Blard T, Cognié J, Deleuze S, Goudet G. Influence of trans-vaginal ultrasound-guided follicular punctures in the mare on heart rate, respiratory rate, facial expression changes, and salivary cortisol as pain scoring. Theriogenology. June 15, 2016;**86**(7):1757-1763. DOI: 10.1016/j.theriogenology.2016.05.040

[116] Schönbom H, Kassens A, Hopster-Iversen C, Klewitz J, Piechotta M, Martinsson G, Kißler A, Burger D, Sieme H. Influence of transrectal and transabdominal ultrasound examination on salivary cortisol, heart rate, and heart rate variability in mares. Theriogenology. mAR 1, 2015:**83**(4):749-756. DOI: 10.1016/j.theriogenology.2014.11.010

[117] Colborn DR, Thompson Jr DL, Roth TL, Capehart JS, White KL. Responses of cortisol and prolactin to sexual excitement and stress in stallions and geldings. Journal of Animal Science. 1991;**69**(6):2556-2562. DOI: 10.2527/1991.6962556x

[118] Erber R, Wulf M, Aurich J, Rose-Meierhöfer S, Hoffmann G, von Lewinski M, Möstl E, Aurich C. Stress response of three-year-old horse mares to changes in husbandry system during initial equestrian training. Journal of Equine Veterinary Science 2013;**33**:1088-1094. DOI: http://dx.doi.org/10.1016/j.jevs.2013.04.008

[119] Leal BB, Geraldo ES, Douglas RH, Bringel B, Young RJ, Haddad JP, Viana WS, Faleiros RR. Cortisol circadian rhythm ratio: A simple method to detect stressed horses at higher risk of colic? Journal of Equine Veterinary Science 2011;**31**:188-190. DOI: http://dx.doi.org/10.1016/j.jevs.2011.02.005

[120] McFarlane D. Equine pituitary pars intermedia dysfunction. The Veterinary Clinics of North America. Equine Practice. 2011;**27**:93. DOI: 10.1016/j.cveq.2010.12.007

[121] van der Kolk JH, Ijzer J, Overgaauw PA, van der Linde-Sipman JS. Pituitary-independent Cushing's syndrome in a horse. Equine Veterinary Journal. 2001;**33**:110-2.93. DOI: 10.2746/042516401776767368

[122] Durham AE. Endocrine disease in aged horses. Veterinary Clinics of North America, Equine Practice. 2016;**32**:301-315. DOI: https://doi.org/10.1016/j.cveq.2016.04.007

[123] Marik PE. Critical illness-related corticosteroid insufficiency. Chest. 2009;**135**:181-193. DOI: 10.1378/chest.08-1149

[124] Sharshar T, Annane D, de la Grandmaison G, Brouland P, Hopkinson NS, Gray F. The neuropathology of septic shock. Brain Pathology. 2004;**14**:21-33. DOI: 10.1111/j.1750-3639.2004.tb00494.x

[125] Couetil LL, Hoffman AM. Adrenal insufficiency in a neonatal foal. Journal of the American Veterinary Medical Association. 1998;**212**:1594-1596 9604031

[126] Gold JR, Divers TJ, Barton MH, Lamb SV, Place NJ, Mohammed HO, Bain FT. Plasma adrenocorticotropin, cortisol, and adrenocorticotropin/ cortisol ratios in septic and normal-term foals. Journal of Veterinary Internal Medicine. 2007;**21**:791-796. DOI: 10.1111/j.1939-1676.2007.tb03023.x

[127] Hurcombe SD, Toribio RE, Slovis N, Kohn CW, Refsal K, Saville W, Mudge MC. Blood arginine vasopressin, adrenocorticotropin hormone, and cortisol concentrations at admission in septic and critically ill foals and their association with survival. Journal of Veterinary Internal Medicine. 2008;**22**(3):639-647. DOI: 10.1111/j.1939-1676.2008.0090.x

[128] Wong DM, Vo DT, Alcott CJ, Stewart AJ, Peterson AD, Sponseller BA, Hsu WH. Adrenocorticotropic hormone stimulation tests in healthy foals from birth to 12 weeks of age. Canadian Journal of Veterinary Research. 2009;**73**(1):65-72. PMC: 2613599

[129] Dowling PM, Williams MA, Clark TP. Adrenal insufficiency associated with long-term anabolic steroid administration in a horse. Journal of the American Veterinary Medical Association. Oct 15, 1993;**203**(8):1166-1169

[130] Martos N, Ayala I, Hernández J, Gutiérrez C. Determinación de los niveles plasmáticos de cortisol en diferentes patologías de los équidos. Anales de Veterinaria de Murcia. 2003; **19**:129-140

[131] Mair TS, Sherlock CE, Boden LA. Cortisol concentrations in horses with colic. Veterinary Journal. 2014;**201**:370-377. DOI: 10.1016/j.tvjl.2014.06.005

[132] Niinistö KE, Korolainen RV, Raekallio MR, Mykkänen AK, Koho NM, Ruohoniemi MO, Leppäluoto J, Pösö AR. Plasma levels of heat shock protein 72 (HSP72) and beta-endorphin as indicators of stress, pain and prognosis in horses with colic. Veterinary Journal 2010;**184**:100-104. DOI: 10.1016/j.tvjl.2009.01.011

[133] Lawson AL, Knowles EJ, Mair TS. Correlation of composite equine pain scores with plasma adrenocorticotropic hormone and serum cortisol concentrations in horses with colic. Equine Veterinary Education. 2017;**29**(S8):22. DOI: 10.1111/eve.46_12792

[134] Keating DL, Lehman JL, Burk SV. Cross-sectional analysis of salivary cortisol and strongyle-type egg shedding levels in horses. Journal of Equine Veterinary Science 2017;**52**. 51-52. DOI: http://dx.doi.org/10.1016/j.jevs.2017.03.039

3

Management of Atopic Dermatitis in Children: A Pediatrician State of the Art

Sanela Domuz Vujnović and Adrijana Domuz

Abstract

Atopic dermatitis (AD) is one of the most common skin conditions in children and adolescents. This disease is characterized by acute and chronic lesions. Acute lesions can occur at any age and have a recurring character. Localization of acute lesions is a characteristic for a certain age of the child. Chronic lesions are present after the second year of life and characterized by pruritus and lichenification. Ichthyosis and xerosis are also characteristics of chronic lesions. The authors represent two hypotheses about pathophysiology of atopic dermatitis: "inside-out" hypothesis suggests that pathophysiological process is the result of an inflammatory response, while the "outside-inside" hypothesis suggests that changes of the epidermal barrier are responsible for the process in lesions in atopic dermatitis. There is no gold standard, clinical or laboratory, for the diagnosis of atopic dermatitis. The diagnosis should be based on anamnesis, clinical features and laboratory results. The therapeutic approach includes general and specific measures. General measures including topical moisturizers, bathing and bathing practices and wet-wrap therapy. Specific measures include topical corticosteroids and topical calcineurin inhibitors. Systemic immunosuppressant agents and phototherapy are a second-line treatment and used when the atopic dermatitis is not controlled. These patients must be treated by a dermatologist or pediatricians.

Keywords: atopic dermatitis, children, corticosteroids, emollients, topical moisturizers, skin care, eczema

1. Introduction

Atopic dermatitis (AD) is one of the most common skin conditions in children and adolescents. This disease is characterized by chronic eczematous and itchy lesions with typical distributions, and relapsing [1, 2]. Atopic dermatitis has a tendency to spontaneous withdrawal, so the incidence of this disease diminished with increasing age. The basic pathophysiological features of this disease are an epidermal barrier dysfunction and an altered immunoallergic profile [3]. Firsthand contact due to their symptoms, these patients have with the primary healthcare team, most often pediatricians and general practitioners. The diagnosis of atopic dermatitis can be defined with standardized clinical criteria and scoring systems [4]. It is important to notice that this disorder can be a major therapeutic challenge for the physician and patient, especially intense and incessant itching. The therapeutic approach includes general and specific measures. General measures include topical moisturizers, bathing and bathing practices and wet-wrap therapy. Children more likely have food-induced exacerbations. If a specific food is suspected to cause an exacerbation of atopic dermatitis, certain dietary interventions can be used. Specific measures include topical corticosteroids and topical calcineurin inhibitors. Systemic immunosuppressant agents and phototherapy are a second-line treatment and used when the atopic dermatitis is not controlled. These patients must be treated by a dermatologist or pediatricians.

2. Pathophysiology of atopic dermatitis

The lack of filaggrin plays an important role in the pathophysiology of atopic dermatitis. The large *polyprotein profilaggrin degraded* to produce monomeric *filaggrin* in the stratum corneum of the skin. Profilaggrin and filaggrin contribute to the structure of the epidermis and the functional barrier (profilaggrin and filaggrin each make different contributions to epidermal structure and barrier function) [5].

Filaggrins with intermediate filaments form solid connections in cornified leyers contributing to formation of a water loss barrier, maintaining epidermal hydration and form so-called "natural moisturizing factor" [5, 6]. Beside damaged skin barrier, in the pathophysiology of atopic dermatitis, numerous cells of innate and adaptive immune cells are involved. Keratinocytes in typical lesions release a large amount of several different proinflammatory cytokines, chemokines, and high levels of TSLP (thymic stromal lipoprotein) which promote Th2 immune response [7]. The Th2 immune response releases a large number of cytokines (IL-4, IL-13, IL-25, IL-33), which cause keratinocyte dysfunction and secondary changes in epidermal barrier. The authors state that Th2 immune response contributes to downregulation of filaggrin expression in differentiated keratinocytes [8]. Beside the filaggrin, Th2 cytokines (IL-17, IL-22, IL-25 and IL-31) significantly downregulate the expression of other proteins of stratum corneum like loricrin and involucrin [6, 8, 9].

There is an increased number of inflammatory cells such as T lymphocytes, dendritic cells, macrophages, mast cells and eosinophils in lesions characteristic for atopic dermatitis [7, 10].

Acute lesions in atopic dermatitis have a significantly higher number of Th2 cytokines (IL-4, IL-5, IL-13), while chronic lesions contain IL-4, IL-13, and numerous interferons of Th1 cells [11]. That is so-called biphasic Th cell response.

Environmental factors such as skin irritation, mechanical damage, low skin moisture and colonizing microorganisms also contribute to filaggrin expression changes [10].

Keratinocytes in patients with atopic dermatitis show increased IFN-induced apoptosis [10]. Also, in patients with atopic dermatitis, smaller keratinocytes in lesions are verified.

Inflammatory response leads to variations in epidermal thickness and the size of corneocytes in stratum corneum in region specific flares and atopic dermatitis [9].

The authors represent two hypotheses about pathophysiology of atopic dermatitis: "inside-out" hypothesis suggests that pathophysiological process is the result of an inflammatory response, while the "outside-inside" hypothesis suggests that changes of the epidermal barrier are responsible for the process in lesions in atopic dermatitis [9].

3. Clinical features

The two basic characteristics of atopic dermatitis are [4]:

- specific localization of skin lesions with areas of the clean skin and
- chronic recurring character, with periods when there is no skin lesions at all and with periods of exacerbation of skin symptoms

First, clinical symptoms of atopic dermatitis occur during the first 6 months of life in 45% of children, during the first year of life in 60%, and before the age of 5 years in at least 85% of affected individuals [4]. But it never occurs in the first week of life [12]. The clinical pattern of atopic dermatitis has a characteristic age-dependent distribution and is commonly associated with elevated IgE, peripheral eosinophilia, *Staphylococcus aureus* colonization and comorbidity with other allergic diseases [4, 12].

Atopic dermatitis as a chronic recurrent disease is characterized by acute and chronic lesions. Acute lesions predominantly occur in infants, while chronic lesions are characteristic of the later age [13, 14]. Acute lesions are characterized by erythematous papules or papulovesicules with oozing, as well as plaque and dry skin. Patients with atopic dermatitis commonly have different intensity of itch.

Acute lesions can occur at any age and have a recurring character. Localization of acute lesions is characteristic for a certain age of the child [12].

Chronic lesions are present after the second year of life and characterized by pruritus and lichenification. Ichthyosis and xerosis are also characteristics of chronic lesions [1, 4, 12].

Pruritus is a typical hallmark in all stages, except during the first weeks of life. Itching itself has different intensity and accompanied by excoriations and fibrotic nodules [1, 4].

Atopic dermatitis can cover a wide spectrum in terms of severity, ranging from very mild to very severe phenotypes. For severity assessment of atopic dermatitis, a diagnostic scoring system such as SCORAD or ECZEMA AREA AND SEVERITY INDEX SCORES is often used [1, 4].

3.1. Atopic dermatitis clinical phenotypes

Atopic dermatitis phenotypes in childhood can be divided into two groups: IgE associated and non-IgE associated atopic dermatitis. Group of children with IgE associated atopic dermatitis can be with or without another allergic diseases, especially with allergic respiratory diseases [13, 14]. Clinical phenotypes of atopic dermatitis define according to [2, 12–14].

A. Age-related clinical pictures with age off onset

B. Diseases severity

C. Non-IgE and IgE associated form

Amat et al. in their ORCA cohort study defined three phenotypes of early onset atopic dermatitis: infant with moderate atopic dermatitis severity and low sensitization, infant with a higher atopic dermatitis severity and frequent multiple sensitization and third phenotype children with moderate atopic dermatitis severity and moderate sensitization with parental familial history of asthma [15]. This phenotypic classification was used only for the epidemiological study, while its use was not verified for clinical practice.

3.2. Infantile atopic dermatitis (under 2 years of age)

First symptoms of atopic dermatitis never appear in first 2 weeks of life. First symptoms commonly appear at the age of 3 months [1, 2, 12, 16]. Typical localization of infantile atopic dermatitis is cheeks with characteristic dry skin, erythema and papules with oozing. Lesions can form large plaques with oozing and crusts. Lesions can appear on the forehead, scalp, neck and extensor surface of the extremities, rarely on the trunk. The diaper area is usually spared. Lesions in this phase may be mild, which make it difficult to diagnose. When there are no erythematous lesions in typical places, the skin is dry, rough, and desquamated [1, 2, 16].

A substantial portion of patients can go into complete remission before 2 years of age [16].

3.3. Childhood atopic dermatitis (age 2–12 years)

Chronic skin lesions with lichenification and exacerbation of acute lesions are characteristic for atopic dermatitis in this age. Children have lichenified papules and plaques involving the hands, feet, wrists, ankles, periorificial areas on the head, antecubital and popliteal regions. Xerosis becomes dominant at this stage. These patients have a high risk of chronic illness [16].

3.4. Atopic dermatitis in adolescents (age 12–18 years)

In this period of life, the lesions are more fixed to classical areas such as the head, neck, and flexural areas. Lesions in the form of chronic dermatitis can also be seen on the hands [16].

3.5. Stratification based on disease severity

Atopic dermatitis covers a wide spectrum of clinical phenotypes. Most authors classify atopic dermatitis according to the severity of the clinical features into four groups: dry skin only, mild, moderate and severe atopic dermatitis. It is the best to use a valid scoring system, such as SCORAD (Scoring atopic dermatitis) or Eczema Area and Severity Index Scores, for assessing the severity of atopic dermatitis [16]. The most commonly used scoring system in clinical practice is SCORAD, for which there is an application for Apple, Mac, PC and android system. This scoring system was created and validated by the European Task Force on Atopic Dermatitis (ETFAD) [1, 2, 16].

4. Diagnosis and trigger factors

4.1. Diagnostic criteria

It is not possible to define the gold standard for diagnosis of atopic dermatitis due to its heterogeneity. Diagnosis of atopic dermatitis cannot be set without skin examination [17]. Some diagnostic criteria developed for use in hospital, while others developed for community settings [17]. The ISAAC proposed the full questionnaire-based protocol where a positive response to all three questions is required for the diagnosis of atopic dermatitis. These ISAAC diagnostic criteria are not for daily use, but for epidemiological studies became the gold standard.

The standard diagnostic tool in a community setting is the Hanifin and Rajka criteria [18] (**Figure 1**). Their criteria are adequate for physicians to make a diagnosis of atopic dermatitis. The diagnosis of atopic dermatitis by Hanifin and Rajka criteria requires the existence at least three major characteristics and at least three minor characteristics [1, 12, 18]. Some other atopic dermatitis diagnostic criteria are more practical for use in a hospital setting such as UK criteria and American Academy of Dermatology (AAD) criteria.

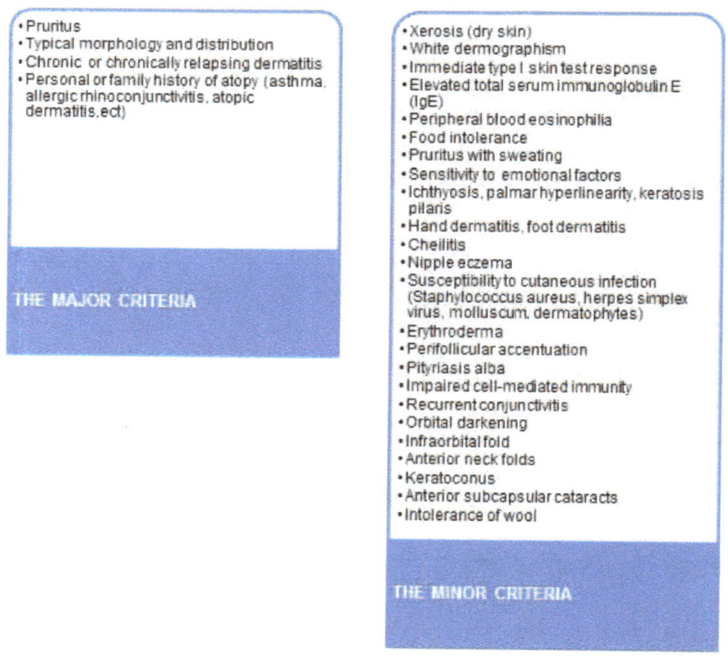

Figure 1. Diagnostic criteria by Hanifin and Rajka [18].

It is very important to use well-defined diagnostic criteria for the diagnosis of atopic dermatitis, especially for those patients who lack the typical phenotype of the disease [4]. Using visible eczema as the only criterion may lead to overdiagnosis of the disease [4].

The following diagnostic algorithm should be applied:

1. Clinical diagnosis based on well-defined diagnostic criteria
2. Patient medical history
3. Positive family history of atopic diseases
4. Blood tests (total IgE, specific IgE)
5. Specific skin test (prick test, prick to prick test, patch test)
6. Exacerbating factors or common triggers in atopic dermatitis
7. Challenge tests

Some facts about the diagnosis of atopic dermatitis should be emphasized:

- the atopy patch test is primarily a way to investigate the mechanisms of eczema
- sensitization can be detected by prick or patch tests or by measuring specific IgE antibodies in the blood
- the decision to make a challenge test should be individualized for each patient
- during the challenge test, children should be supervised for 48 h. In the case of a negative test, it is necessary to examine the child's skin after 24 h [12].

There is no gold standard, clinical or laboratory, for the diagnosis of atopic dermatitis. Diagnosis should be based on anamnesis, clinical features and laboratory results [1, 2, 12, 16].

Although Hanifin and Rajka developed the gold criteria for the clinical diagnosis of atopic dermatitis, in clinical practice, physician also needs to use a valid scoring system to define the severity of clinical features [1].

4.2. Common triggers

Atopic dermatitis exacerbations can be triggered by allergens that are inhaled, ingested or in direct contact with the skin. Most commonly triggers are sweat, contact allergens, aeroallergens and microbial agents.

Sensitization to food allergens (cow's milk and hen's eggs) is associated with infantile atopic dermatitis and related to disease severity [4]. Exposure to aeroallergens (pets, mites, and pollen) has been clearly shown to increase the risk factors for atopic dermatitis and atopic dermatitis severity [1, 4].

Children with atopic dermatitis are at high risk of allergic asthma and allergic rhinitis [4, 12].

4.3. Differential diagnosis

Differential diagnosis of atopic dermatitis is shown in **Figure 2**.

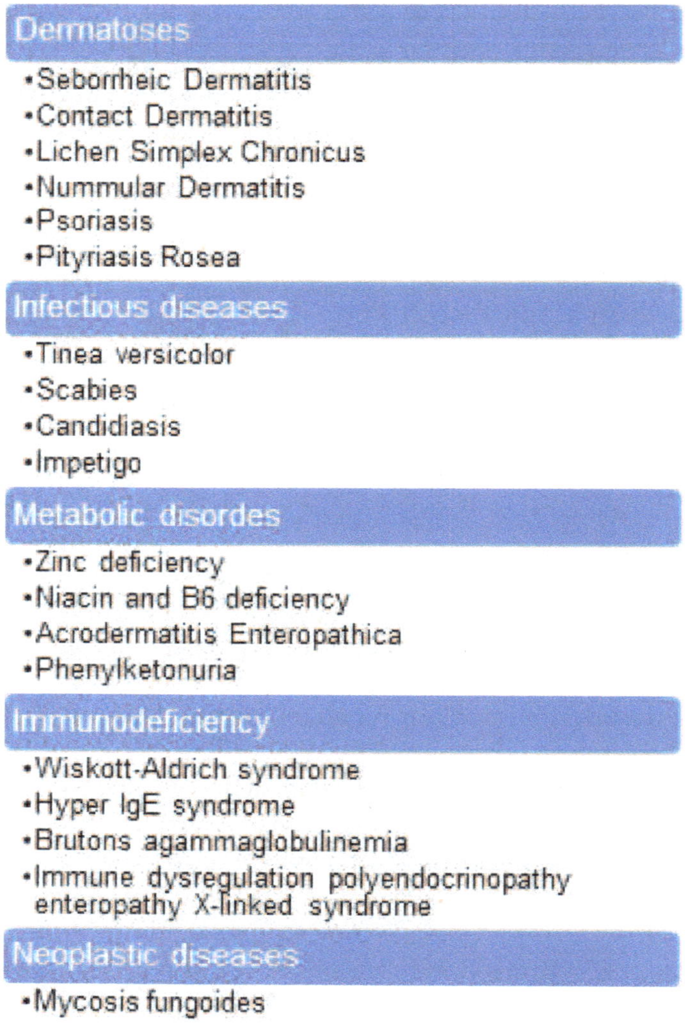

Figure 2. Differential diagnosis of atopic dermatitis [1, 4, 19].

5. Management

The management of atopic dermatitis presents a clinical challenge [4, 12, 20].

Some studies emphasize that the breastfeeding at least 4–6 months reduced the incidence of atopic dermatitis in infants, but this effect is most probably transient and last to the 3rd year of life [4]. Some studies on high-risk infants population demonstrate that using different partially and extensively hydrolyzed casein formulas for the first 6 months of life has the capacity to reduce atopic dermatitis by 50% in the first year of life [21].

Management of atopic dermatitis should be adapted to the severity of the clinical manifestation of atopic dermatitis [1]. Therapeutic modalities include basic treatment of the skin, topical and systemic drug application.

5.1. General measures

Basic treatment [1, 22, 23] means to use a skin hydration on a regular base, avoided hot water during showering or bathing, and contact with water should be minimized. Synthetic or wool material clothes should be avoided. Also, detergents and soaps designed for sensitive skin should be used. Further treatment should be adapted to the disease severity. It is very important to educate child's parent/guardian about atopic dermatitis, and treatment challenges.

Topical treatment [1, 22] includes emollients, topical glucocorticosteroids, topical antimicrobial therapy, topical calcineurin inhibitors, wet-wrap therapy. A combination of two different topical agents can be used.

Systemic treatment [22] needs to be considered if topical treatment cannot control the severity of atopic dermatitis. Systemic treatment includes antihistamines, antimicrobial treatment, systemic corticosteroids, Cyclosporin A, Azathioprine, and so on. In a case where the physician has a negative or poor therapeutic response, another specialist (dermatologist, pediatrician, etc.) should be involved in the diagnostic and treatment management to get optimal results.

Also, in some cases, hospitalization in centers with a multidisciplinary team approach might be the best option for the patient.

People with atopic dermatitis should not work in the area with high humidity, places where they need to wash their hands often or use stronger disinfectants/irritants [1, 22].

5.1.1. Hydration, topical moisturizers and emollients

Xerose is a leading clinical sign of atopic dermatitis. Emollient creams represent the basic therapy of atopic dermatitis [23]. The basic mechanism of their effect is to maintain satisfactory skin hydration, preserve the skin barrier and reduce transdermal loss of water. It is recommended that they can be used daily. They can be different in composition: lotions, oils, creams or gels. Studies have shown that one form of emollient has no advantage over others [22, 23]. Oily preparations usually do not contain preservatives, which has advantages in terms of adverse effects. Lotions contain a high concentration of water, which speeds up their evaporation from the skin [22, 23].

The choice of a moisture can be left to the patient, which may be associated with increased *adherence* to recommended *therapy* [22, 24]. Selected moistures should be effective, safe, without additional additives and perfumes. The efficiency of the selected moisture should be reviewed frequently. It can be used 2–4 times a day, which depends on the frequency of bathing/showering. It is recommended to apply immediately after bathing/showering, plus 2–3 a day [23].

5.1.2. Effectiveness and application technique

Original packaging emollients should be carefully stored because of possible contamination with bacteria. The most practical use is the pump-dispenser because there is the smallest risk for contamination [1, 23].

There is no accord in order to use the determined quantity of the applied layer and the surface to be covered with the emollients (the whole body surface or only the affected areas of the skin). The rule of fingertip unit is not generally accepted for them as for corticosteroids.

In principle, in the treatment of atopic dermatitis, a moisturizer or skin care product should be applied to a mild eczematous lesion or dry skin on the facial surface without applying any topical steroids. It is reported that twice a day, external application of a moisturizer significantly inhibits the relapse of inflammation of atopic dermatitis compared with the untreated group [1].

5.1.3. Wet-wrap therapy

Wet-wrap therapy is a method for administering topical corticosteroids in order to increase their absorption [1, 2]. It can be used on the recommendation of a specialist pediatrician or dermatologist. It should be applied for a short period of time (7–14 days), once daily at exclusively restricted area in children with severe atopic dermatitis who did not have an adequate therapeutic response to conventional therapy [22].

In wet-wrap therapy, it is recommended to use low potency and extremely mild corticosteroid preparations [19, 22]. Some authors recommend 5–10% dilution of potency topical corticosteroid preparation.

The application technique: a topical corticosteroid is applied to the affected skin, which then covers with a wet layer of tubular bandages, a gauze or a cotton suit, then placed a second dry layer. The recommended duration of a wet-wrap therapy is 12 h, so it is better to apply it overnight [2].

5.1.4. Dietary interventions

Recent studies did not show relation between food allergies and *outbreaks* or exacerbations in atopic dermatitis in children. If parents or a child notice that child's symptoms of atopic dermatitis *aggravated* by *eating some foods,* a provocation test for that food should be considered. Studies show that this deficient nutrition did not have a positive therapeutic effect on atopic dermatitis in children [24].

What is certainly recommended for infants with atopic dermatitis is exclusive breastfeeding and later transitioning to *solids foods* [1, 24].

5.2. Topical corticosteroids

Topical corticosteroids represent the basic antiinflammatory, immunosuppressive and antiproliferative therapy in atopic dermatitis. Topical corticosteroids are categorized into *four groups* based on their potency (**Table 1**) [1, 2, 22, 24]. The outbreak of topical corticosteroid therapy should be based on the severity of the clinical picture [1]. For mild atopic dermatitis, we use low potency topical corticosteroid preparations, for severe atopic dermatitis we use high potency topical corticosteroids [22].

Ultra high potency topical corticosteroids	Moderate potency topical corticosteroids
• **Group I** • Clobetasol propionate cream (0.05%) • Diflorasone diacetate ointment (0.05%)	• **Group IV** • Desoximetasone cream (0.05%) • Fluocinonide acetonide ointment (0.025%) • Hydrocortisone valerate ointment (0.2%) • Triamcinolone acetonide cream (0.1%) • **Group V** • Betamethasone dipropionate lotion (0.02%) • Betamethasone valerate cream (0.1%) • Fluocinonide acetonide cream (0.025%) • Hydrocortisone butyrate cream (0.1%) • Hydrocortisone valerate cream (0.2%) • Triamcinolone acetonide lotion (0.1%)
High potency topical corticosteroids	**Low potency topical corticosteroids**
• **Group II** • Amcinonide ointment (0.1%) • Betamethasone dipropionate ointment (0.05%) • Desoximetasone (cream or ointment) (0.025%) • Fluocinonide (cream, ointment, or gel) (0.05%) • Halcinonide cream (0.1%) • **Group III** • Betamethasone dipropionate cream (0.05%) • Betamethasone valerate ointment (0.1%) • Diflorasone diacetate cream (0.05%) • Triamcinolone acetonide ointment (0.1%)	• **Group VI** • Betamethasone valerate lotion (0.05%) • Desonide cream (0.05%) • Fluocinolone acetonide solution (0.01%) • **Group VII** • Dexamethasone sodium phosphate cream (0.1%) • Hydrocortisone acetate cream (1%) • Methylprednisolone acetate cream (0.25%)

Table 1. Topical corticosteroids potency classification [1, 2].

Also, for areas such as face, neck, axillary and groin, it should be used a mild topical corticosteroid preparations. In these areas, a moderate or potent topical corticosteroid should not be used for more than 3–5 days [24]. Topical corticosteroids can be used once or twice a day. Start the therapy with a single daily application, and if there is no adequate therapeutic response, introduce twice daily application [1, 22, 24]. This simple therapy mode will increase patients adherence to recommended therapy and reduce the fear of side effects of topical corticosteroids by parents and GPs.

The application technique: the topical corticosteroid preparations dosage according to the finger type unit (FTU) rule. One FTU is the amount of a cream which can be applied from the distal skin-crease to the tip of the index finger of an adult and represents approximately 0.5 g. This amount of cream is enough to cover the surface of *two hand* areas (hand area is surface you are *covering with* hand palm down with your fingers closed together) [2, 22]. Topical corticosteroids should be applied half an hour before or after emollient creams.

Keep in mind that children have a proportionally larger body surface compared to body weight, which results in a higher absorption of topical corticosteroids for the same cream amount compared to adults [4, 24].

There are two different approaches to choose a topical corticosteroids, one recommending to start therapy with low potency TCS then use moderate potency TCS ("set up approach"), while others recommend reverse access from moderate to low potency topical corticosteroids ("set down approach"). These recommendations are primarily related to mild and moderate atopic dermatitis [1, 2, 24].

There are two forms of TCS therapy for atopic dermatitis: proactive and reactive therapy [1]. Proactive therapy is defined as using of topical corticosteroids in the acute phase, with intermittent use of topical corticosteroids and a moisturizer during the remission period. Reactive therapy means the using of topical corticosteroids only in case of exacerbation of symptoms, and using only the moisture in the remission phase [1].

5.2.1. Potency and adverse effects

Potency and adverse effects are described in **Tables 1** and **2**.

5.2.2. Effectiveness and application technique

A fingertip unit (FTU) is the *amount* of topical steroid that is *squeezed* out from a standard tube along an adult's *fingertip*. It should be enough to treat an area of skin double the size of the flat of your hand with your fingers together. The recommended dosage will depend on what part of the body is being treated [2, 22, 24].

For adults, the recommended FTUs to be applied in one single dose are, for example, 1 FTU for hands, elbows and knees, 2.5 FTUs for the face and neck, 3 FTUs for the scalp, or 4 FTUs for a hand and arm together, or the buttocks [25].

The following dosages are recommended for a child aged 3–6 months: entire face and neck 1 FTU, an entire arm and hand 1 FTU, an entire leg and foot 1.5 FTUs, the entire front of chest and tummy (abdomen) 1 FTU, and the entire back including buttocks 1.5 FTUs [25].

For a child aged 1–2 years, entire face and neck 1.5 FTUs, an entire arm and hand 1.5 FTUs, an entire leg and foot 2 FTUs, the entire front of chest and abdomen 2 FTUs, the entire back including buttocks 3 FTUs [25].

For a child aged 3–5 years, entire face and neck 1.5 FTUs, an entire arm and hand 2 FTUs, an entire leg and foot 3 FTUs, the entire front of chest and abdomen 3 FTUs, the entire back including buttocks 3.5 FTUs [25].

- Acne-like rash, including folliculitis and rosacea
- Eyelid and perioral dermatitides
- Epidermal-dermal atrophy, dermal vulnerability (most likely to occur on the geriatric or sunlight damaged skin, intertriginous zone, or facial surface)
- Delay in wound healing
- Gluteal granuloma
- Purpura
- Telangiectasia and erythema
- Skin striae
- Depigmentation
- Hypertrichosis
- Hidden or exacerbated dermatophyte infection
- Secondary infection or exacerbation of existing infection
- Contact dermatitis
- May be caused by an ingredient of the preservative or other base material.
- May be caused by a corticosteroid molecule. In this case, the skin may crossreact with a corticosteroid molecule of similar structure.
- Others

Table 2. Topical corticosteroids adverse effects [1].

For older children aged 6–10 years, entire face and neck 2 FTUs, an entire arm and hand 2.5 FTUs, an entire leg and foot 4.5 FTUs, the entire front of chest and abdomen 3.5 FTUs, and the entire back including buttocks 5 FTUs [25].

5.3. Topical calcineurin inhibitors

Topical calcineurin inhibitors are non-steroidal immunomodulatory agents. The use of topical calcineurin inhibitors preparations *should* be *under supervision by* specialist *dermatologists or* pediatricians and for short time of period.

There are three preparations available [1, 22, 24]:

(1) 0.03% tacrolimus ointment,

(2) 0.1% tacrolimus ointment and

(3) 1% pinecrolimus cream.

Tacrolimus ointment 0.03% is approved for use in children over 2 years, while at a higher concentration (0.1%), it can be used only in children over 16 years of age [24]. Evidence from clinical trials supports the safe use of topical tacrolimus 0.03% in infants and younger children [22]. These drugs presents the second line of therapy, and only in case of acute exacerbation that do not respond to TCS.

Their use is recommended for the acute phase of moderate or severe atopic dermatitis in sensitive areas of the skin (e.g., the face, the folds) and in areas where steroid-induced atrophy is present [1, 24]. Numerous studies show that different combinations of TCI and TCS given together have sometimes a better effect than individual treatment [22, 24]. Some combinations did not show an expected effect than single administration. The combination of preparations should be personalized for each individual patient [24]. The TCS recommended to use first, and in inadequate response to therapy switched to low potent TCS with TCI.

The application technique: an intermittent application 2–3 times a week according to the recommendation of a specialist dermatologist or pediatrician is recommended.

Side effects: the most common side effect of TCI is a transient burning that passes after several days of use [1, 22, 24]. These preparations cannot be used on the skin with signs of infection and uneroded surface.

5.4. Antimicrobial treatments

Regular administration of systemic or topical antibiotics is not recommended in patients with atopic dermatitis [2, 22, 24]. In patients with atopic dermatitis, affected skin is usually colonized with *Staphylococcus aureus* [1, 2]. Previous studies show that there is no benefit from using topical antibiotics, antiseptics, antibacterial soaps or antibacterial bath additives [22, 24]. Also, the use of these agents can cause contact dermatitis or skin colonization with multiresistant strains of bacteria. In children aged 6 months to 17 years with moderate/severe atopic dermatitis and secondary *S. aureus* infection, the use of diluted bleach baths twice weekly with administration of intranasal mupirocin twice daily (5 days per month) is more affected. This treatment should be repeated for 3 months [1, 2, 22, 24].

In children with frequent skin infections with *S. aureus*, a nasopharyngeal *culture test for whole family* should be done due to frequent intranasal colonization with this bacterium. It should be noted that the regular use of moisturizer and TCS significantly reduces skin colonization with *S. aureus* [22–24].

Eczema herpeticum is a potentially life-threatening infection in children with atopic dermatitis. Herpes infection should always be considered in patients with painful erosions and vesicles. In these patients, systemic antiviral ther`apy and supportive therapies are required [1, 2].

5.5. Systemic anti-inflammatory therapy

Oral and injectable *systemic* corticosteroids are not recommended for long-term treatment in children with atopic dermatitis because of the possible side effects [1, 2, 22]. But their use as short-term therapy is effective to interrupt acute exacerbation in children with severe atopic dermatitis [22, 24]. Duration of these intermittent therapies should be between 3 days and 3 weeks.

Beclomethasone dipropionate and Flunisolide should be limited for treatment of severe atopic dermatitis in children with atopic dermatitis refractory to standard therapies [19, 20, 26].

Immunosuppressants, such as Cyclosporine A (6–8 weeks), Methotrexate, and Azathioprine, could be used in children older than 16 years with severe atopic dermatitis refractory to standard therapies [1, 20, 24]. Only Cyclosporine A licensed for use in clinical practice for the treatment of atopic dermatitis. Prescriptions and using of systemic immunosuppressive therapy should be supervised by a specialist pediatrician [1, 20, 22]. Recommendations for the use of these drugs are short durations of therapy and severe atopic dermatitis refractory to standard therapies. Systemic side effects always should be kept in mind.

5.6. Phototherapy

Phototherapy is a second-line therapy for severe atopic dermatitis, and administration should be supervised by a dermatologist [2, 24].

It represents the use of ultraviolet light (UVA or UVB). In atopic dermatitis, UVB narrowband and long-wave UVA are use. The phototherapy is usually applied in elderly children with chronic atopic dermatitis or severe atopic dermatitis or intractable severe atopic dermatitis.

5.7. Antihistamines

The use of antihistamines can be considered in older children with acute flares where there is significant sleep disturbance [24]. Recent studies show that administration of fexofenadine hydrochloride has effects in the treatment of itch and nocturnal pruritus. Application should be limited to 1 week [22, 24].

The use of oral antihistamines is not recommended in the treatment of atopic dermatitis [2]. It is recommended to use a more potent TCS in children with itch or nocturnal pruritus in a short period of time [1, 2, 22].

5.8. Reasons for treatment failure

There are many reasons for tretment failure, most commonly are presented below [1, 27–30].

5.8.1. Incorrect diagnosis

Many skin conditions can present with eczema and make confusion in diagnosis, such as psoriasis, skin infection and impetigo, fungal skin infections, seborrheic dermatitis, drug reactions, skin T cell lymphoma, and keratosis pilaris.

5.8.2. Inconvenience of patients

Some patients believe that skin lesions are results of the infectious due to poor hygiene and feel uncomfortable to show such lesions to the doctor. In some countries and regions, there is a stigma for people with skin lesions. These patients often do not have adequate therapeutic treatment.

5.8.3. Poor understanding

Patients sometimes do not clearly understand the instructions given by physician about the therapy and the goals of the therapy. Sometimes child's parents believe that traditional medicines are better than recommended therapy. Also, they expect a quick therapeutic effect. They have no understanding that the disease is a chronic character.

5.8.4. Psycho-social factors

Chronic itch and sleep deprivation can lead to anxiety and depression in patients with atopic dermatitis.

5.8.5. Lack of education

Inadequate drug administration is most likely a reason for treatment failure. Patients sometimes are not informed enough about the correct application of creams and ointments. Patients sometimes are unable to abide by a prescribed therapeutic regimen due to their daily duties. The higher the number of daily applications, the less the chance that the patient will take them. Also, instructions given to child's parents must be appropriate to their intellectual abilities.

5.8.6. Fear of adverse drug effects and steroid phobia

Topical corticosteroid phobia is especially affecting parents of pediatric patients with atopic dermatitis [27]. Establishing the trust-based doctor-patient/parents relationship can help overcome parents' fears about therapy [28, 30]. This fear is commonly caused by misinformation or misadvice given by friends, relatives, other parents and the media. A corticosteroid phobia can lead to poor patient therapy compliance.

5.8.7. Hypersensitivity reactions to treatment

Moisturizers can contain different chemicals which may cause irritation or hypersensitivity reactions. Urea containing emollients may cause stinging. Pimecrolimus cream may cause erythema. Chemical stabilizers of sun topical corticosteroids can cause delayed hypersensitivity responses [20].

5.8.8. Economic

The cost of therapy may be more expensive than the patient expects. Also, long-term therapy increases the cost of treatment. This can affect the patient's adherence to therapy.

5.8.9. Lack of bonding and communication with a doctor

The physician should empathize with the patient and parents, be aware of patient's fears, anxieties and beliefs. Communication with the patient should be in language which patient and parents can understand. During the examination, the doctor should be patient, talk to a patient without haste and listen to the patient without interruption. Also, the doctor during the repeated visits should create a trust-based relationship with the patient.

More frequent visits to the doctor increase adherence to treatment. Studies show that shorter periods between physicians control increase the patient's compliance with the recommended therapy. Available consultation with well-educated nurse can also improve treatment adherence.

6. Conclusion

Atopic dermatitis (AD) is one of the most common skin conditions in children and adolescents. This disease is characterized by chronic eczematous and itchy lesions with typical distributions, and relapsing. The clinical pattern of atopic dermatitis has a characteristic age-dependent distribution and is commonly associated with elevated IgE, peripheral eosinophilia, *Staphylococcus aureus* colonization and comorbidity with other allergic diseases. There is no gold standard, clinical or laboratory, for the diagnosis of atopic dermatitis. Diagnosis should be based on anamnesis, clinical features and laboratory results.

Xerose is a leading clinical sign of atopic dermatitis; therefore, emollient creams represent the basic therapy of atopic dermatitis. The basic mechanism of their effect is to maintain satisfactory skin hydration, preserve the skin barrier and reduce transdermal loss of water.

Topical corticosteroids represent the basic anti-inflammatory, immunosuppressive and antiproliferative therapy in atopic dermatitis. The outbreak of topical corticosteroid therapy should be based on the severity of the clinical picture. For mild atopic dermatitis, we use low potency topical corticosteroid preparations; for severe atopic dermatitis, we use high potency topical corticosteroids. There are two different approaches to choose a topical corticosteroids, one recommends to start therapy with low potency TCS than using moderate potency TCS ("set up approach"). While others recommend reverse access from moderate to low potency topical corticosteroids ("set down approach"). These recommendations are primarily related to mild and moderate atopic dermatitis.

The expectations of patients and parental expectations in children with atopic dermatitis should always be determined, and the specific concerns of the parents should be sought and addressed.

Abbreviations

AAD	American Academy of Dermatology
ETFAD	the European Task Force on Atopic Dermatitis
FTU	finger type unit
IFN	interferon
IgE	immunoglobulin E
IL	interleukins
ISAAC	International Study of Asthma and Allergies in Childhood
SCORAD	Scoring atopic dermatitis
TCI	topical calcineurin inhibitors
TCS	topical corticosteroids
TSLP	thymic stromal lipoprotein
UVA	ultraviolet light A
UVB	ultraviolet light B

Author details

Sanela Domuz Vujnović[1]* and Adrijana Domuz[2]

*Address all correspondence to: drdomuz@gmail.com

1 School of Applied Medical Sciences, Prijedor, Republic of Srpska, Bosnia and Herzegovina

2 Primary Health Center, Srbac, Republic of Srpska, Bosnia and Herzegovina

References

[1] Katayama I, Aihara M, Ohya Y, Saeki H, Shimojo N, Shoji S, Taniguchi M, Yamada H. Japanese Society of Allergology. Japanese guidelines for atopic. Dermatitis 2017. Allergology International. 2017;**66**(2):230-247. DOI: 10.1016/j.alit. 2016.12.003

[2] Leung TNH, Chow CM, Chow MPY, Luk DCK, Ho KM, Hon KL, et al. Clinical guidelines on Management of Atopic Dermatitis. HK J Paediatr (new series). 2013;**18**(2):96-104

[3] Cork MJ, Danby SG, Vasilopoulos Y, Hadgraft J, Lane ME, Moustafa M, et al. Epidermal barrier dysfunction in atopic dermatitis. The Journal of Investigative Dermatology. 2009;**129**(8):1892-1908. DOI: 10.1038/jid.2009.133

[4] Akdis CA, Akdis M, Bieber T, Bindslev-Jensen C, Boguniewicz M, Eigenmann P, et al. Diagnosis and treatment of atopic dermatitis in children and adults: European academy of Allergology and clinical immunology/American Academy of allergy, asthma and immunology/PRACTALL consensus report. Allergy. 2006;**61**(8):969-987. DOI: 10.1111/j.1398-9995.2006.01153.x

[5] Brown SJ, McLean WH. One remarkable molecule: Filaggrin. The Journal of Investigative Dermatology. 2012;**132**(3 Pt 2):751-762. DOI: 10.1038/jid.2011.393

[6] Denecker G, Ovaere P, Vandenabeele P, Declercq W. Caspase-14 reveals its secrets. The Journal of Cell Biology. 2008;**180**(3):451-458. DOI: 10.1083/jcb.200709098

[7] Eyerich K, Novak N. Immunology of atopic eczema: Overcoming the Th1/Th2 paradigm. Allergy. 2013;**68**(8):974-982. DOI: 10.1111/all.12184

[8] De Benedetto A, Agnihothri R, McGirt LY, Bankova LG, Beck LA. Atopic dermatitis: A disease caused by innate immune defects? The Journal of Investigative Dermatology. 2009;**129**(1):14-30. DOI: 10.1038/jid.2008.259

[9] Cork MJ, Robinson DA, Vasilopoulos Y, Ferguson A, Moustafa M, Mac Gowan A, et al. New perspectives on epidermal barrier dysfunction in atopic dermatitis: Gene-environment interactions. The Journal of Allergy and Clinical Immunology. 2006;**118**(1):3-21. DOI: 10.1016/j.jaci.2006.04.042

[10] Peng W, Novak N. Pathogenesis of atopic dermatitis. Clinical and Experimental Allergy. 2015;**45**(3):566-574. DOI: 10.1111/cea.12495

[11] Furue M, Chiba T, Tsuji G, Ulzii D, Kido-Nakahara M, Nakahara T, et al. Atopic dermatitis: Immune deviation, barrier dysfunction, IgE autoreactivity and new therapies. Allergology International. 2017;**66**(3):398-403. DOI: 10.1016/j.alit.2016.12.002

[12] Lyons JJ, Milner JD, Stone KD. Atopic dermatitis in children: Clinical features, pathophysiology, and treatment. Immunology and Allergy Clinics of North America. 2015;**35**(1):161-183. DOI: 10.1016/j.iac.2014.09.008

[13] Ricci G, Dondi A, Neri I, Ricci L, Patrizi A, Pession A. Atopic dermatitis phenotypes in childhood. Italian Journal of Pediatrics. 2014;**40**:46. DOI: 10.1186/1824-7288-40-46

[14] Werfel T, Schwerk N, Hansen G, Kapp A. The diagnosis and graded therapy of atopic dermatitis. Deutsches Ärzteblatt International. 2014;**111**(29-30):509-520. DOI: 10.3238/arztebl.2014

[15] Amat F, Saint-Pierre P, Bourrat E, Nemni A, Couderc R, Boutmy-Deslandes E, et al. Early-onset atopic dermatitis in children: Which are the phenotypes at risk of asthma? Results from the ORCA cohort. PLoS One. 2015;**10**(6):e0131369. DOI: 10.1371/journal.pone.0131369

[16] Bieber T, D'Erme AM, Akdis CA, Traidl-Hoffmann C, Lauener R, Schäppi G, et al. Clinical phenotypes and endophenotypes of atopic dermatitis: Where are we, and where should we go? The Journal of Allergy and Clinical Immunology. 2017;**139**(4S):S58-S64. DOI: 10.1016/j.jaci.2017.01.008

[17] Lee HJ, Lee SH. Epidermal permeability barrier defects and barrier repair therapy in atopic dermatitis. Allergy, Asthma & Immunology Research. 2014;**6**(4):276-287. DOI: 10.4168/aair.2014.6.4.276

[18] Hanifin JM, Rajka G. Diagnostic features of atopic dermatitis. Acta Derm Venereol (Stockh). 1980;**92**(suppl):44-47. DOI: 10.2340/00015555924447

[19] Eichenfield LF, Tom WL, Chamlin SL, Feldman SR, Hanifin JM, Simpson EL, et al. Guidelines of care for the management of atopic dermatitis: Section 1. Diagnosis and assessment of atopic dermatitis. Journal of the American Academy of Dermatology. 2014;**70**(2):338-351. DOI: 10.1016/j.jaad.2013.10.010

[20] Arkwright PD, Motala C, Subramanian H, Spergel J, Schneider LC, Wollenberg A, et al. Management of difficult-to-treat atopic dermatitis. The Journal of Allergy and Clinical Immunology. In Practice. 2013;**1**(2):142-151. DOI: 10.1016/j.jaip.2012.09.002

[21] von Berg A, Koletzko S, Grübl A, Filipiak-Pittroff B, Wichmann HE, Bauer CP, et al. The effect of hydrolyzed cow's milk formula for allergy prevention in the first year of life: The German infant nutritional intervention study, a randomized double-blind trial. The Journal of Allergy and Clinical Immunology. 2003;**111**(3):533-540. DOI: 10.1067/mai.2003.101

[22] Eichenfield LF, Tom WL, Berger TG, Krol A, Paller AS, Schwarzenberger K, et al. Guidelines of care for the management of atopic dermatitis: Section 2. Management and treatment of atopic dermatitis with topical therapies. Journal of the American Academy of Dermatology. 2014;**71**(1):116-132. DOI: 10.1016/j.jaad.2014.03.023

[23] Simpson EL, Chalmers JR, Hanifin JM, Thomas KS, Cork MJ, McLean WH, et al. Emollient enhancement of the skin barrier from birth offers effective atopic dermatitis prevention. The Journal of Allergy and Clinical Immunology. 2014;**134**(4):818-823. DOI: 10.1016/j.jaci.2014.08.005

[24] Scottish Intercollegiate Guidelines Network (SIGN). Management of Atopic Eczema in Primary Care. Edinburgh: SIGN; 2011

[25] Kalavala M, Mills CM, Long CC, Finlay AY. The fingertip unit: A practical guide to topical therapy in children. The Journal of Dermatological Treatment. 2007;**18**(5):319-320. DOI: 10.1080/09546630701441723

[26] Leung DY, Guttman-Yassky E. Deciphering the complexities of atopic dermatitis: Shifting paradigms in treatment approaches. The Journal of Allergy and Clinical Immunology. 2014;**134**(4):769-779. DOI: 10.1016/j.jaci.2014.08.008

[27] Smith SD, Stephens AM, Werren JC, Fischer GO. Treatment failure in atopic dermatitis as a result of parental health belief. The Medical Journal of Australia. 2013;**199**(7):467-469. DOI: 10.5694/mja12.10802

[28] Ohya Y, Williams H, Steptoe A, Saito H, Iikura Y, Anderson R, et al. Psychosocial factors and adherence to treatment advice in childhood atopic dermatitis. The Journal of Investigative Dermatology. 2001;**117**(4):852-857. DOI: 10.1046/j.0022-202x.2001.01475.x

[29] Uldahl-Curiac A, Björk AK, Lundahl L, Aberg-Gullstrand E, Aurell G, Svensson A, et al. Compliance difficulties in atopic children, reflections from an eczema School in Sweden. Journal of Clinical & Experimental Dermatology Research. 2016;**7**:350. DOI: 10.4172/2155-9554.1000350

[30] El Hachem M, Gesualdo F, Ricci G, Diociaiuti A, Giraldi L, Ametrano O, et al. Topical corticosteroid phobia in parents of pediatric patients with atopic dermatitis: A multicentre survey. Italian Journal of Pediatrics. 2017;**43**(1):22. DOI: 10.1186/s13052-017-0330-7

4

Cortisol in Correlation to Other Indicators of Fish Welfare

Hanna Kalamarz-Kubiak

Abstract

Cortisol is the major corticosteroid in teleost fish, secreted and released by interrenal cells of the head kidney during activation of the hypothalamic-pituitary-interrenal (HPI) axis. Although cortisol is universally recognized as a key mediator of stress-associated responses, other hormones are also involved in the stress response, e.g., arginine vasotocin (AVT), isotocin (IT), urotensins, dopamine, serotonin or β-endorphin. Cortisol affects AVT and IT secretion from nerve endings in gilthead sea bream (*Sparus aurata)* and round goby (*Neogobius melanostomus*). Moreover, it is pointed out that different mechanisms are involved in the regulation of AVT and IT release from the hypothalamic-pituitary complex in round goby. In the case of AVT, both genomic and nongenomic pathways are mediating the effect of cortisol while in the case of IT, it is only the nongenomic pathway. In turn, urotensin I instead of corticotropin-releasing factor (CRF) may contribute to the regulation of HPI axis and regulate AVT in *Sparus aurata*. In this species, urotensin II together with AVT and IT may control stress response to different salinities. Therefore, AVT, IT and urotensins, and their interactions with cortisol, seem to be significant in response to stress in fish.

Keywords: stress, cortisol, AVT, IT, UI, UII, *in vitro* techniques, fish

1. Introduction

Stress triggers reactions in all living organisms, and fish are no exception to this rule. It is known that fish are exposed to stress, not only in nature but also in aquaculture, fish markets and laboratories. In the past decades, knowledge and understanding of stress in fish has increased, particularly in the field of physiological mechanisms and responses that lead to changes in metabolism, growth, immune function, reproductive capacity and natural behavior. Interestingly, fish have proved to be more sensitive to stressors than many other vertebrates and responded to stressors at the intensity levels that are often far below those that can be detected by terrestrial animals [1–4]. The stress response in fish has been widely categorized into the primary, secondary and tertiary responses [5–11]. The primary response (the neuroendocrine response) includes the rapid release of stress hormones, catecholamines and corticosteroids, into the circulation [1, 12, 13]. This physiological response to stressors encompasses activation of the brain-sympathetic-chromaffin cell (BSC) axis and the hypothalamic-pituitary-interrenal (HPI) axis [1] (**Figure 1**). During the BSC axis activation, chromaffin cells of the head kidney release catecholamines (adrenaline and noradrenaline) from sympathetic nerve terminals. Catecholamines are controlled by factors released from sympathetic nerve terminals, mainly acetylcholine and angiotensin. The action of catecholamines includes increased hemoglobin oxygen affinity, arterial blood pressure [14] and glucose mobilization from liver and muscles [1]. The activation of HPI axis comprises the corticotropin-releasing factor (CRF) release from the hypothalamus, which in turn stimulates the corticotrophic cells in the anterior pituitary to secrete adrenocorticotropic hormone (ACTH). Following that, the interrenal cells of the head kidney synthesize and release cortisol into the circulatory system. In teleosts, the head kidney a major endocrine, hematopoietic and lymphatic tissue, are the equivalent of the adrenal gland in mammals [1, 12]. The secondary response comprises the various biochemical and physiological effects such as metabolic changes (increased glucose and lactate in blood and decreased tissue glycogen), osmoregulatory disturbance (water/ion balance), changes in hematological features (hematocrit, leukocrit and hemoglobin), cellular changes (increased heat shock or stress protein production) and changes in the immune response (lysozyme activity and antibody production) [13, 15–17]. The tertiary response represents changes in whole-animal performance characteristic (growth, swimming capacity and disease resistance) and modified behavioral patterns (feeding, aggression and reproduction) ("for review [9, 11, 18]").

In fish, cortisol acts as a regulatory factor for a wide range of physiological functions under normal conditions and also to allow for rapid physiological adjustments in the face of exposure to stressors [13]. Cortisol appears to play a pivotal role in the aerobic and anaerobic

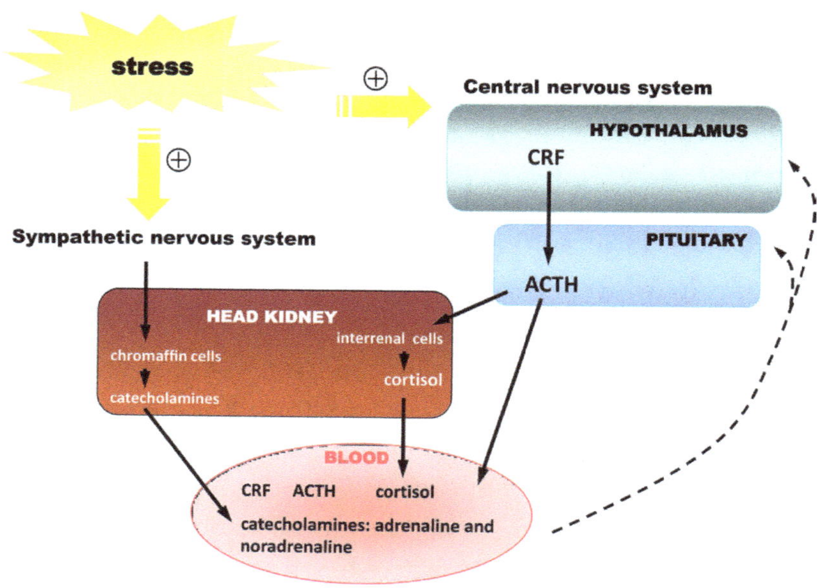

Figure 1. The stimulation of BSC axis and HPI axis in response to stress in fish.

metabolism, stimulating several aspects of intermediary energy metabolism, elevating oxygen uptake, increasing gluconeogenesis and inhibiting synthesis of glycogen synthesis [1, 13, 19–21]. Furthermore, increases in plasma corticosteroids have a wide range of other metabolic effects including increases in protein turnover, regulation of amino acid metabolism, ammonia output and increased lipolysis ("reviewed in [13]"). This hormone also performs an osmoregulatory function in teleosts, being the main hormone for seawater adaptation and ion uptake [22, 23]. Moreover, cortisol may regulate the immune response in fish [1, 13, 24]. Cortisol modulates, among others, the tissue inflammatory response through inhibitory effects on cytokine production [25] and appears to attenuate the cellular heat shock protein response to thermal insult [26, 27]. Corticosteroid hormones may highly participate in the modulation of the reproductive endocrine control in both sexes [18].

It should be noted that cortisol dramatically rises during stress and seems to be a key mediator of stress-associated responses [13, 28]. There is considerable variability in the magnitude of the corticosteroid response among species [9, 29, 30]. Among teleosts, some species exhibit high cortisol concentrations (10^{-7}–10^{-6} M) in response to acute stress [9], while some species reveal low cortisol levels (10^{-9}–10^{-8} M) in response to the same stress [31–33]. Most fish species show their increase in plasma cortisol within about 0.5–1 hour after a stressful disturbance [34, 35], but there are exceptions to the role. In the sea raven (*Hemitripterus americanus*), circulating cortisol takes up to 4 hours to reach its peak level following an acute stressor [36]. Probably, the slow rate of response to the stressor may help conserve energy in a normally inactive, sedentary, benthic marine species having a slow metabolic rate [36]. Corticosteroid responses to stress also vary within species according to the duration or severity of the stressor ("for review: [9]"). What is more, differences in corticosteroid stress responses may exist among strains or stocks within the same fish species [37, 38], their hybrids [39], and between wild and hatchery fish [40]. It should be noted that the variation in stress responses within a single strain or population may indicate genetic determinants [41–43]. Beyond genetic and environmental factors, the developmental stage of the fish can also affect its responsiveness to a stressor ("for review: [9]").

2. How does cortisol interact with other hormones in fish?

Although cortisol is universally recognized as a critical component of the endocrine response to stress, other hormones are also involved in the stress response, e.g., arginine vasotocin (AVT), isotocin (IT), urotensins, dopamine, serotonin or β-endorphin [13, 44–48]. However, other hormones, such as thyroxine, prolactin and somatolactin can also elevate during stress but they have not yet been demonstrated to be useful stress indicators *per se* [49–51]. Our interest has focused on nonapeptides AVT, IT and urotensins, and their interactions with cortisol, in response to stress.

2.1. Arginine vasotocin, isotocin and urotensin I

Nonapeptides, such as AVT and IT, are fish homologs of the mammalian arginine vasopressin (AVP) and oxytocin (OT) [52]. In fish, AVT and IT are synthesized in separate parvo- and magnocellular neurons of the preoptic area (POA), stored in axon terminals in neurohypophysis and released into the circulatory system after proper stimulation [53–55]. Only mature nonapeptides, after dissociation from the noncovalent complex, play an active role as peripheral hormones and neurotransmitters or neuromodulators in the central nervous system (CNS). The physiological role of AVT involves cardiovascular activity and maintenance of water/ ion homeostasis. Both nonapeptides interact with other endocrine systems and control social and reproductive behavior [56–59]. More importantly, there is evidence that AVT and IT are engaged in physiological stress response in fish. Changes in hypothalamic, pituitary and plasma AVT and IT concentrations were found in many fish species subjected to various unfavorable situations such as confinement, disturbance, high density, food deprivation or osmoregulatory stress [33, 47, 60]. Therefore, AVT and IT are important components of stress axis in fish [61]. Moreover, AVT neurons are colocalized with CRF in the preoptic nucleus (NPO) [62, 63], and the expression of AVT and CRF mRNAs increases simultaneously in response to various stressors in many fish spices [56, 64, 65]. *In vitro* studies have shown that independently or in synergy with CRF, AVT stimulates ACTH release from fish pituitary cells [44, 66, 67]. In gilthead sea bream (*Sparus aurata*), unlike other teleosts, CRF is not a releasing factor for ACTH and cortisol, because there are no anatomical connections between CRF perikarya and ACTH cells in the adenohypophysis [68–70]. Therefore, it is possible that urotensin I (UI) instead of CRF regulates AVT and IT release in *S. aurata*.

It has been known that UI is implicated in the regulation of neuroendocrine, autonomic and behavioral responses to stressors in fish [71, 72]. Gene expression of UI was found not only in urophysis but also in the telencephalon-preoptic, hypothalamic, optic tectum-thalamus and posterior brain regions, which indicates the regulatory action of this peptide in CNS [73–75]. The structural similarity of UI with CRF suggests similar hypophysiotropic roles of both hormones in HPI axis in fish [76–78]. It has been established that UI modulates cortisol secretion either directly by acting on steroidogenic cells of an interrenal tissue or indirectly via the hypothalamic-pituitary axis [71, 77, 79, 80]. In many fish species, UI-immunoreactive (UI-ir) fibers from the nucleus lateral tuberalis (NLT) extend to the pituitary where they may interact with AVT and IT nerve terminals [81–84].

The effect of cortisol on AVT has been examined *in vivo* in gilthead sea bream. The application of cortisol implants enhanced the hypothalamic expression of AVT mRNA and subsequently hypophysial AVT content in this species [85]. Although IT studies are very limited, they suggest that IT potentiates ACTH release from fish pituitary cells [44]. The *in vitro* effect of cortisol or UI on AVT and IT secretion in fish has been studied only by Kalamarz-Kubiak et al. [86]. In this study, primary cultures of pituitary cells were prepared by a modification of the method described by Levavi-Sivan et al. [87, 88]. Pituitary cells were cultured with medium supplemented with cortisol (1.4×10^{-8}, 1.4×10^{-7} and 0.4×10^{-6} M) or UI (10^{-12}, 10^{-10} and 10^{-8} M). The doses of cortisol were chosen taking into account different cortisol responses to stress in various fish species [9, 29, 30]. The doses of UI used in the cell culture were determined based on the literature, considering its concentration in different tissues [29, 30, 80, 89, 90]. After 6, 24 and 48 hours, the media were collected and stored at −70°C until AVT and IT analysis. AVT and IT concentrations were determined in incubation media by HPLC with fluorescence and UV detection according to a modified procedure by Kulczykowska [91].

The study performed by Kalamarz-Kubiak et al. [86] demonstrated that AVT and IT secretion from nerve ending of *S. aurata* pituitary was influenced by cortisol and UI. In this study,

cortisol showed a stimulatory action on pituitary cells of *S. aurata* inducing AVT secretion at all doses. Dose-dependent effect of cortisol on AVT secretion has been manifested after 24 hours of cell culture. In mammals, the influence of cortisol on AVP secretion was studied by *in vivo* and *in vitro* methods [92, 93]. In turn, other findings indicate that the expression of AVP in parvocellular neurons of the paraventricular nucleus (PVN) and AVP secretion into the pituitary portal circulation increase under chronic stress in rats [94–97]. It is also shown that stress upregulates the number of AVP receptors in rat anterior pituitary [96]. The results presented by Kalamarz-Kubiak et al. [86] demonstrated that the stimulatory effect of cortisol on AVT secretion from nerve ending of *S. aurata* pituitary diminishes after 48 hours of culture. The most likely explanation for the decline seems to be the depletion of AVT stores without subsequent supplementation of secretory granules from AVT-ergic nerves. However, corticoid receptor (CR) desensitization could be another cause. In mammals, desensitization of CRs is the result of physiological processes, as well as stress, and disease [98–100]. On the other hand, the reduction of AVT secretion after 48 hours of cortisol exposure could be also linked with an increase of aminopeptidase activity responsible for nonapeptide metabolism as it was shown in rats and chickens [101–103]. As in the case of AVT, *in vitro* cortisol action on IT secretion in teleosts was not known. Results presented by Kalamarz-Kubiak et al. [86] showed that cortisol decreased IT secretion from nerve ending of *S. aurata* pituitary. In mammals, cortisol action on OT was investigated by *in vitro* and *in vivo* experiments. It was found that glucocorticoids exert an inhibitory effect on the neurosecretory activity of parvocellular OT-ergic neurons of rats [104]. In rats, the increase in plasma OT levels after intravenous injection of isotonic or hypertonic saline was blocked by dexamethasone [105].

For the reasons mentioned above, it was presumed that UI, instead of CRF, might regulate AVT and IT release in *S. aurata*. In the *in vitro* study presented by Kalamarz-Kubiak et al. [86], the dose-dependent stimulatory effect of UI on AVT secretion from nerve ending of *S. aurata* pituitary was observed after 6 hours of culture. In rats, it has been shown that UI slightly increases the hypothalamus AVP secretion *in vitro*, indicating the probable stimulatory effect of this peptide on AVT production [106]. In turn, the presented *in vitro* results [86] have demonstrated that after 24 hours only the highest dose of UI elevates AVT secretion from *S. aurata* pituitary cells. Moreover, this stimulatory effect of UI completely expires after 48 hours of pituitary cell culture. Since UI is a natural ligand of CRF receptors (CRFRs) [78, 107], the later desensitization of CRFRs may be an explanation of these results. A number of *in vitro* studies demonstrate desensitization of CRFRs [108–111]. Moreover, it is also known that UI increases cortisol secretion [108–111]. Thus, UI may also influence AVT secretion indirectly, stimulating cortisol release. In gilthead sea bream, UI did not affect IT secretion from pituitary cells. Note that the influence of UI on IT or OT secretion had never been investigated before. The opposite response of AVT and IT to UI or cortisol exposure in pituitary cell culture is in accordance with other data showing an independent regulation of nonapeptide secretion [58, 112]. In a summary, the following conclusions were formulated:

- Cortisol affects AVT and IT secretion from nerve endings in *S. aurata* pituitary.
- Cortisol stimulates AVT secretion in a dose-dependent manner and inhibits IT secretion in *S. aurata* pituitary cell culture.

- UI stimulates AVT secretion but does not influence IT secretion from nerve endings in *S. aurata* pituitary.
- UI instead of CRF may contribute to the regulation of HPI axis and regulate AVT secretion.
- AVT and IT are essential components of stress response in fish.

2.2. Urotensin II

At the beginning of this chapter, it was noticed that besides cortisol, urotensins are also involved in the response to stress in fish. UI action has already been discussed. In turn, urotensin II (UII), a cyclic peptide originally isolated from the urophysis of the goby (*Gillichthys mirabilis*) [113], appears to be involved in the control of osmoregulatory and metabolic functions and also in the cardiovascular and gastrointestinal activities, and immune response in teleosts [114–118]. In the European flounder (*Platichthys flesus*), urophysial UII content rose over the 24 hours following a transfer from seawater to fresh water, whereas plasma UII content and UII receptor expression in kidney and gill decreased, implying downregulation of the UII system [115, 119]. It should be noted that in fish, hormonal regulation of water and ion homeostasis requires participation and interaction of many endocrine systems at the various functional levels of the organism [58]. In teleosts, also AVT and IT seem to be involved in the maintenance of water and ion homeostasis [57, 58]. What is more, there is also evidence of the role of AVT and IT in response to different osmotic stimuli [47, 60]. It has been observed that the synthesis of AVT and IT and their release from the neurohypophysis are sensitive to changes in water salinity. In teleosts, an acute change in water salinity results in altered pro-AVT and pro-IT mRNA expression in hypothalamic neurons [120–122] and in the altered content of AVT and IT in the pituitary [119, 122, 123]. It should be emphasized that the potential relationship between AVT and other hormonal systems such as UII contributing to the osmoregulation in fish has been suggested before [119, 124, 125]. As already mentioned, AVT and IT are synthesized in the POA and transported to the neurohypophysis for storage and release into the vascular system via axon terminals. UII has been identified in teleost and nonteleost fish not only in the urophysis but also in the CNS [126–129]. Moreover, UII and UII receptor mRNA expression has been detected in all brain regions of European flounder, including the telencephalon-preoptic region, hypothalamus and pituitary [115]. These results indicate the probable site of interaction between the UII and AVT/IT systems within the POA, hypothalamus and pituitary. In the European flounder, it was found that both UII and AVT are engaged in the hyper- and hypo-osmotic stress In the European flounder [119, 124, 125]. However, to the best of our knowledge, the influence of UII on AVT and IT secretion in teleosts has been studied only by Kalamarz-Kubiak and coworkers [130]. The aim of this study was to determine whether AVT and IT release from nerve endings is affected by UII in the pituitary of gilthead sea bream. Three-year-old gilthead sea bream of both sexes were used for *in vitro* study. Primary cultures of pituitary cells were prepared by a modification of the method described by Levavi-Sivan et al. [87, 88]. Pituitary cells were cultured with medium supplemented with UII (10^{-12}, 10^{-10} and 10^{-8} M). The doses of UII used in this *in vitro* study were determined based on the literature, considering its concentration in different fish tissues [30, 125, 131]. After 6, 24 and 48 hours of incubation, the media were collected and stored at –70°C until HPLC analysis of AVT and IT. The results of this *in vitro* study indicate that UII inhibits AVT secretion in pituitary cell culture. It has been shown that AVT is an antidiuretic hormone reducing urine production in fish [132, 133]. Thus, by inhibiting AVT secretion, UII may have a diuretic effect. Furthermore, it is known that UII administrated *in vivo* increases renal blood flow and glomerular filtration rate and consequently enhances diuresis and natriuresis in the rat [134, 135]. This mammalian paradigm could be helpful in the interpretation of fish data. The *in vitro* study in *S. aurata* indicated that UII's strong inhibitory action on AVT release from nerve endings in the pituitary is independent of tested doses and exposure time. What is more, after 24 hours of incubation, AVT inhibition was lower and persisted to the end of culture. This disinhibition of AVT secretion after a long time of incubation may indicate the desensitization of UII receptors as it was proved in human cell lines [136, 137]. In contrast to AVT, UII significantly increased IT release from nerve endings after 24 hours of culture. This stimulatory effect of UII appeared to be independent of tested doses. In mammals, UII is a naturally occurring somatostatin analog sharing some functional similarities with somatostatin [113, 138]. The results in fish are consistent with data in mammals that show that the intracerebroventricular somatostatin infusion significantly increases plasma OT secretion in virgin and pregnant rats [139]. Moreover, the opposite response of AVT and IT to UII exposure in pituitary cell culture showed an independent regulation of nonapeptide secretion. This idea was documented previously in rainbow trout (*Oncorhynchus mykiss*) [47, 112, 140].

From those results, the following conclusions were formulated:

- UII affects AVT and IT release from nerve endings in the pituitary of gilthead sea bream.
- UII inhibits AVT release and stimulates release of IT in *S. aurata* pituitary cell culture.
- UII together with AVT and IT may control response to different salinities in fish.

The hormonal interactions between UII and AVT and IT are presented in **Figure 2**.

3. What is the mechanism of cortisol action in fish?

It has been established that cortisol has both a corticosteroid and a mineralocorticoid function in fish [1]. An involvement of both classes of corticoid receptors (CRs), mineralocorticoid (MRs) and glucocorticoid (GRs), was widely demonstrated during adaptation to different salinities and osmoregulatory stress [141–144], fish reproduction [145, 146] and expression of social behavior [147–149]. It is worth noting that both MRs and GRs were engaged in tilapia's response to handling stress [150] and expressed in rainbow trout organs with slow-release cortisol implants [151].

Glucocorticoid and mineralocorticoid receptors are involved in the genomic and nongenomic mechanisms of cortisol action in fish [149, 152, 153]. Corticosteroid-intracellular receptor complex binds to the nuclear glucocorticoid response elements (GRE) to modulate transcription and protein synthesis (genomic pathway) [13, 25, 154]. The nongenomic effect is mediated through either nonspecific physicochemical interaction with the plasma membrane [155] or specific membrane receptors such as the G protein–coupled receptor (GPCR) [156] or the

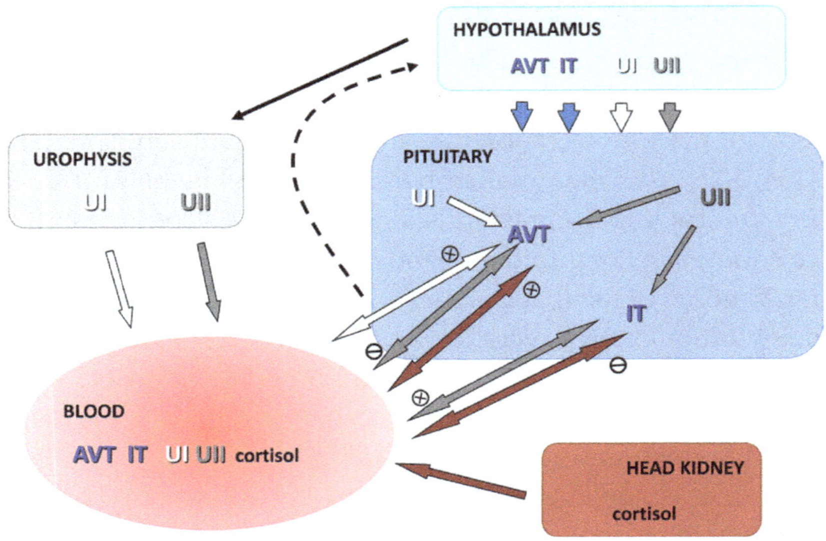

Figure 2. The effect of cortisol, urotensin I and urotensin II on arginine vasotocin and isotocin secretion in gilthead sea bream.

plasma membrane-bound form of GR (mGRs) (nongenomic pathway) [157]. ("Nongenomic steroid action is presented in accordance with Mannheim classification [155].")

3.1. What method can investigate the mechanism of action of cortisol?

Recently, there is growing concern about effects of farming and environmental pollution on fish well-being; thus, there is the need for new tests to study the endocrine responses in fish [158]. Furthermore, fish are increasingly being used as substitutes for mammalian model organisms in fundamental research and as a research model for chemical testing. Hence, research must remain focused on the discovery of new alternative techniques or on an adaptation of methods established for mammalian models for use as fish models [159].

The mechanism presented in this section requires a method that allows monitoring the dynamic hormone secretion and registering even small and short-term fluctuations in their release. Only perfusion culture method allows detailed examination of changes in the release of hormones while ensuring optimal culture conditions. Kalamarz-Kubiak et al. [160] developed a new procedure for the unique gradient perfusion technique (3D) of brain and pituitary explants collected from three-spined stickleback (*Gasterosteus aculeatus*) and round goby (*Neogobius melanostomus*). So far, organ perfusion methods have not been often used in fish for lack of suitable techniques. Simple organ perfusion systems were applied in pituitary [161–165] and pineal gland [166–168] studies. However, an innovative system for organ perfusion (MINUCELLS and MINUTISSUE Vertriebs GmbH, Germany), proposed by Minuth in early 1990s, gives more options for this kind of technique. This gradient perfusion technique meets the requirements for studies of nervous tissues, blood-brain barrier, retina and blood-retina, regeneration of blood vessels, skin renewal, bone and muscular tissue in mammals [169]. Thus, Kalamarz-Kubiak et al. [160] presented the first application of the MINUCELLS and MINUTISSUE tissue engineering technique for perfusion of fish brain tissues. In this study, tissues were placed on the membrane between rings of tissue carriers inside the gradient container. A specific construction of this container facilitated the uniform supply of medium to the luminal and basal sides to avoid the dead space. The methods of medium transport into the gradient container were tested using three perfusion sets. *Set 1* and *set 2* allow the supply of one medium from the top without aeration or with aeration, respectively. *Set 3* allows the supply of one or two aerated media from the top and bottom, simultaneously. Moreover, *set 1* was used to determine the time required to achieve a stable basal level of AVT and IT release during tissue explant perfusion. The stable basal level of AVT and IT release was achieved between 60 and 80 minutes of perfusion for both fish species. *Set 2* equipped with gas exchange module was aerated by an air pump (0.3% CO_2) or a mixture of 95% O_2 and 5% CO_2 at a pressure of 127.51 mmHg. The results indicated that only usage of a mixture of 95% O_2 and 5% CO_2 provided the proper conditions for perfusion and tissue reactivity in the medium supplemented with high K^+ concentration (60 mM KCl) (**Figure 3**). In order to optimize the conditions of perfusion, the various pressure of gas mixture (127.51, 255.02 and 315.03 mmHg at the outlet of the gas bottle) was tested. The gas pressure of 127.51 mmHg provides optimal conditions for perfusion in the *set 2* with one gas exchange module. To ensure the same pressure conditions in *set 3*, with two gas exchange modules, higher pressure of 315.03 mmHg at the outlet of the gas bottle must be applied. Concentrations of AVT and IT in the media collected after perfusion were determined by HPLC with fluorescence and UV detection according to the modified procedure by Gozdowska et al. [170]. Although the presented procedure has been elaborated for studies of AVT and IT in fish explants, after only minor modification, if any, it can serve many other purposes. From those results, the following conclusions were drawn and the recommendations were formulated:

- *Set 1* is preferable only for short-term research.
- *Set 2*, where the medium is aerated with a mixture of 95% O_2 and 5% CO_2 at a pressure of 127.51 mmHg, is recommended for long-term studies.
- *Set 3* is also preferable for long-term studies but requires aeration with a mixture of 95% O_2 and 5% CO_2 at a pressure of 315.03 mmHg.
- *Sets 1* and *2* allow the supply of only one type of medium at the same time to the gradient perfusion container. *Set 3* allows the transport of two different media from the top and bottom to the perfusion container at the same time.

The schemes of sets used for gradient perfusion and graphs of AVT and IT release during tests of those sets are presented in **Figure 3**.

3.2. How does cortisol affect the release of AVT and IT and what kind of pathway, genomic or nongenomic, is involved in this regulation?

In teleost, two different GR coding genes (GR1 and GR2) and one MR gene were found [171, 172]. The expression of GR1, GR2 and MR genes, as well as the immunoreactivity of GRs (GRs-ir), was noted in most of the magno- and parvocellular neurons of the preoptic nucleus

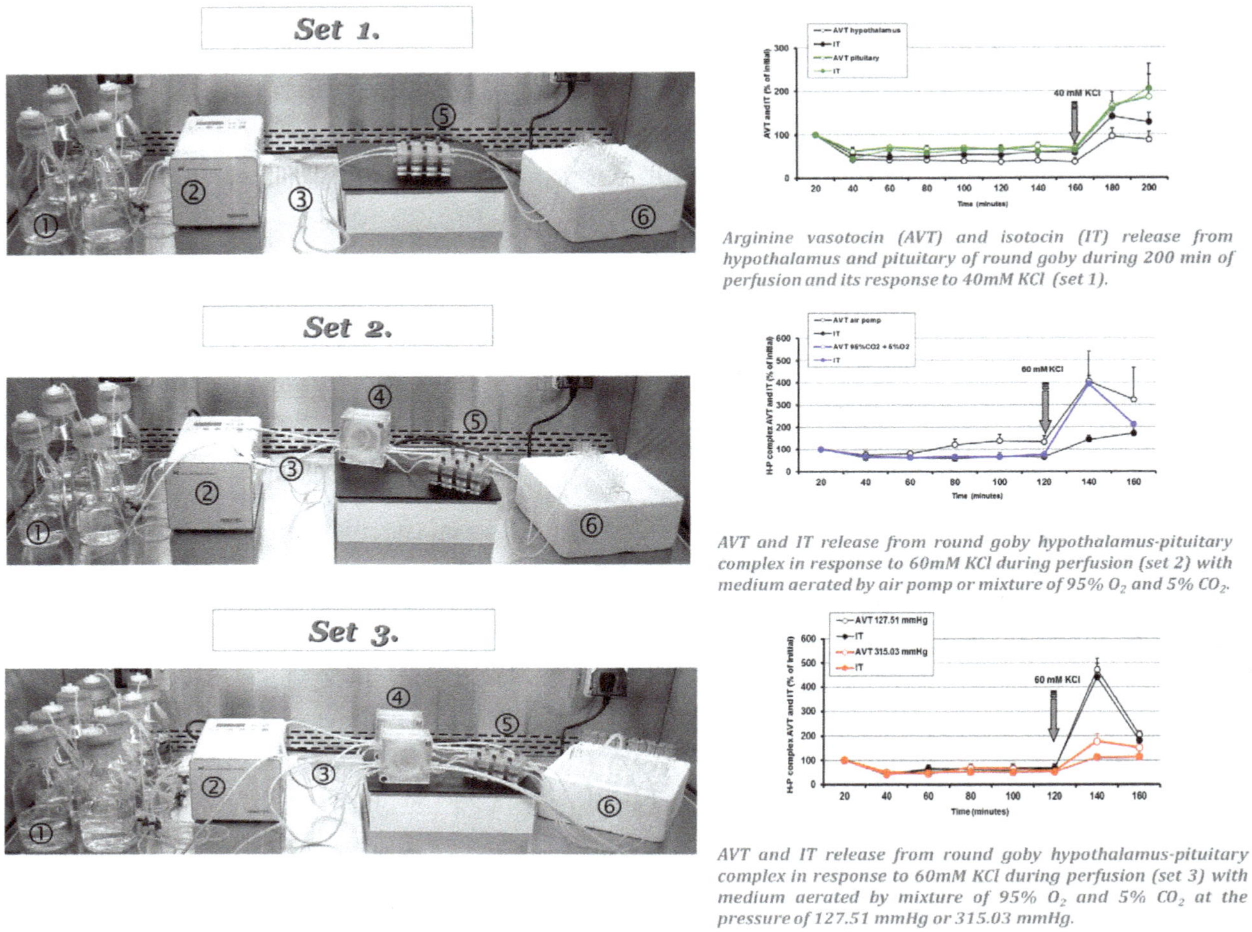

Figure 3. The schemes of culture sets used for gradient perfusion. Components of perfusion culture set: (1) storage medium bottles, (2) peristaltic pumps, (3) connecting fittings, (4) gas exchange modules, (5) gradient culture container, (6) sampling vials. The release of arginine vasotocin and isotocin during tests of these sets (graphs).

(NPO), known for synthesizing AVT, IT and CRF, in tilapia (*Oreochromis mossambicus*), rainbow trout and common carp (*Cyprinus carpio*) [173–175]. In the pituitary, GR1, GR2 and MR mRNA expression and GRs-ir have localized in *pars distalis* and *pars intermedia* where AVT-ergic fibers give their projections [173–175].

As it was mentioned earlier, AVT and IT are engaged in physiological stress response and seem to be important components of stress axis in fish [33, 47, 61]. In gilthead sea bream, the application of cortisol implants in this species enhanced the hypothalamic expression of provasotocin mRNA and pituitary AVT content [85]. What is more, an *in vitro* study indicated that cortisol affects AVT and IT release from the *nerve terminalis* in *S. aurata* pituitary [86]. However, to the best of the authors' knowledge, the mechanism of cortisol action on AVT and IT release in teleosts has been studied only by Kalamarz-Kubiak and coworkers [176]. This *in vitro* perfusion study was performed to determine which class of receptors, GRs or MRs, participated in cortisol regulation of AVT and IT release from the hypothalamic-pituitary (H-P) complex of round goby (*Neogobius melanostomus*). Moreover, this *in vitro* study allowed to determine which pathways, genomic or nongenomic, are engaged in the aforementioned process. Adult round gobies of both sexes were used in this in vitro study.

Hypothalamic-pituitary explants were perfused using *set 2* of gradient perfusion technique (for details see Section 3.2). The explants were perfused with medium supplemented with different treatments (cortisol, mifepristone [RU486], spironolactone [C03DA01] and actinomycin D). Mifepristone is a glucocorticoid receptor antagonist, which affects a wide range of physiological and behavioral traits (metabolism, reproduction, osmotic stress, vocalizations and aggression in fish) [13, 177]. Spironolactone is a mineralocorticoid receptor antagonist, which blocks the ion uptake in osmoregulation [142, 152] and reduces aggression during social interaction [149, 178]. Actinomycin D is a transcription inhibitor, which binds DNA at the transcription initiation complex and prevents elongation by RNA polymerase [179–181]. Cortisol was tested at three doses (1.4×10^{-7} M, 2.8×10^{-7} M and 0.4×10^{-6} M). Cortisol doses were selected based on our previous experiments and literature [9, 86, 182–185]. The doses of inhibitors were selected on the basis of available data [186–190]. Finally, cortisol at 0.4×10^{-6} M dose in combination with RU486 (0.3×10^{-6} M) or C03DA01 (0.36×10^{-6} M) or actinomycin D (1×10^{-7} M) was used in experiments. Concentrations of AVT and IT in the media collected after perfusion were determined by HPLC with fluorescence and UV detection according to the modified procedure by Gozdowska et al. [170]. In this study, cortisol showed a dose-dependent stimulatory effect on AVT release from H-P explants similar to the one presented previously in pituitary cells of *S. aurata*. In rats, corticosterone also affected AVP release from hypothalamic slices containing paraventricular and supraoptic nuclei in a dose-dependent manner [191]. The results presented by Kalamarz-Kubiak et al. [176] indicate that cortisol, most likely acting through GRs, stimulates the release of AVT from the H-P complex of round goby. It has been suggested that cortisol preferentially binds to GR2 in teleosts, in response to low or mild stress, and to both GR2 and GR1 in response to extreme stress [192, 193]. Therefore, it is probable that both isoforms of GRs are engaged in cortisol action on AVT release from the H-P complex of round goby [176]. However, a biphasic AVT response may depict an initial release of mature AVT from the pool stored in the secretory granules, followed by the release of newly matured AVT molecules just after their dissociation from the noncovalent complex. Cortisol may exert biphasic effects on the release of inflammatory mediators, e.g., the plasma macrophage migration inhibitory factor and the tumor necrosis factor-α, interleukin-6 and acute-phase proteins in vertebrates, including fish [194, 195]. The results of presented *in vitro* study indicate that cortisol affects AVT release through GRs via genomic and nongenomic pathways in round goby. The biphasic response of AVT to cortisol was hindered by both the GR antagonist RU486 and the transcription inhibitor actinomycin D [176]. In the marine medaka (*Oryzias dancena*), RU486 blocked the transcriptional activity of both GR isoforms in response to cortisol action [193]. However, RU486 blocks some rapid, nongenomic effects of cortisol mediated via plasma membrane receptors in fish [181, 196, 197]. Probable mGRs are engaged in the first phase of the biphasic AVT response to cortisol in *Neogobius melanostomus*. Alternatively, cortisol may demonstrate nongenomic action through specific membrane receptors such as the GPCRs or without receptor engagement through the nonspecific action that alters the plasma membrane's physicochemical properties, as it has been shown in mammals [155] and fish [153, 180]. It is worth noting that in higher vertebrates and fish, the mechanism of corticosteroid action may integrate nongenomic and genomic pathways [25, 156, 198]. For instance, in rodents, such integration between nongenomic and genomic mechanisms has been shown in the neurons of the amygdala, hippocampus and cortex in response to stress and the administration of corticosterone ("for a review: [198]").

In results presented by Kalamarz-Kubiak et al. [176], the stimulation of IT secretion by cortisol appeared within 20 minutes and persisted for the next 100 minutes, similarly as in the case of AVT, but did not disclose a biphasic character. The nongenomic, stimulatory effect of cortisol *in vivo* on Na^+ -K^+ and Ca^{2+} -ATPase activity in gills of tilapia occurred after 30 minutes and persisted for 120 minutes. [180]. Similar observations, i.e., fast and long-lasting effects of corticosteroids *in vitro* on the excitability of different brain areas, were noted in rodents ("for a review: [198]"). In round goby, cortisol probably influenced IT release by GRs via the nongenomic pathway because cortisol action was inhibited by RU486, but not by actinomycin D. In contrast to the data in round goby, *in vitro* study of pituitary cells in *S. aurata* showed that cortisol decreased the IT release from nerve endings [86]. It should be noted that gilthead sea breams approached the reproductive season, while round gobies were out of their spawning season. Therefore, the IT responses to cortisol may be dependent on their physiological status and/or differ in various species.

In fish, the cortisol effects are mediated through both the GRs but also through MRs [1]. However, the *in vitro* study suggests that cortisol effect on AVT and IT release from the H-P complex in round goby is not mediated by MRs because the MRs' antagonist, C03DA01, does not hinder AVT and IT release caused by cortisol.

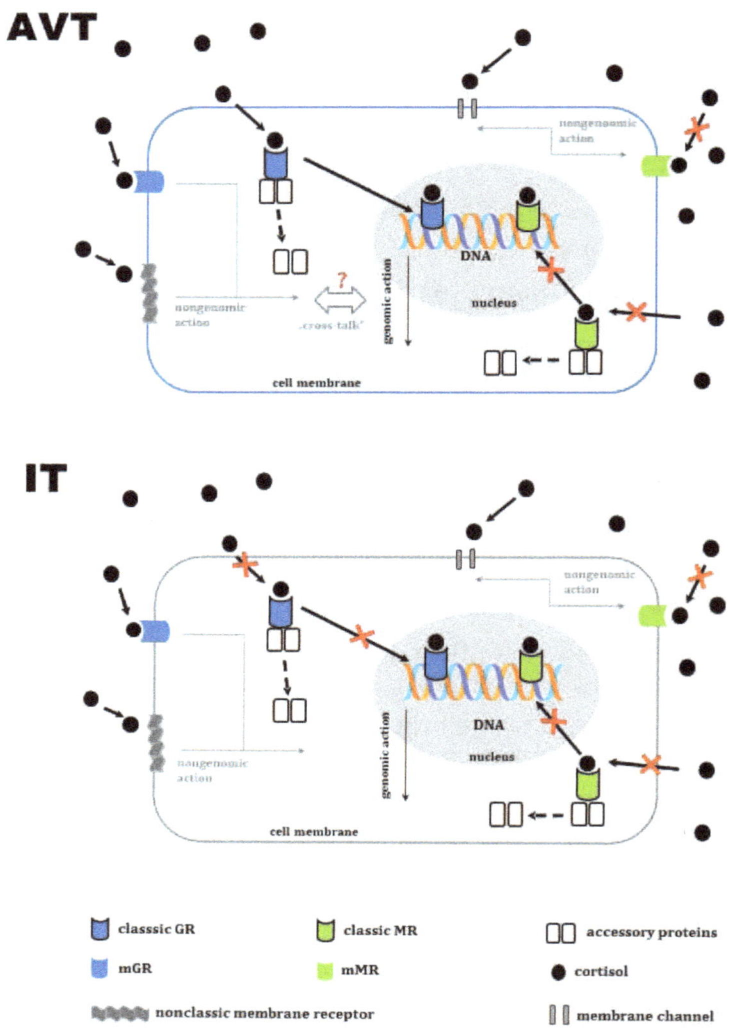

Figure 4. The mechanism of cortisol action on arginine vasotocin and isotocin release in round goby.

Outside the scope of this study, an opposite effect, i.e., the stimulation of cortisol secretion by AVT, should also be considered. There is evidence that AVT neurons innervate corticotrophic cells in green molly (*Poecilia latipinna*) pituitary [199] and that AVT synergizes with CRH/CRF (corticotrophin-releasing hormone/factor) to promote ACTH secretion from the pituitary in rainbow trout [66]. Consequently, AVT can stimulate cortisol release, and thus relationships between AVT and cortisol may be more complicated.

From those data, the following conclusions were formulated:

- Cortisol affects AVT and IT secretion from the H-P complex in round goby.
- Cortisol stimulates the release of both nonapeptides. However, the effect of cortisol on AVT release is dose-dependent.
- Cortisol has biphasic effects on the release of AVT, while this effect on IT is monophasic.
- GRs but not MRs are involved in cortisol regulation of AVT and IT release.
- In the case of AVT, both genomic and nongenomic pathways mediate the effect of cortisol.
- In the case of IT, only the nongenomic pathway mediates the effect of cortisol.

The mechanism of cortisol action on AVT and IT release in round goby are presented in **Figure 4**.

4. Summary

The purpose of this chapter was to gain new knowledge on the involvement of cortisol and other indicators of fish welfare in the regulation of stress response in fish. The basis of the subject was to assume that both nonapeptides and urotensins are essential components of stress response in fish. So far, nobody has attempted to check if there is a functional relationship between cortisol and both nonapeptides and urotensins using *in vitro* technique of cell culture and gradient perfusion. For the first time, MINUCELLS and MINUTISSUE tissue engineering technique (3D) has been applied for the gradient perfusion of fish brain and pituitary by Kalamarz-Kubiak et al. [160]. Although the presented procedure has been elaborated for studies of AVT and IT in fish explants, after only minor modification, if any, it can serve many other purposes. It has been confirmed that AVT and IT are essential components of stress response in fish. Presented results showed an independent regulation of nonapeptide secretion. Cortisol affects AVT and IT secretion from nerve endings in gilthead sea bream and round goby. Therefore, the cortisol effect may be different in various species and/or dependent on their physiological status. *S. aurata* is a very interesting species for this type of research. In gilthead sea bream, unlike other teleosts, CRF is not a releasing factor for ACTH, because there are no anatomical connections between CRF perikarya and ACTH cells. It has been investigated that urotensin I instead of CRF may contribute to the regulation of HPI axis and regulate AVT. In turn, urotensin II together with AVT and IT may control response to different salinities in fish. The results confirm that urotensins together with nonapeptides are involved in the regulation of stress response in fish. Here, the first feasible mechanism of cortisol action on AVT and IT release from the H-P complex has been presented in round goby.

The different mechanisms have been pointed out, where GRs are involved, whereas MRs are not. In the case of AVT, both genomic and nongenomic pathways mediate the effect of cortisol. In the case of IT, only the nongenomic pathway mediates the effect of cortisol. Therefore, AVT and IT seem to be good candidates for welfare indicators. Probably, the examination of cortisol in relation to other welfare indicators in the regulation of stress response will allow the separation of (physiological) stress from (psychological) distress, the separation of chronic stress from acclimation and the interactions between feelings, mood and behavior.

In conclusion, it is worth to quote the statement of Victoria Braithwaite [200], about the pain and stress in fish, for The Los Angeles Times dated October 8, 2006: "Their brains are not as different from ours as we once thought. Although less anatomically complex than our own brain, the function of two of their forebrain areas is very similar to the mammalian amygdala and hippocampus – areas associated with emotion, learning and memory. If these regions are damaged in fish, their learning and emotional capacities are impaired; they can no longer find their way through mazes, and they lose their sense of fear".

Author details

Hanna Kalamarz-Kubiak

Address all correspondence to: hkalamarz@iopan.gda.pl

Genetic and Marine Biotechnology Department, Institute of Oceanology Polish Academy of Sciences, Sopot, Poland

References

[1] Wendelaar Bonga SE. The stress response in fish. Physiological Reviews. 1997;**77**:591-625

[2] Dunlop R, Laming P. Mechanoreceptive and nociceptive responses in the central nervous system of goldfish (*Carassius auratus*) and trout (*Oncorhynchus mykiss*). The Journal of Pain. 2005;**6**:561-568

[3] Nordgreen J, Horsberg TE, Ranheim B, Chen AC. Somatosensory evoked potentials in the telencephalon of Atlantic salmon (*Salmo salar*) following galvanic stimulation of the tail. Journal of Comparative Physiology. A, Neuroethology, Sensory, Neural, and Behavioral Physiology. 2007;**193**:1235-1242

[4] Sneddon LU. Pain perception in fish: Evidence and implications for the use of fish. Journal of Consciousness Studies. 2012;**18**:209-229

[5] Mazeaud MM, Mazeaud F. Adrenergic responses to stress in fish. In: Pickering AD, editor. Stress and Fish. London: Academic Press; 1981. pp. 50-75

[6] Donaldson EM. The pituitary-interrenal axis as an indicator of stress in fish. In: Pickering AD, editor. Stress and Fish. New York: Academic Press; 1981. pp. 11-47

[7] Wedemeyer GA, Barton BA, McLeay DJ. Stress and acclimation. In: Schreck CB, Moyle PB, editors. Methods for Fish Biology. Bethesda, Maryland: Am Fish Soc; 1990. pp. 451-489

[8] Anderson DP. Immunological indicators: Effects of environmental stress on immune protection and disease outbreaks. American Fisheries Society Symposium. 1990;**8**:38-50

[9] Barton BA. Stress in fishes: A diversity of responses with particular reference to changes in circulating corticosteroids. Integrative and Comparative Biology. 2002;**42**:517-525

[10] Iwama GK, Afonso LOB, Vijayan MM. Stress in Fish. AquaNet Workshop on Fish Welfare. B.C. Canada: Campbell River; 2004. pp. 1-4

[11] Ellis T, Yildiz HY, López-Olmeda J, Spedicato MT, Tort L, Øverli Ø, Martins CI. Cortisol and finfish welfare. Fish Physiology and Biochemistry. 2012;**38**:163-188

[12] Reid SG, Bernier NJ, Perry SF. The adrenergic stress response in fish: Control of catecholamine storage and release. Comparative Biochemistry and Physiology. 1998;**120C**:1-27

[13] Mommsen TP, Vijayan MM, Moon TW. Cortisol in teleosts: Dynamics, mechanisms of action, and metabolic regulation. Reviews in Fish Biology and Fisheries. 1999;**9**:21-268

[14] Perry SF, Bernier NJ. The acute humoral adrenergic stress response in fish: Facts and fiction. Aquaculture. 1999;**177**:285-295

[15] Pickering AD. Introduction: The concept of biological stress. In: Pickering AD, editor. Stress and Fish. New York: Academic Press; 1981. pp. 2-9

[16] Iwama GK, Pickering AD, Sumpter JP, Schreck CB. Fish stress and health in aquaculture. In: Soc. Exp. Biol. Sem. Ser. 62. Cambridge, UK: Cambridge Univ. Press; 1997. pp. 223-246

[17] Iwama GK, Thomas PT, Forsyth RB, Vijayan MM. Heat shock protein expression in fish. Reviews in Fish Biology and Fisheries. 1998;**8**:35-56

[18] Milla S, Wang N, Mandiki SN, Kestemont P. Corticosteroids: Friends or foes of teleost fish reproduction? Comparative Biochemistry and Physiology. Part A, Molecular & Integrative Physiology. 2009;**153**:242-251

[19] Barton BA, Schreck CB, Barton LD. Effects of chronic cortisol administration and daily acute stress on growth, physiological conditions, and stress responses in juvenile rainbow trout. Diseases of Aquatic Organisms. 1987;**2**:173-185

[20] Morgan JD, Iwama GK. Cortisol-induced changes in oxygen consumption and ionic regulation in coastal cutthroat trout (*Oncorhynchus clarki clarki*) parr. Fish Physiology and Biochemistry. 1996;**15**:385-394

[21] Tort L. Stress in farmed fish: Its consequences in health and performance. In: Koumoundouros G, editor. Recent Advances in Aquaculture Research. Trivandrum: Transworld Research Network; 2010. pp. 55-84

[22] McCormick SD. Effects of growth hormone and insulin-like growth factor I on salinity tolerance and gill Na^+, K^+-ATPase in Atlantic salmon (*Salmo salar*): Interaction with cortisol. General and Comparative Endocrinology. 1996;**101**:3-11

[23] McCormick MD. Endocrine control of osmoregulation in Teleost fish. American Zoologist. 2001;**41**:781-794

[24] Vizzini A, Vazzana M, Cammarata M, Parrinello N. Peritoneal cavity phagocytes from the teleost sea bass express a glucocorticoid receptor (cloned and sequenced) involved in genomic modulation of the in vitro chemiluminescence response to zymosan. General and Comparative Endocrinology. 2007;**150**:114-123

[25] Aluru N, Vijayan MM. Stress transcriptomics in fish: A role for genomic cortisol signalling. General and Comparative Endocrinology. 2009;**164**:142-150

[26] Ackerman PA, Forsyth RB, Mazur CF, Iwama GK. Stress hormones and the cellular stress response in salmonids. Fish Physiology and Biochemistry. 2000;**23**:327-336

[27] Basu N, Nakano T, Grau EG, Iwama GK. The effects of cortisol on heat shock protein 70 levels in two fish species. General and Comparative Endocrinology. 2001;**24**:97-105

[28] Vijayan MM, Pereira C, Grau EG, Iwama GK. Metabolic responses associated with confinement stress in tilapia: The role of cortisol. Comparative Biochemistry and Physiology. 1997;**116C**:89-95

[29] Arnold-Reed DE, Balment RJ. Steroidogenic role of the caudal neurosecretory system in the flounder, *Platichthys flesus*. General and Comparative Endocrinology. 1989;**76**:267-273

[30] Kelsall CJ, Balment RJ. Native urotensins influence cortisol secretion and plasma cortisol concentration in the euryhaline flounder, *Platichthys flesus*. General and Comparative Endocrinology. 1998;**112**:210-219

[31] Alderman SL, Raine JC, Bernier NJ. Distribution and regional stressor-induced regulation of corticotrophin-releasing factor binding protein in rainbow trout (*Oncorhynchus mykiss*). Journal of Neuroendocrinology. 2008;**20**:347-358

[32] Bernier NJ, Alderman SL, Bristow EN. Heads or tails? Stressor-specific expression of corticotropin-releasing factor and urotensin I in the preoptic area and caudal neurosecretory system of rainbow trout. The Journal of Endocrinology. 2008;**196**:637-648

[33] Mancera JM, Vargas-Chacoff L, García-López A, Kleszczyńska A, Kalamarz H, Martínez-Rodríguez G, Kulczykowska E. High density and food deprivation affect arginine vasotocin, isotocin and melatonin in gilthead sea bream (*Sparus auratus*). Comparative Biochemistry and Physiology Part A. 2008;**149**:92-97

[34] Barton BA, Iwama GK. Physiological changes in fish from stress in aquaculture with emphasis on the response and effects of corticosteroids. Annual Review of Fish Diseases. 1991;**1**:3-26

[35] Pankhurst NW. The endocrinology of stress in fish: An environmental perspective. General and Comparative Endocrinology. 2011;**170**:265-275

[36] Vijayan MM, Moon TW. The stress-response and the plasma disappearance of corticosteroid and glucose in a marine teleost, the sea raven. Canadian Journal of Zoology. 1994;**72**:379-386

[37] Iwama GK, McGeer JC, Bernier NJ. The effects of stock and rearing density on the stress response in juvenile coho salmon (*Oncorhynchus kisutch*). ICES Marine Science Symposia. 1992;**194**:67-83

[38] Pottinger TG, Moran TA. Differences in plasma cortisol and cortisone dynamics during stress in two strains of rainbow trout (*Oncorhynchus mykiss*). Journal of Fish Biology. 1993;**43**:121-130

[39] Noga EJ, Kerby JH, King W, Aucoin DP, Giesbrecht F. Quantitative comparison of the stress response of striped bass (*Morone saxatilis*) and hybrid striped bass (*Morone saxatilis* x *Morone chrysops* and *Morone saxatilis* x *Morone americana*). American Journal of Veterinary Research. 1994;**55**:405-409

[40] Woodward CC, Strange RJ. Physiological stress responses in wild and hatchery-reared rainbow trout. Transactions of the American Fisheries Society. 1987;**116**:574-579

[41] Heath DD, Bernier NJ, Heath JW, Iwama GK. Genetic, environmental, and interaction effects on growth and stress response of chinook salmon (*Oncorhynchus tshawytscha*) fry. Canadian Journal of Fisheries and Aquatic Sciences. 1993;**50**:435-442

[42] O'Leary DB, Coughlan J, Dillane E, McCarthy TV, Cross TF. Microsatellite variation in cod *Gadus morhua* throughout its geographic range. Journal of Fish Biology. 2007;**70**:1095-8649

[43] Kijewska A, Kalamarz-Kubiak H, Arciszewski B, Guellard T, Petereit C, Wenne R. Adaptation to salinity in Atlantic cod from different regions of the Baltic Sea. Journal of Experimental Marine Biology and Ecology. 2016;**478**:62-67

[44] Fryer J, Lederis K, Rivier J. ACTH-releasing activity of urotensin I and ovine CRF: Interactions with arginine vasotocin, isotocin and arginine vasopressin. Regulatory Peptides. 1985;**11**:11-15

[45] Winberg S, Nilsson A, Hylland P, Söderstöm V, Nilsson GE. Serotonin as a regulator of hypothalamic-pituitary-interrenal activity in teleost fish. Neuroscience Letters. 1997;**230**:113-116

[46] Arends RJ, Mancera JM, Muñoz JL, Wendelaar Bonga SE, Flik G. The stress response of the gilthead sea bream (*Sparus aurata* L.) to air exposure and confinement. The Journal of Endocrinology. 1999;**163**:149-157

[47] Kulczykowska E, Warne JM, Balment RJ. Day-night variations in plasma melatonin and arginine vasotocin concentrations in chronically cannulated flounder (*Platichthys flesus*). Comparative Biochemistry and Physiology Part A. 2001;**130**:827-834

[48] Gesto M, Lopez-Patiño MA, Hernandez J, Soengas JL, Míguez JM. The response of brain serotonergic and dopaminergic systems to an acute stressor in rainbow trout: A time course study. The Journal of Experimental Biology. 2013;**216**:4435-4442

[49] Pottinger TG, Prunet P, Pickering AD. The effects of confinement stress on circulating prolactin levels in rainbow trout (*Oncorhynchus mykiss*) in fresh water. General and Comparative Endocrinology. 1992;**88**:454-460

[50] Kakizawa S, Kaneko T, Hasegawa S, Hirano T. Effects of feeding, fasting, background adaptation, acute stress, and exhaustive exercise on the plasma somatolactin concentrations in rainbow trout. General and Comparative Endocrinology. 1995;**98**:137-146

[51] Geven EJ, Verkaar F, Flik G, Klaren PH. Experimental hyperthyroidism and central mediators of stress axis and thyroid axis activity in common carp (*Cyprinus carpio* L.). Journal of Molecular Endocrinology. 2006;**37**:443-452

[52] Acher R. Neurohypophysial peptide systems: Processing machinery, hydroosmotic regulation, adaptation and evolution. Regulatory Peptides. 1993;**45**:1-13

[53] Van den Dungen HM, Buijs RM, Pool CW, Terlou M. The distribution of vasotocin and isotocin in the brain of the rainbow trout. The Journal of Comparative Neurology. 1982;**212**:146-157

[54] Holmqvist BI, Ekström P. Hypophysiotrophic systems in the brain of the Atlantic salmon. Neuronal innervation of the pituitary and the origin of pituitary dopamine and nonapeptides identified by means of combined carbocyanine tract tracing and immunocytochemistry. Journal of Chemical Neuroanatomy. 1995;**8**:125-145

[55] Saito D, Komatsuda M, Urano A. Functional organization of preoptic vasotocin and isotocin neurons in the brain of rainbow trout: Central and neurohypophysial projections of single neurons. Neuroscience. 2004;**124**:973-984

[56] Balment RJ, Lu W, Weybourne E, Warne JM. Arginine vasotocin a key hormone in fish physiology and behaviour: A review with insights from mammalian models. General and Comparative Endocrinology. 2006;**147**:9-16

[57] McCormick SD, Bradshaw D. Hormonal control of salt and water balance in vertebrates. General and Comparative Endocrinology. 2006;**147**:3-8

[58] Kulczykowska E. Arginine vasotocin and isotocin: Towards their role in fish osmoregulation. In: Baldisserotto B, Romero Mancera JM, Kapoor BG, editors. Fish Osmoregulation. Durham, NH: Science Publisher; 2007. pp. 151-176

[59] Goodson JL. Nonapeptides and the evolutionary patterning of sociality. Progress in Brain Research. 2008;**170**:3-15

[60] Kleszczyńska A, Vargas-Chacoff L, Gozdowska M, Kalamarz H, Martìnez-Rodrìguez G, Mancera JM, Kulczykowska E. Arginine vasotocin, isotocin and melatonin responses following acclimation of gilthead sea bream (*Sparus aurata*) to different environmental salinities. Comparative Biochemistry and Physiology Part A. 2006;**145**:268-273

[61] Kulczykowska E. Arginine vasotocin and isotocin as multifunctional hormones, neurotransmitters and neuromodulators in fish. In: Munoz-Cueto JA, Mancera JM, Martínez-Rodríguez G, editors. Avances en Endocrinología Comparada. Vol. IV. Servicio de Publicaciones. Spain: Universidad de Cádiz; 2008. pp. 41-47

[62] Yulis CR, Lederis K. Co-localization of the immunoreactivities of corticotropin-releasing factor and arginine vasotocin in the brain and pituitary system of the teleost *Catostomus commersoni*. Cell and Tissue Research. 1987;**247**:267-273

[63] Olivereau M, Moons L, Olivereau J, Vandesande F. Coexistence of corticotropin-releasing factor-like immunoreactivity and vasotocin in perikarya of the preoptic nucleus in the eel. General and Comparative Endocrinology. 1988;**70**:41-48

[64] Ando H, Hasegawa M, Ando J, Urano A. Expression of salmon corticotropin-releasing hormone precursor gene in the preoptic nucleus in stressed rainbow trout. General and Comparative Endocrinology. 1999;**113**:87-95

[65] Gilchriest BJ, Tipping DR, Hake L, Levy A, Baker BI. The effects of acute and chronic stresses on vasotocin gene transcripts in the brain of the rainbow trout (*Oncorhynchus mykiss*). Journal of Neuroendocrinology. 2000;**12**:795-801

[66] Baker BI, Bird DJ, Buckingham JC. In the trout, CRH and AVT synergize to stimulate ACTH release. Regulatory Peptides. 1996;**67**:207-210

[67] Pierson PM, Guibbolini ME, Lahlou BA. V1-type receptor for mediating the neurohypophysial hormone-induced ACTH release in trout pituitary. The Journal of Endocrinology. 1996;**149**:109-115

[68] Quesada J, Lozano MT, Ortega A, Agulleiro B. Immunocytochemical and ultrastructural characterization of the cell types in the adenohypophysis of *Sparus aurata* L. (Teleost). General and Comparative Endocrinology. 1988;**72**:209-225

[69] Mancera JM, Fernandez-Lebrez P. Localization of corticotropin-releasing factor immunoreactivity in the brain of the teleost *Sparus aurata*. Cell and Tissue Research. 1995;**281**: 569-572

[70] Duarte G, Segura-Noguera MM, Martín del Río MP, Mancera JM. The hypothalamo-hypophyseal system of the white seabream *Diplodus sargus*: Immunocytochemical identification of arginine-vasotocin, isotocin, melanin-concentrating hormone and corticotropin-releasing factor. The Histochemical Journal. 2001;**33**:569-578

[71] Lovejoy DA, Balment RJ. Evolution and physiology of the corticotrophin-releasing factor (CRF) family of neuropeptides in vertebrates. General and Comparative Endocrinology. 1999;**115**:1-22

[72] Flik G, Klaren PH, Van den Burg EH, Metz JR, Huising MOCRF. stress in fish. General and Comparative Endocrinology. 2006;**146**:36-44

[73] Bernier NJ, Lin X, Peter RE. Differential expression of corticotropin-releasing factor (CRF) and urotensin I precursor genes, and evidence of CRF gene expression regulated by cortisol in goldfish brain. General and Comparative Endocrinology. 1999;**116**:461-477

[74] Lu W, Dow L, Gumusgoz S, Brierley MJ, Warne JM, McCrohan CR, Balment RJ, Riccardi D. Coexpression of corticotropin-releasing hormone and urotensin I precursor genes in the caudal neurosecretory system of the euryhaline flounder (*Platichthys flesus*): A possible shared role in peripheral regulation. Endocrinology. 2004;**145**:5786-5797

[75] Alderman SL, Bernier NJ. Localization of corticotropin-releasing factor, urotensin I, and CRF-binding protein gene expression in the brain of the zebrafish, *Danio rerio*. The Journal of Comparative Neurology. 2007;**502**:783-793

[76] Ichikawa T, McMaster D, Lederis K, Kobayashi H. Isolation and amino acid sequence of urotensin I, a vasoactive and ACTH-releasing neuropeptide, from the carp (*Cyprinus carpio*) urophysis. Peptides. 1982;**3**:859-867

[77] Fryer J, Lederis K, Rivier J. Urotensin I, a CRF-like neuropeptide, stimulates ACTH release from the teleost pituitary. Endocrinology. 1983;**113**:2308-2310

[78] Lederis K, Fryer JN, Okawara Y, Schonrock CHR, Richter D. Corticotropin-releasing factors acting on the fish pituitary: Experimental and molecular analysis. In: Farrell AP, Randall DJ, editors. Fish Physiology. San Diego, CA: Academic Press Inc.; 1994;**13**:67-110

[79] Fryer J, Lederis K, Rivier J. Cortisol inhibits the ACTH-releasing activity of urotensin I, CRF and sauvagine observed with superfused goldfish pituitary cells. Peptides. 1984;**5**:925-930

[80] Arnold-Reed DE, Balment RJ. Peptide hormones influence in vitro interrenal secretion of cortisol in the trout, *Oncorhynchus mykiss*. General and Comparative Endocrinology. 1994;**96**:85-91

[81] Yulis CR, Lederis K, Wong KL, Fisher AW. Localization of urotensin I- and corticotropin-releasing factor-like immunoreactivity in the central nervous system of *Catostomus commersoni*. Peptides. 1986;**7**:79-86

[82] McMaster D, Lederis K. Urotensin I- and CRF-like peptides in *Catostomus commersoni* brain and pituitary HPLC and RIA characterization. Peptides. 1988;**9**:1043-1048

[83] Fryer J. Neuropeptides regulating the activity of goldfish corticotropes and melanotropes. Fish Physiology and Biochemistry. 1989;**7**:21-27

[84] Mathieu M, Vallarino M, Trabucchi M, Chartrel N, Vaudry H, Conlon JM. Identification of an urotensin I-like peptide in the pituitary of the lungfish *Protopterus annectens*: Immunocytochemical localization and biochemical characterization. Peptides. 1999;**20**: 1303-1310

[85] Cádiz L, Roman-Padilla J, Gozdowska M, Kulczykowska E, Martínez-Rodríguez G, Mancera JM, Martos-Sitcha JA. Cortisol modulates vasotocinergic and isotocinergic pathways in the gilthead sea bream. The Journal of Experimental Biology. 2015;**218**:1-10

[86] Kalamarz-Kubiak H, Meiri-Ashkenazi I, Kleszczyńska A, Rosenfeld H. In vitro effect of cortisol and urotensin I on arginine vasotocin and isotocin secretion from pituitary cells of gilthead sea bream *Sparus aurata*. Journal of Fish Biology. 2014;**84**:448-458

[87] Levavi-Sivan B, Ofir M, Yaron Z. Possible sites of dopaminergic inhibition of gonadotropin release from the pituitary of a teleost fish, tilapia. Molecular and Cellular Endocrinology. 1995;**109**:87-97

[88] Levavi-Sivan B, Safarian H, Rosenfeld H, Elizur A, Avitan A. Regulation of gonadotropin-releasing hormone (GnRH)-receptor gene expression in tilapia: Effect of GnRH and dopamine. Biology of Reproduction. 2004;**70**:1545-1555

[89] Suess U, Lawrence J, Ko D, Lederis K. Radioimmunoassays for fish tail neuropeptides: I. Development of assay and measurement of immunoreactive urotensin I in Catostomus commersoni brain, pituitary, and plasma. Journal of Pharmacological Methods. 1986;**15**:335-346

[90] Backström T, Pettersson A, Johansson V, Winberg S. CRF and urotensin I effects on aggression and anxiety-like behavior in rainbow trout. The Journal of Experimental Biology. 2011;**214**:907-914

[91] Kulczykowska E. Solid-phase extraction of arginine vasotocin and isotocin in fish samples and subsequent gradient reversed-phase high-performance liquid chromatographic separation. Journal of Chromatography B. 1995;**673**:289-293

[92] Engler D, Pham T, Fullerton MJ, Ooi G, Funder JW, Clarke IJ. Studies of the secretion of corticotropin-releasing factor and arginine vasopressin into the hypophysial-portal circulation of the conscious sheep. I. Effect of an audiovisual stimulus and insulin-induced hypoglycemia. Neuroendocrinology. 1989;**49**:367-381

[93] Parker AJ, Hamlin GP, Coleman CJ, Fitzpatrick LA. Excess cortisol interferes with a principal mechanism of resistance to dehydration in *Bos indicus* steers. Journal of Animal Science. 2004;**82**:1037-1045

[94] Holmes MC, Antoni FA, Catt KJ, Aguilera G. Predominant release of vasopressin vs. corticotropin-releasing factor from the isolated median eminence after adrenalectomy. Neuroendocrinology. 1986;**43**:245-251

[95] de Goeij DC, Jezova D, Tilders FJ. Repeated stress enhances vasopressin synthesis in corticotropin-releasing factor neurons in the paraventricular nucleus. Brain Research 1992;**577**:165-168.

[96] Aguilera G. Regulation of pituitary ACTH secretion during chronic stress. Frontiers in Neuroendocrinology. 1994;**15**:321-350

[97] Chowdrey HS, Larsen PJ, Harbuz MS, Jessop DS, Aguilera G, Eckland DJ, Lightman SL. Evidence for arginine vasopressin as the primary activator of the HPA axis during adjuvant-induced arthritis. British Journal of Pharmacology. 1995;**16**:2417-2424

[98] Meaney MJ, Viau V, Aitken DH, Bhatnagar S. Glucocorticoid receptors in brain and pituitary of the lactating rat. Physiology & Behavior. 1989;**45**:209-212

[99] Modell S, Yassouridis A, Huber J, Holsboer E. Corticosteroid receptor function is decreased in depressed patients. Neuroendocrinology. 1997;**65**:216-222

[100] Cole SW, Mendoza SP, Capitanio JP. Social stress desensitizes lymphocytes to regulation by endogenous glucocorticoids: Insights from *in vivo* cell trafficking dynamics in rhesus macaques. Psychosomatic Medicine. 2009;**71**:591-597

[101] Wang XC, Burbach JP, Verhoef JC, De Wied D. Proteolytic conversion of arginine-vasotocin by synaptic membranes from rat and chicken brain. Brain Research. 1983;**275**:83-90

[102] Burbach JPH, Terwel D, Lebouille JL. Measurement and distribution of vasopressin-converting aminopeptidase activity in rat brain. Biochemical and Biophysical Research Communications. 1987;**144**:726-731

[103] Burbach JP, Schoots O, Hernando F. Biochemistry of vasopressin fragments. Progress in Brain Research. 1998;**119**:127-136

[104] Di S, Malcher-Lopes R, Halmos KC, Tasker JG. Nongenomic glucocorticoid inhibition via endocannabinoid release in the hypothalamus: A fast feedback mechanism. The Journal of Neuroscience. 2003;**23**:4850-4857

[105] Durlo FV, Castro M, Elias LL, Antunes-Rodrigues J. Interaction of prolactin, ANP-ergic, oxytocinergic and adrenal systems in response to extracellular volume expansion in rats. Experimental Physiology. 2004;**89**:541-548

[106] Bagosi Z, Csaba K, Telegdi G, Szabó G. The actions of the urocortins on the mediators of stress response. In: Világi I, editor. 13th Conference of the Hungarian Neuroscience Society. Lausanne: Frontiers Media; 2011. p. 145

[107] Arai M, Assil IQ, Abou-Samra AB. Characterization of three corticotrophin releasing factor receptors in catfish: A novel third receptor is predominantly expressed in pituitary and urophysis. Endocrinology. 2001;**142**:446-454

[108] Hauger RL, Dautzenberg FM, Flaccus A, Liepold T, Spiess J. Regulation of corticotropin-releasing factor receptor function in human Y-79 retinoblastoma cells: Rapid and reversible homologous desensitization but prolonged recovery. Journal of Neurochemistry. 1997;**68**:2308-2316

[109] Aguilera G, Nikodemova M, Wynn PC, Catt KJ. Corticotropin releasing hormone receptors: Two decades later. Peptides. 2004;**25**:319-329

[110] Hauger RL, Risbrough V, Brauns O, Dautzenberg FM. Corticotropin releasing factor (CRF) receptor signaling in the central nervous system: New molecular targets. CNS & Neurological Disorders Drug Targets. 2006;**5**:453-479

[111] Teli T, Markovic D, Levine MA, Hillhouse EW, Grammatopoulos DK. Regulation of corticotropin-releasing hormone receptor type 1α signaling: Structural determinants for G protein-coupled receptor kinase-mediated phosphorylation and agonist mediated desensitization. Molecular Endocrinology. 2008;**19**:474-490

[112] Saito D, Urano A. Synchronized periodic Ca^{2+} pulses define neurosecretory activities in magnocellular vasotocin and isotocin neurons. The Journal of Neuroscience. 2001;**21**:RC178

[113] Pearson D, Shively JE, Clark BR, Geschwind II, Barkley M, Nishioka RS, Bern HA. Urotensin II: A somatostatin-like peptide in the caudal neurosecretory system of fishes. Proceedings of the National Academy of Sciences of the United States of America.1980;**77**:5021-5024

[114] Sheridan MA, Plisetskaya EM, Bern HA, Gorbman A. Effects of somatostatin-25 and urotensin II on lipid and carbohydrate metabolism of coho salmon, *Oncorhynchus kisutch*. General and Comparative Endocrinology. 1987;**66**:405-414

[115] Lu W, Greenwood M, Dow L, Yuill J, Worthington J, Brierley MJ, McCrohan CR, Riccardi D, Balment RJ. Molecular characterization and expression of urotensin II and its receptor in the flounder (*Platichthys flesus*): A hormone system supporting body fluid homeostasis in euryhaline fish. Endocrinology. 2006;**147**:3692-3708

[116] Le Mével JC, Lancien F, Mimassi N, Leprince J, Conlon JM, Vaudry H. Central and peripheral cardiovascular, ventilatory, and motor effects of trout urotensin-II in the trout. Peptides. 2008;**29**:830-837

[117] Nobata S, Donald JA, Balment RJ, Takei Y. Potent cardiovascular effects of homologous urotensin II (UII)-related peptide and UII in unanesthetized eels after peripheral and central injections. American Journal of Physiology. Regulatory, Integrative and Comparative Physiology. 2011;**300**:R437-R446

[118] Singh R, Rai U. Immunomodulatory role of urotensins in teleost *Channa punctatus*. General and Comparative Endocrinology. 2011;**170**:613-621

[119] Bond H, Winter MJ, Warne JM, McCrohan CR, Balment RJ. Plasma concentrations of arginine vasotocin and urotensin II are reduced following transfer of the euryhaline flounder (*Platichthys flesus*) from seawater to fresh water. General and Comparative Endocrinology. 2002;**125**:113-120

[120] Hyodo S, Kato Y, Ono M, Urano A. Cloning and sequence analyses of cDNA encoding vasotocin and isotocin precursors of chum salmon, *Oncorhynchus keta*: Evolutionary relationships of neurohypophysial hormone precursors. Journal of Comparative Physiology. B. 1991;**160**:601-608

[121] Urano A, Kubokawa K, Hiraoka S. Expression of the vasotocin and isotocin gene family in fish. In: Sherwood NM, Hew CL, editors. Fish Physiology. New York: Academic Press; 1994. pp. 101-132

[122] Martos-Sitcha JA, Wunderink YS, Gozdowska M, Kulczykowska E, Mancera JM, Martínez-Rodríguez G. Vasotocinergic and isotocinergic systems in the gilthead sea bream (*Sparus aurata*): An osmoregulatory story. Comparative Biochemistry and Physiology. Part A, Molecular & Integrative Physiology. 2013;**166**:571-581

[123] Haruta K, Yamashita T, Kawashima S. Changes in arginine vasotocin content in the pituitary of the medaka (*Oryzias latipes*) during osmotic stress. General and Comparative Endocrinology. 1991;**83**:327-336

[124] Warne JM, Balment RJ. Effect of acute manipulation of blood volume and osmolality on plasma [AVT] in seawater flounder. The American Journal of Physiology. 1995;**269**:R1107-R1112

[125] Winter MJ, Hubbard PC, McCrohan CR, Balment RJ. A homologous radioimmunoassay for the measurement of urotensin II in the euryhaline flounder, *Platichthys flesus*. General and Comparative Endocrinology. 1999;**114**:249-256

[126] Yulis CR, Lederis KL. Extraurophyseal distribution of urotensin II immunoreactive neuronal perikarya and their processes. Proceedings of the National Academy of Sciences of the United States of America. 1986;**83**:7079-7083

[127] Yulis CR, Lederis KL. Occurrence of an anterior spinal, cerebrospinal fluid-contacting, urotensin II neuronal system in various fish species. General and Comparative Endocrinology. 1988;**70**:301-311

[128] Waugh D, Conlon JM. Purification and characterization of urotensin II from the brain of a teleost (trout, *Oncorhynchus mykiss*) and an elasmobranch (skate, *Raja rhina*). General and Comparative Endocrinology. 1993;**92**:419-427

[129] Waugh D, Youson J, Mims SD, Sower S, Conlon JM, Urotensin II. from the River lamprey (*Lampetra fluviatilis*), the Sea lamprey (*Petromyzon marinus*), and the Paddlefish (*Polyodon spathula*). General and Comparative Endocrinology. 1995;**99**:323-332

[130] Kalamarz-Kubiak H, Meiri-Ashkenazi I, Kleszczyńska A, Rosenfeld H. Urotensin II inhibits arginine vasotocin and stimulates isotocin release from nerve endings in the pituitary of gilthead sea bream (*Sparus aurata*). Journal of Experimental Zoology. Part A, Ecological Genetics and Physiology. 2014;**321**:467-471

[131] Kobayashi Y, Lederis K, Rivier J, Ko D, McMaster D, Poulin P. Radioimmunoassay for fish tail neuropeptides. II: Development of a specific and sensitive assay for and the occurrence of immunoreactive urotensin II in the central nervous system and blood of *Catostomus commersoni*. Journal of Pharmacological Methods. 1986;**15**:321-333

[132] Henderson IW, Wales NA. Renal diuresis and antidiuresis after injections of arginine vasotocin in the freshwater eel (*Anguilla anguilla* L.). The Journal of Endocrinology. 1974;**61**:487-500

[133] Babiker MM, Rankin JC. Neurohypophysial hormonal control of kidney function in the European eel (*Anguilla anguilla* L.) adapted to sea-water or fresh water. The Journal of Endocrinology. 1978;**76**:347-358

[134] Zhang AY, Chen YF, Zhang DX, Yi F-X, Qi J, Andrade-Gordonm P, de Garavilla L, Li P-L, Zou A-P. Urotensin II is a nitric oxide-dependent vasodilator and natriuretic peptide in the rat kidney. The American Journal of Physiology 2003;**285**:F792–F798.

[135] Abdel-Razik AES, Forty EJ, Balment RJ, Ashton N. Renal haemodynamic and tubular actions of urotensin II in the rat. The Journal of Endocrinology 2008;**198**:617-624.

[136] Proulx CD, Holleran BJ, Lavigne P, Escher E, Guillemette G, Leduc R. Biological properties and functional determinants of the urotensin II receptor. Peptides. 2008;**29**:691-699

[137] Batuwangala MS, Calo G, Guerrini R, Ng LL, McDonald J, Lambert DG. Desensitisation of native and recombinant human urotensin-II receptors. Naunyn-Schmiedeberg's Archives of Pharmacology. 2009;**380**:451-457

[138] Conlon JM, Tostivint H, Vaudry H. Somatostatin- and urotensin II-related peptides: Molecular diversity and evolutionary perspectives. Regulatory Peptides. 1997;**69**:95-103

[139] Meddle SL, Bull PM, Leng G, Russell JA, Ludwig M. Somatostatin actions on rat supraoptic nucleus oxytocin and vasopressin neurones. Journal of Neuroendocrinology. 2010;**22**:438-445

[140] Kulczykowska E. Response of circulating arginine vasotocin and isotocin to rapid osmotic challenge in rainbow trout. Comparative Biochemistry and Physiology Part A. 1997;**118**:772-778

[141] Takahashi H, Sakamoto T. The role of 'mineralocorticoids' in teleost fish: Relative importance of glucocorticoid signaling in the osmoregulation and 'central' actions of mineralocorticoid receptor. General and Comparative Endocrinology. 2013;**181**:223-228

[142] McCormick SD, Regish A, O'Dea MF, Shrimpton JM. Are we missing a mineralocorticoid in teleost fish? Effects of cortisol, deoxycorticosterone and aldosterone on osmoregulation, gill Na^+, K^+-ATPase activity and isoform mRNA levels in Atlantic salmon. General and Comparative Endocrinology. 2008;**157**:35-40

[143] Kiilerich P, Milla S, Sturm A, Valotaire C, Chevolleau S, Giton F, Terrien X, Fiet J, Fostier A, Debrauwer L, Prunet P. Implication of the mineralocorticoid axis in rainbow trout osmoregulation during salinity acclimation. The Journal of Endocrinology. 2011;**209**:221-235

[144] Aruna A, Nagarajan G, Chang CF. Differential expression patterns and localization of glucocorticoid and mineralocorticoid receptor transcripts in the osmoregulatory organs of tilapia during salinity stress. General and Comparative Endocrinology. 2012;**179**:465-476

[145] Consten D, Lambert JG, Komen H, Goos HJ. Corticosteroids affect the testicular androgen production in male common carp (*Cyprinus carpio* L.). Biology of Reproduction. 2002;**66**:106-111

[146] Milla S, Terrien X, Sturm A, Ibrahim F, Giton F, Fiet J, Prunet P, Le Gac F. Plasma 11 deoxycorticosterone (DOC) and mineralocorticoid receptor testicular expression during rainbow trout *Oncorhynchus mykiss* spermiation: Implication with 17alpha, 20beta dihydroxyprogesterone on the milt fluidity? Reproductive Biology and Endocrinology. 2008;**19**:6-19

[147] Overli O, Kotzian S, Winberg S. Effects of cortisol on aggression and locomotor activity in rainbow trout. Hormones and Behavior. 2002;**42**:53-61

[148] Di Battista JD, Anisman H, Whitehead M, Gilmour KM. The effects of cortisol administration on social status and brain monoaminergic activity in rainbow trout *Oncorhynchus mykiss*. The Journal of Experimental Biology. 2005;**208**:2707-2718

[149] Schjolden J, Basic D, Winberg S. Aggression in rainbow trout is inhibited by both MR and GR antagonists. Physiology & Behavior. 2009;**98**:625-630

[150] Aruna A, Nagarajan G, Chang CF. Involvement of corticotrophin-releasing hormone and corticosteroid receptors in the brain-pituitary-gill of tilapia during the course of seawater. Journal of Neuroendocrinology. 2012;**24**:818-830

[151] Teles M, Tridico R, Callol A, Fierro-Castro C, Tort L. Differential expression of the corticosteroid receptors GR1, GR2 and MR in rainbow trout organs with slow release cortisol implants. Comparative Biochemistry and Physiology Part A. 2013;**164**:506-511

[152] Sloman KA, Desforges PR, Gilmour KM. Evidence for a mineralocorticoid-like receptor linked to branchial chloride cell proliferation in freshwater rainbow trout. The Journal of Experimental Biology. 2001;**204**:3953-3961

[153] Dindia L, Faught E, Leonenko Z, Thomas R, Vijayan MM. Rapid cortisol signaling in response to acute stress involves changes in plasma membrane order in rainbow trout liver. American Journal of Physiology. Endocrinology and Metabolism. 2013;**304**:E1157

[154] Prunet P, Sturm A, Milla S. Multiple corticosteroid receptors in fish: From old ideas to new concepts. General and Comparative Endocrinology. 2006;**147**:17-23

[155] Falkenstein E, Tillmann HC, Christ M, Feuring M, Wehling M. Multiple actions of steroid hormones, a focus on rapid, nongenomic effects. Pharmacological Reviews. 2000;**52**:513-556

[156] Tasker JG, Di S, Malcher-Lopes R. Minireview: Rapid glucocorticoid signaling via membrane-associated receptors. Endocrinology. 2006;**147**:5549-5556

[157] Bartholome B, Spies CM, Gaber T, Schuchmann S, Berki T, Kunkel D, Bienert M, Radbruch A, Burmester GR, Lauster R, Scheffold A, Buttgereit F. Membrane glucocorticoid receptors [mGCR] are expressed in normal human peripheral blood mononuclear cells and up-regulated after in vitro stimulation and in patients with rheumatoid arthritis. The FASEB Journal 2004;**18**:70-80.

[158] Freshney RI. Culture of Animal Cells: A Manual of Basic Technique. 5th revised ed. Hoboken, NJ: JohnWiley & Son; 2005

[159] Schaeck M, Van den Broeck W, Hermans K, Decostere A. Fish as research tools: Alternatives to in vivo experiments. Alternatives to Laboratory Animals. 2013;**41**:219-229

[160] Kalamarz-Kubiak H, Gozdowska M, Nietrzeba M, Kulczykowska E. A novel approach to AVT and IT studies in fish brain and pituitary: In vitro perfusion technique. Journal of Neuroscience Methods. 2011;**199**:56-61

[161] Habibi HR, Marchant TA, Nahorniak CS, Van der Loo H, Peter RE, Rivier JE, Vale WW. Functional relationship between receptor binding and biological activity for analogs of mammalian and salmon gonadotropin-releasing hormones in the pituitary of goldfish (*Carassius auratus*). Biology of Reproduction. 1989;**40**:1152-1161

[162] Rotllant J, Balm PH, Ruane NM, Pérez-Sánchez J, Wendelaar-Bonga SE, Tort L. Pituitary proopiomelanocortin-derived peptides and hypothalamus-pituitary-interrenal axis activity in gilthead sea bream (*Sparus aurata*) during prolonged crowding stress: Differential regulation of adrenocorticotropin hormone and alpha-melanocyte-stimulating hormone release by corticotropin-releasing hormone and thyrotropin-releasing hormone. General and Comparative Endocrinology. 2000;**119**:152-163

[163] Moriyama S, Ito T, Takahashi A, Amano M, Sower SA, Hirano T, Yamamori K, Kawauchi HA. homolog of mammalian PRL-releasing peptide (fish arginyl-phenylalanyl-amide peptide) is a major hypothalamic peptide of PRL release in teleost fish. Endocrinology. 2002;**143**:2071-2079

[164] Metz JR, Huising MO, Meek J, Taverne-Thiele AJ, Wendelaar Bonga SE, Flik G. Localization, expression and control of adrenocorticotropic hormone in the nucleus preopticus and pituitary gland of common carp (*Cyprinus carpio* L.). The Journal of Endocrinology. 2004;**182**:23-31

[165] Weber GM, Seale AP, Richman IIINH, Stetson MH, Hirano T, Grau EG. Hormone release is tied to changes in cell size in the osmoreceptive prolactin cell of a euryhaline teleost fish, the tilapia, *Oreochromis mossambicus*. General and Comparative Endocrinology. 2004;**138**:8-13

[166] Falcón J, Marmillon JB, Claustrat B, Collin JP. Regulation of melatonin secretion in a photoreceptive pineal organ: An in vitro study in the pike. The Journal of Neuroscience. 1989;**9**:1943-1950

[167] Yáñez J, Meissl H. Secretion of the methoxyindoles melatonin, 5-methoxytryptophol, 5-methoxyindoleacetic acid, and 5-methoxytryptamine from trout pineal organs in superfusion culture: Effects of light intensity. General and Comparative Endocrinology. 1996;**101**:165-172

[168] Okimoto DK, Stetson MH. Presence of an intrapineal circadian oscillator in the teleostean family *Poeciliidae*. General and Comparative Endocrinology. 1999;**114**:304-312

[169] Minuth WW, Denk L, Glashauser AA. modular culture system for the generation of multiple specialized tissues. Biomaterials. 2010;**31**:2945-2954

[170] Gozdowska M, Kleszczyńska A, Sokołowska E, Kulczykowska E. Arginine vasotocin (AVT) and isotocin (IT) in fish brain: Diurnal and seasonal variations. Comparative Biochemistry and Physiology. B. 2006;**143**:330-334

[171] Bury NR, Sturm A. Evolution of the corticosteroid receptor signalling pathway in fish. General and Comparative Endocrinology. 2007;**153**:47-56

[172] Greenwood AK, Butler PC, White RB, et al. Multiple corticosteroid receptors in a teleost fish: Distinct sequences, expression patterns, and transcriptional activities. Endocrinology. 2003;**144**:4226-4236

[173] Teitsma CA, Anglade I, Toutirais G, Muñoz-Cueto J-A, Saligaut D, Ducouret B, Kah O. Immunohistochemical localization of glucocorticoid receptors in the forebrain of the rainbow trout (*Oncorhynchus mykiss*). The Journal of Comparative Neurology. 1998;**401**:395-410

[174] Pepels PP, Van Helvoort H, Wendelaar Bonga SE, Balm PH. Corticotropin-releasing hormone in the teleost stress response: Rapid appearance of the peptide in plasma of tilapia (*Oreochromis mossambicus*). The Journal of Endocrinology. 2004;**180**:425-438

[175] Stolte EH, de Mazon AF, Leon-Koosterziel KM, Jesiak M, Bury NR, Sturm A, Savelkoul HFJ, Lidy Verburg van Kemenade BM, Flik G. Corticosteroid receptors involved in stress regulation in common carp, *Cyprinus carpio*. The Journal of Endocrinology 2008;**198**:403-417

[176] Kalamarz-Kubiak H, Kleszczyńska A, Kulczykowska E. Cortisol stimulates arginine vasotocin and isotocin release from the hypothalamo-pituitary complex of round goby (*Neogobius melanostomus*): Probable mechanisms of action. Journal of Experimental Zoology. Part A, Ecological Genetics and Physiology. 2015;**323**:616-626

[177] Ros AF, Vullioud P, Bshary R. Treatment with the glucocorticoid antagonist RU486 reduces cooperative cleaning visits of a common reef fish, the lined bristletooth. Hormones and Behavior. 2012;**61**:37-43

[178] Sakamoto T, Mori C, Minami S, Takahashi H, Abe T, Ojima D, Ogoshi M, Sakamoto H. Corticosteroids stimulate the amphibious behavior in mudskipper: Potential role of mineralocorticoid receptors in teleost fish. Physiology & Behavior. 2011;**104**:923-928

[179] Sobell HM. Actinomycin and DNA transcription. Proceedings of the National Academy of Sciences of the United States of America. 1985;**82**:5328-5331

[180] Sunny F, Oommen OV. Rapid action of glucocorticoids on branchial ATPase activity in *Oreochromis mossambicus*: An in vivo and in vitro study. Comparative Biochemistry and Physiology. B. 2001;**130**:323-330

[181] Prevoo B, Miller DS, van de Water FM, Wever KE, Russel FGM, Flik G, Masereeuw R. Rapid, nongenomic stimulation of multidrug resistance protein 2 (Mrp2) activity by glucocorticoids in renal proximal tubule. The Journal of Pharmacology and Experimental Therapeutics. 2011;**338**:362-371

[182] Rotllant J, Balm PH, Pérez-Sánchez J, Wendelaar-Bonga SE, Tort L. Pituitary and interrenal function in gilthead sea bream (*Sparus aurata* L., Teleostei) after handling and confinement stress. General and Comparative Endocrinology. 2001;**121**:333-342

[183] Van der Salm AL, Martínez M, Flik G, Wendelaar Bonga SE. Effects of husbandry conditions on the skin colour and stress response of red porgy, *Pagrus pagrus*. Aquaculture. 2004;**241**:371-386

[184] Martínez-Porchas M, Martínez-Cordova LR, Ramos-Enriquez R. Cortisol and glucose: Reliable indicators of stress? Pan-American Journal of Aquatic Sciences. 2009;**4**:158-178

[185] Marentette JR, Tong S, Balshine S. The cortisol stress response in male round goby (*Neogobius melanostomus*): Effects of living in polluted environments? Environmental Biology of Fishes. 2013;**96**:723-733

[186] Aluru N, Vijayan MM. Hepatic transcriptome response to glucocorticoid receptor activation in rainbow trout. Physiological Genomics. 2007;**31**:483-491

[187] Sathiyaa R, Vijayan MM. Autoregulation of glucocorticoid receptor by cortisol in rainbow trout hepatocytes. American Journal of Physiology. Cell Physiology. 2003;**284**:C1508

[188] Mazon AF, Nolan DT, Lock RA, Fernandes MN, Wendelaar Bonga SE. A short-term in vitro gill culture system to study the effects of toxic (copper) and non-toxic (cortisol) stressors on the rainbow trout, *Oncorhynchus mykiss* (Walbaum). Toxicology In Vitro. 2004;**18**:691-701

[189] Kiilerich P, Kristiansen K, Madsen SS. Cortisol regulation of ion transporter mRNA in Atlantic salmon gill and the effect of salinity on the signaling pathway. The Journal of Endocrinology. 2007;**194**:417-427

[190] Shaw JR, Gabor K, Hand E, Lankowski A, Durant L, Thibodeau R, Stanton CR, Barnaby R, Coutermarsh B, Karlson KH, Sato JD, Hamilton JW, Stanton BA. Role of glucocorticoid receptor in acclimation of killifish (*Fundulus heteroclitus*) to seawater and effects of arsenic. American Journal of Physiology. Regulatory, Integrative and Comparative Physiology. 2007;**292**:R1052

[191] Liu X, Wang CA, Chen YZ. Nongenomic effect of glucocorticoid on the release of arginine vasopressin from hypothalamic slices in rats. Neuroendocrinology. 1995;**62**: 628-633

[192] Bury NR, Sturm A, Le Rouzic P, Lethimonier C, Ducouret B, Guiguen Y, Robinson-Rechavi M, Laudet V, Rafestin-Oblin ME, Prunet P. Evidence for two distinct functional glucocorticoid receptors in teleost fish. Journal of Molecular Endocrinology. 2003;**31**:141-156

[193] Kim MA, Kim DS, Sohn YC. Characterization of two functional glucocorticoid receptors in the marine medaka *Oryzias dancena*. General and Comparative Endocrinology. 2011;**171**:341-349

[194] Sapolsky RM, Romero LM, Munck AU. How do glucocorticoids influence stress responses? Integrating permissive, suppressive, stimulatory, and preparative actions. Endocrine Reviews. 2000;**21**:55-89

[195] Yeager MP, Pioli PA, Wardwell K, Beach ML, Martel P, Lee HK, Rassias AJ, Guyre PM. In vivo exposure to high or low cortisol has biphasic effects on inflammatory response pathways of human monocytes. Anesthesia & Analgesia. 2008;**107**:1726-1734

[196] Roy B, Rai U. Genomic and non-genomic effect of cortisol on phagocytosis in freshwater teleost *Channa punctatus*: An *in vitro* study. Steroids. 2009;**74**:449-455

[197] Johnstone 3rd WM, Mills KA, Alyea RA, Thomas P, Borski RJ. Characterization of membrane receptor binding activity for cortisol in the liver and kidney of the euryhaline teleost, Mozambique tilapia (*Oreochromis mossambicus*). General and Comparative Endocrinology 2013;**192**:107-114.

[198] Groeneweg FL, Karst H, de Kloet ER, Joëls M. Rapid non-genomic effects of corticosteroids and their role in the central stress response. The Journal of Endocrinology 2011;**209**:153-167

[199] Batten TF, Cambre ML, Moons L, Vandesande F. Comparative distribution of neuropeptide immunoreactive systems in the brain of the green molly, *Poecilia latipinna*. The Journal of Comparative Neurology. 1990;**302**:893-919

[200] Braithwaite V. Hooked on a myth [Internet]. Los Angeles Times. October 8, 2006. Available from: http://articles.latimes.com/2006/oct/08/opinion/oe-braithwaite8

5

Glucocorticoid-Mediated Regulation of Circadian Rhythms: Interface with Energy Homeostasis and Reproduction

Silvia Graciela Ruginsk, Ernane Torres Uchoa,
Cristiane Mota Leite, Clarissa Silva Martins,
Leonardo Domingues de Araujo,
Margaret de Castro, Lucila Leico Kagohara Elias and
José Antunes Rodrigues

Abstract

All living organisms have evolved by developing concomitant physiological and behavioral adaptations to environment. Through these processes, biological rhythms, such as reproduction, can be synchronized by environmental cues, which include not only the light/dark cycle itself but also the feeding pattern. These adaptations depend on two highly conserved and interrelated systems: an endogenous timing system and the hypothalamic-pituitary-adrenal (HPA) axis. In mammals, the biological circadian rhythms are controlled by a "master oscillator," the suprachiasmatic nucleus of the hypothalamus (SCN). Through neural signals to paraventricular nucleus of hypothalamus (PVN), the SCN also modulates the activation of the HPA axis, ultimately resulting in the circadian rhythm of glucocorticoid secretion by the adrenal cortex. Glucocorticoids, in turn, are well known for their important role in the regulation of energy homeostasis. Accordingly, obese animals exhibit increased glucocorticoid levels and are more susceptible to glucocorticoid-induced anabolic effects. In parallel, glucocorticoids modulate reproductive function and fertility: at physiological levels, glucocorticoids control the timing of puberty onset and gonadal steroidogenesis, as well modulate the immune system, which determines conception and pregnancy progression. However, stress-induced glucocorticoid secretion may exert a dual effect on reproductive function.

Keywords: glucocorticoids, hypothalamus, energy homeostasis, reproductive function, circadian rhythm

1. Introduction

Glucocorticoids are steroid hormones produced by the intermediate layer of the adrenal gland cortex (fasciculate zone) under the stimulation by the adrenocorticotropic hormone (ACTH), released from the anterior pituitary. ACTH secretion, in turn, is stimulated by corticotrophin-releasing hormone (CRH), produced by hypothalamic neurons and released into the portal pituitary capillary system. CRH, ACTH, and glucocorticoids (mainly cortisol in humans) integrate the hypothalamus-pituitary-adrenal (HPA) axis [1], whose activity influences a broad range of physiological functions such as metabolism, immune and inflammatory responses, as well as central nervous system activity [2].

The intracellular actions of glucocorticoids are mediated by the interaction with glucocorticoid (GR) and mineralocorticoid (MR) nuclear receptors, which hold great structural homology and are both ligand-driven transcription factors. In the cytoplasm of target cells, MRs and GRs exist at their unbound form; upon hormone binding, the receptor-ligand complex then translocates to the nucleus to modulate gene transcription [3]. It has been assumed that GR primarily mediates the reactive feedback during stressful episodes, whereas MR mediates the axis feedback during the nadir phase of the circadian rhythm [4].

MR and GR have also been identified in association with neuronal membranes [5], a signaling mechanism that is apparently shared by other steroid receptors [6]. Supporting this evidence, Evanson and coworkers [7] showed that stress-induced corticosterone secretion in rats is rapidly inhibited by the intrahypothalamic dexamethasone administration and that previous conjugation of dexamethasone to bovine serum albumin did not prevent dexamethasone-induced inhibition of ACTH release in stressed animals. Therefore, besides MR and GR being mostly known for their intracellular, delayed genomic role, these results make increasingly evident that these receptors can also mediate rapid, nongenomic signaling.

Indeed, transmembrane GRs seem to be upstream of a complex network controlling neuronal activity. It has been demonstrated that dexamethasone-induced activation of postsynaptic G-protein coupled receptors produces a rapid suppression of excitatory postsynaptic inputs in neurosecretory hypothalamic neurons [8, 9]. These effects were shown to be dependent upon the activation of nonconventional retrograde neurotransmission, mediated by the production of membrane-derived lipid mediators (endocannabinoids) and a gaseous modulator [nitric oxide (NO)]. These nongenomic glucocorticoid actions would accomplish, within the hypothalamus, for rapid, retrograde inhibition of glutamatergic (by endocannabinoids) and stimulation of GABAergic (by NO) signaling. Therefore, this simultaneous and rapid glucocorticoid-mediated and synapse-specific inhibition potentially impacts all the homeostatic responses initiated within hypothalamic nuclei in response to stress.

2. Glucocorticoids and the circadian rhythm

All living organisms have evolved by developing concomitant physiological and behavioral adaptations to environment. Through these processes, biological rhythms, such as reproduction, can be synchronized by environmental cues or "zeitgebers," which include not only the light/dark cycle itself but also the feeding pattern. These adaptations depend on two highly conserved and interrelated systems: an endogenous timing system and the HPA axis [10, 11].

The HPA axis circadian maturation may occur at early ages, influenced by prenatal and postnatal environmental synchronizers [12, 13]. In mammals, the biological circadian rhythms are controlled by a "master clock," the suprachiasmatic nucleus of the hypothalamus (SCN), which receives external information via the retinohypothalamic tract and synchronizes the "peripheral clocks," located in almost all organs and tissues [14].

The interaction between the circadian timing system and the HPA axis occurs at different signaling levels. Through neural signals to paraventricular nucleus of hypothalamus (PVN), the SCN also modulates the secretion of CRH, arginine vasopressin [(AVP), an ACTH secretagogue], and ACTH, ultimately resulting in the circadian rhythm of glucocorticoids secretion by the adrenal cortex [15]. The SCN also influences adrenal sensitivity to ACTH through the autonomic nervous system, in a second level of interaction [16].

The molecular machinery for the cell-autonomous circadian clock depends on transcriptional feedback loops. The two core clock proteins—CLOCK and BMAL1—form a heterodimer that activates the transcription of their target genes, *Period* (*Per*) and *Cryptochrome* (*Cry*). The proteins encoded by the genes *Pers* and *Crys* interact with the heterodimer CLOCK/BMAL1, inhibiting their own transcription. The genes *Rev-erbα* and *Rorα* also modulate this transcriptional loop, creating a repetitive and self-sustainable cycle of almost 24 h [17].

At transcriptional level, glucocorticoids synchronize central oscillators in some areas of the brain [18], influencing the expression of clock genes in response to a series of conditions. Glucocorticoids also modulate the circadian rhythm of peripheral oscillators [19–21], regulating the expression of clock genes through genomic actions mediated by activated GR [22]. *Per1* and *Per2* contain glucocorticoid-responsive elements (GREs), whereas *Rev-erbα* and *Rorα* are negatively regulated by glucocorticoids [23].

Additionally, the transcriptional activity of GR is reduced in response to acetylation of multiple lysine residues mediated by the CLOCK protein [24]. The CLOCK/BMAL1 heterodimer physically interacts with the ligand-binding domain (LBD) of the α-subunit of the glucocorticoid receptor (GRα) and represses the transcription of glucocorticoid-responsive genes [24, 25]. Furthermore, the posttranslational acetylation of GRα by CLOCK appears to repress the activation of genes targeted by GRα [25]. Taken together, these findings suggest that CLOCK/BMAL1 heterodimer behaves as a negative regulator of GRα in peripheral tissues, antagonizing the physiological actions of circulating glucocorticoids [24].

An interesting example of the complex interaction between the HPA axis and peripheral oscillators is provided by the modification of the daily dietary pattern, which is considered a powerful "zeitgeber" for the diurnal rhythm of glucocorticoid secretion [26, 27]. In rats, which are nocturnal animals, the change in dietary schedule to the light period results in the inversion of the circadian rhythm of the HPA axis, producing a corticosterone peak in the morning. This evidence reinforces the hypothesis that HPA axis activity is influenced not only by photic synchronizers such as the light/dark cycle but also by nonphotic clues, such as feeding episodes [28, 29].

Therefore, it is quite reasonable to assume that glucocorticoid signaling might somehow reset peripheral clocks in response to changes in feeding pattern [22]. However, larger phase shifts were observed in adrenalectomized (ADX) mice and rats submitted to daytime feeding, suggesting that glucocorticoids in fact inhibit rather than promote phase adjustments of peripheral oscillators to daytime feeding [20]. Based on this finding, it has been hypothesized that nutrient-sensing molecules, such as sirtuin-1 (SIRT1) and AMP-activated protein kinase (AMPK) may also act as clock-resetting signals in response to altered feeding time [30].

The literature clearly reveals feeding as a potent synchronizer of HPA axis activity in murines and the insight into this relationship for humans is not so clear. A study performed in male volunteers before and during Ramadan, the ninth month of the Muslim calendar, during which food intake is restricted to 9 p.m., showed that serum cortisol levels rose in the afternoon, whereas the morning cortisol rise was delayed, with a higher morning peak and a sharper decline, suggesting mealtime as a synchronizer also in humans [31]. A recent report reinforced this hypothesis, demonstrating profound changes in the diurnal expression of CLOCK in Ramadan practitioners [32]. On the other hand, obese women submitted to hypocaloric diet in different restricted feeding patterns demonstrated no significant changes in the circadian rhythm of cortisol secretion regardless the meal timing [33]. These conflicting results could be related to gender differences as well as the duration of feeding/restriction protocol, possibly indicating that a longer duration of altered feeding pattern could be also necessary to evoke those HPA axis changes.

Another line of evidence that has been recently revisited is the relative importance of environmental light (either natural or artificial) as one important "zeitgeber" for cortisol circadian rhythm in humans. Indeed, occasional or sustained (i.e., shift work, exposure to artificial light from electronic devices, etc.) alterations in the timing of the sleep-wake cycle or light exposure can lead to changes in circadian hormonal organization (including cortisol and melatonin secretion) and may contribute to negative health outcomes, such as obesity [34].

In summary, the endogenous timing system and the HPA axis modulate each other's activity through multilevel interactions, which ultimately coordinate homeostasis with the various environmental challenges. Therefore, uncoupling of these systems alters internal regulatory mechanisms and promotes pathologic changes in virtually all organs and tissues, especially those implicated in energy metabolism. Despite the significant progress that has been made during the past few years on the knowledge of molecular mechanisms underlying this multilevel communication, most of the physiologic and pathophysiologic aspects of this interplay remain to be elucidated.

3. Glucocorticoids and energy homeostasis

Energy homeostasis is basically defined as the balance between energy intake and expenditure, being regulated by central and peripheral factors. Feeding behavior is homeostatically controlled by peripheral factors (such as leptin and insulin, known as adiposity signals), as well as by gut-derived signals, classically known as satiety signals [35]. Leptin and insulin mediate the long-term control of energy homeostasis, by acting primarily in hypothalamic neurons that express orexigenic or anorexigenic neuropeptides [35]. Neuropeptide Y (NPY) and agouti-related protein (AgRP) in the arcuate nucleus of the hypothalamus (ARC), and orexins and melanin-concentrating hormone in the lateral hypothalamic area, constitute the classical hypothalamic orexigenic pathway. The hypothalamic anorexigenic circuit, in turn, includes proopiomelanocortin (POMC) and cocaine and amphetamine-regulated transcript (CART) in the ARC, and CRH and oxytocin (OT) in the PVN. On the other hand, brainstem areas, mainly the nucleus of the *tractus solitarii* (NTS), receive immediate information about the meal from satiety signals [mechanical and chemical stimulation of stomach and small intestine, as well as hormones released during a meal, as cholecystokinin (CCK)], and thus acutely regulate meal size [36].

Glucocorticoids appear as critical hormones regulating energy balance, given their participation in the metabolism of glucose, lipids, and proteins, as well as in the control of food intake and body weight gain and composition. As evidenced before, feeding also plays a key role as a rhythmicity synchronizer of the HPA axis [37], the amount of food ingested also being related to glucocorticoid secretion [38]. On a reciprocal way, increases in circulating glucocorticoids, in consequence to stress, therapeutic strategy, or Cushing's disease, lead to an enhancement in food intake and body weight gain, in addition to increased glucose production, decreased glucose transport and utilization, decreased protein synthesis, and increased muscular protein degradation [39, 40]. Long-term glucocorticoid treatment in intact rodents also induces the development of obesity, as well as other physiological hallmarks of metabolic syndrome, such as increased plasma leptin and insulin, increased plasma triglycerides, and impaired glucose tolerance [41, 42].

On the other hand, anorexia and body weight loss are typically found in response to chronic glucocorticoid deficiency, as observed in Addison's disease or primary adrenal insufficiency [43]. Similarly, removal of endogenous glucocorticoids by bilateral adrenalectomy (ADX) is a well-established experimental model to investigate the mechanisms underlying the hypophagic effect of human primary adrenal insufficiency [44–46]. An increased expression of the anorexigenic neuropeptides CRH and OT is indeed found in the PVN of ADX rats [45, 46], together with a reduction in the expression of the orexigenic neuropeptides NPY and AgRP in the ARC [47]. Surprisingly, ADX was shown to reduce the expression of POMC and CART in the ARC, suggesting that ADX-induced hypophagia may be somehow dissociated from the expression of these neuropeptides [48].

Interestingly, although serum cortisol levels are not clearly increased in human obesity, circulating corticosterone is enhanced in several murine obesity models, ADX being a very effective way to diminish hyperphagia and obesity under these experimental conditions [49, 50]. Reciprocally, obese animals seem to be more sensitive to the anabolic effects of glucocorticoids, evidenced by a higher response to CRH stimulation, as well as by enhanced basal and stimulated response to stress [51].

It is well established that glucocorticoids stimulate the drive to eat, and thus ADX-induced hypophagia involves, at least in part, a reduction on this stimulatory drive. However, glucocorticoids also seem to participate in the short-term control of food intake, since the anorexigenic effect of ADX is also associated with the increased activation of satiety-related responses in the brainstem, primarily implicated in the control of meal size [44, 45]. In this context, it has been already demonstrated that the hypothalamus and the brainstem are reciprocally interconnected, and OT axonal projections from the PVN to the NTS were also enhanced following ADX [52]. Furthermore, the intracerebroventricular administration of type 2 CRH receptor and OT receptor antagonists reversed ADX-induced hypophagia and the increased activation of NTS neurons induced by feeding [45, 46, 52]. Actually, OT neurons of the PVN may act as downstream mediators of CRH effects on the enhanced meal-induced satiety induced by ADX [53].

Glucocorticoids are also known for their dual effects on lipid metabolism, which vary from lipogenic to lipolytic. White adipose tissue can be found in different regions of the body: in visceral or central depots (omental and mesenteric), found within the abdominal cavity associated with digestive organs, and in subcutaneous depots, located under the skin. In response to excessive energy intake and limited energy expenditure, energy homeostasis is disturbed and subcutaneous adipose tissue is recruited by acting as a metabolic sink, where excess free fatty acids (FFAs) and glycerol are stored as triglycerides (TGs) in adipocytes. If the storage capacity of subcutaneous adipose tissue is exceeded or its ability to generate new adipocytes is impaired, lipid begins to accumulate in areas outside the subcutaneous tissue, originating as visceral adiposity [54].

Indeed, the net effect of glucocorticoids on lipid storage appears to depend on the physiologic context and the type of fat depot. Glucocorticoids increase lipolysis in mature adipocytes as a result of increased transcription and expression of the adipose triglyceride lipase (ATGL) and hormone-sensitive lipase (HSL). ATGL is predominantly responsible for the first step of the process [conversion of triacylglycerol (TAG) to diacylglycerol, with the consequent release of one FFA], whereas HSL converts diacylglycerol to monoacylglycerol [55]. The lipolytic actions of glucocorticoids occur primarily under fasting conditions, characterized by a low-ratio insulin/glucagon, possibly through a permissive role on growth hormone- and catecholamine-induced lipolysis [56].

On the other hand, the lipogenic action of glucocorticoids is composed of several steps, starting with increases in caloric and dietary lipid intake and followed by an increased storage of lipids in the adipose tissue. Glucocorticoids enhance both adipocyte hyperplasia (through increased differentiation of preadipocytes to mature adipocytes) and hypertrophy (through increased synthesis and storage of lipids) [57].

The glucocorticoid-mediated hypertrophic process is accomplished by the deposition of FFA and TAG, originated either from dietary intake (chylomicrons) or from liver secretion [very low-density lipoproteins (VLDL)] and by the parallel stimulation of lipoprotein lipase (LPL), which in turn hydrolyses circulating TAG and increases the amount of FFA available for ectopic lipid accumulation (liver, muscle, and visceral adipocytes) [58]. Interestingly, insulin seems to be crucial for some of these effects, since it potentiates glucocorticoid-induced effects on LPL. Furthermore, treatment with glucocorticoid decreases glucose uptake and metabolism in the absence of insulin [59].

Additionally, glucocorticoids were also demonstrated to increase the secretion of VLDL by the liver (increasing TAG plasma levels), as well as to enhance *de novo* lipid production in hepatocytes and adipocytes by stimulation of the key enzymes acetyl-CoA carboxylase (ACC) and fatty acid synthase (FAS) [55, 56, 58]. Furthermore, glucocorticoids stimulate the enzymatic routes for nicotinamide adenine dinucleotide phosphate (NADPH) generation, required for *de novo* lipogenesis [60].

Interestingly, these lipogenic effects of glucocorticoids are more effective in visceral than in subcutaneous tissue, since both LPL activity and the expression of GRs and MRs are greater in visceral compared to other adipose depots [61, 62]. In addition, elevated levels of type 1 11-beta-hydroxysteroid dehydrogenase (11b-HSD1), the enzyme that generates active glucocorticoid from inactive metabolites, are found in the adipose depots of obese subjects [63, 64]. Accordingly, higher activity of 11b-HSD1 within visceral *versus* subcutaneous adipose tissue suggests that this enzyme may be another target to mediate the site-specific actions of glucocorticoids in the adipose tissue [65]. Indeed, visceral adipose accumulation was observed in mice overexpressing 11b-HSD1, whereas inhibition of this enzyme improved metabolic parameters and reduced body weight in obese animals [66, 67]. Therefore, these results suggest that elevated 11b-HSD1 activity might be one of the causes rather than one of the consequences of visceral adiposity and obesity.

Furthermore, the glucocorticoid-induced increase in the circulating levels of TAG and FFA, besides producing dyslipidemia, is also known to restrict glucose utilization and leads to insulin resistance [68], resulting in other metabolic outcomes such as increased muscle proteolysis and hepatic gluconeogenesis. This impairment of insulin-stimulated glucose uptake in response to chronic exposure to increased levels of glucocorticoids may also be explained by decreased expression of insulin receptor or the insulin receptor substrate 1 (IRS1), with the consequent decrease in insulin binding, and decreased type 4 glucose transporter (GLUT4) translocation to cell membrane [56].

Therefore, it is suggested that the anabolic actions of glucocorticoids in lipid metabolism occur through their effects on the turnover and uptake of FFAs in adipose tissue. Considering that LPL and 11b-HSD1 activities, as well as GR and MR expressions, are higher in visceral fat than in any other adipose depot, glucocorticoids are likely to contribute to central adiposity. This would be also facilitated by an increased insulin/glucagon ratio, exhibited by individuals under positive energy balance and/or elevated glucocorticoid levels. In summary, glucocorticoids act though parallel prolipolytic, antilipolytic, and lipogenic mechanisms, with some of these mechanisms playing more important roles than the others depending on the physiological condition, targeted adipose tissue, and dose and duration of glucocorticoid exposure.

4. Glucocorticoids and reproductive function

In mammals, the capacity to reproduce is crucial to ensure the species perpetuation and is dependent on a functional hypothalamic-pituitary-gonadal (HPG) axis. In males, there is a regular and continuous pulsatile release of gonadotrophin-releasing hormone (GnRH) from hypothalamic neurons into the portal capillary system. In the anterior pituitary of both males and females, GnRH binds to its receptor in gonadotrophs, promoting the production and release of the gonadotrophin-luteinizing hormone (LH) and follicle-stimulating hormone (FSH). The systemically secreted gonadotrophins, in turn, act on ovaries and testis to stimulate hormone production and gametogenesis.

In males, the HPG axis is always under a negative feedback loop control. In females with spontaneous ovulation (such as rodents and women), however, the regulation of reproduction involves more complex mechanisms, including a cyclic and pulsatile GnRH secretion and the occurrence of preovulatory surges of gonadotrophins, which trigger ovulation.

During most of the cycle's duration, the female HPG axis is under the influence of the negative feedback mechanism exerted by low and moderate concentrations of estradiol, which inhibit the synthesis and release of GnRH and gonadotrophins. Just prior to ovulation, when a more acute estradiol peak takes place, together with a gradual increase in progesterone, the feedback loop changes from negative to positive, resulting in increased GnRH/LH synthesis and release.

The activity of GnRH neurons as well as of other HPG axis components is regulated by several factors, including the two newly discovered neuropeptides: kisspeptin and RF (Arg-Phe) amide-related peptide (RFRP). In rodents, kisspeptin neurons comprise two main hypothalamic populations: one located in the anteroventral periventricular (AVPV) nucleus of preoptic area (POA), whose function seems to be crucial for GnRH surge generation [69–71], and a second population localized in the ARC [69, 70].

Kisspeptin and RFRP exert opposing effects on GnRH secretion: the former stimulates GnRH release [69, 72], whereas RFRP inhibits it [73]. Kisspeptin binds to its cognate receptor KISS-1R, which is expressed, in a gender-independent manner [74, 75], in approximately 70% of GnRH neurons [74]. RFRP effects on GnRH secretion, in turn, seem to be mediated by a G protein-coupled receptor 147 (GPR147) (also known as NPFF1R). Studies have demonstrated that GPR147 is expressed in 15–33% of mice GnRH neurons, and also in kisspeptidergic neurons of the AVPV (5–16%) and ARC (25%) [76–78]. Furthermore, kisspeptin and RFRP neurons seem to mediate the ER-α-induced effects of estradiol on GnRH release [77, 79, 80]. Taken together, these data support the hypothesis that both kisspeptin and RFRP actively participate as neuroendocrine regulators of reproduction.

As discussed previously in this chapter, the master biological clock in mammals is located in the SCN and regulates the circadian rhythm of most biological functions. Evidence indicates that the SCN also integrates and synchronizes all the neuroendocrine events necessary for the activation of GnRH neurons, thereby controlling the onset of GnRH/LH preovulatory surge [81, 82]. The SCN neural outputs to GnRH neurons would involve two neuropeptides: AVP and vasoactive intestinal peptide (VIP). It has been reported that the VIPergic pathway directly modulates GnRH neurons [81, 83], whereas the circadian signaling of AVP to GnRH neurons would be indirectly mediated by AVPV kisspeptidergic neurons [84, 85]. Moreover, it has been recently suggested that the SCN, through VIPergic signaling, may suppress RFRP activity in the dorsomedial hypothalamus (DMH), allowing a full activation of the LH surge [86]. Therefore, the generation of GnRH/LH surges involves many neuroendocrine events that are dependent upon the positive feedback effects of estradiol (in females) and a circadian neural signal indirectly provided by the SCN [87].

Glucocorticoids are also among the central mechanisms controlling HPG axis function. It is quite clear that exposure to increased glucocorticoid levels, either induced by stress condition or by exogenous administration, may significantly interfere with reproductive function, with massive impacts on fertility [88–90].

In this regard, it has been demonstrated that glucocorticoids inhibit GnRH secretion [91]. In GT1 cells, which synthesize GnRH, glucocorticoids repress GnRH gene expression and hormone release [92]. Glucocorticoids also induce a decrease in gonadotropin synthesis and secretion; however, this effect may be at least partially mediated by the inhibition of GnRH neurons and their neural inputs to gonadotrophs, since GR expression in the anterior pituitary is still controversial [93-95]. Glucocorticoids also decrease GnRH responsiveness in gonadotrophs, a mechanism that apparently underlies glucocorticoid-mediated inhibition of LH secretion [96].

Recently, evidence has been provided on the role of kisspeptin and RFRP also in the mediation of glucocorticoids' actions on the HPG axis. Both kisspeptidergic [97] and RFRP neurons [98] express GR, suggesting that these neuronal populations are responsive to glucocorticoids. Accordingly, corticosterone decreases hypothalamic kisspeptin gene expression and neuronal activity during the estradiol-induced LH surge [99].

The RFRP system has also been implicated in glucocorticoid-mediated effects [98, 100, 101]. Both acute and chronic stress stimulate the RFRP system activation, evidenced by an increase in RFRP mRNA expression [98, 102], which, in turn, suppresses GnRH mRNA levels [102] and LH secretion [98]. Conversely, RFRP expression induced by both acute and chronic immobilization stress is abolished by ADX [98].

In the testis, GR is expressed in both Leydig and Sertoli cells [103, 104], reinforcing the modulation of steroidogenesis, testosterone release, and spermatogenesis by glucocorticoids. Indeed, at physiological levels, glucocorticoids are required for testis development in the postnatal period [105], for the onset and maintenance of spermatogenesis [104, 105], as well as for sperm maturation [104] and erectile function [106]. High circulating levels of glucocorticoids, however, have been associated with disruption of male fertility, with inhibition of testosterone secretion, spermatogenesis, and libido [107, 108]. Indeed, chronic stress was also shown to induce an important reduction in spermatid number in male rats [109]. The induction of Leydig cell and germ cell apoptosis has also been reported in response to high glucocorticoid circulating levels [110]. Another hypothesis is that the LH receptor may be downregulated in Leydig cells in response to stress, thus suppressing testicular response to gonadotropins [111]. There is also evidence showing that glucocorticoids may induce the inhibition of enzymatic machinery required for testosterone biosynthesis [112–114].

In the ovaries, glucocorticoids can modulate the functions of granulosa, cumulus, and luteal cells [99], reducing ovarian response to gonadotropins through the inhibition of LH-induced steroidogenesis [115]. Similar results were obtained in response to dexamethasone in cultured rat preovulatory follicles [116]. Although glucocorticoids seem to impair oocyte development *in vitro* by increasing apoptosis [117], no alterations in oocyte maturation have been reported in response to high circulating levels of glucocorticoids *in vivo* [118]. However, the same study highlighted a decreased blastocyst formation, suggesting that glucocorticoids may alter the oocyte potential for fertilization rather than oocyte maturation.

5. Concluding remarks

Glucocorticoids exert diverse actions throughout the body and remarkably participate in the maintenance of homeostasis. Their importance for energy homeostasis may be illustrated by the fact that obese animals exhibit increased glucocorticoid levels and are more susceptible to glucocorticoid-induced anabolic effects, such as the increase in visceral fat depots. Increased glucocorticoid levels also directly impact food intake, which is consistent with the experimental evidence that the bilateral removal of adrenal glands (ADX) produces hypophagia and also improves other metabolic parameters in obesity models. At physiological levels, glucocorticoids also seem to be crucial for reproductive function, controlling the timing of puberty onset and gonadal steroidogenesis, as well modulating the immune system, which determines conception and pregnancy progression. This broad range of actions is coordinated by the circadian variation of glucocorticoid secretion and is accomplished by both neural interconnections at SCN level and also by the peripheral clocks, which adapt the central oscillator timing to individual organ requirements. This is particularly important for the essential hormone variation in female reproductive cycle. In the case of energy homeostasis, this circadian variation also receives important feed forward information from food intake, one of the most potent synchronizers of the HPA axis activity. Under a broader point of view, the actions mediated by glucocorticoids may permit environmental clues, such as food availability, or stressors, to match internal metabolic priorities, which determine not only individual but also the species survival.

Conflict of interest

All the authors state that they have no conflict of interest to declare.

Abbreviations

ACC	acetyl-CoA carboxylase
ACTH	adrenocorticotropic hormone
ADX	adrenalectomized
AgRP	agouti-related protein
AMPK	adenosine monophosphate-activated protein kinase
ARC	arcuate nucleus of the hypothalamus
ATGL	adipose triglyceride lipase
AVP	arginine vasopressin
AVPV	anteroventral periventricular nucleus

CART	cocaine and amphetamine-regulated transcript
CCK	cholecystokinin
CRH	corticotrophin-releasing hormone
CRHr2	type 2 corticotrophin releasing hormone receptor
DMH	dorsomedial hypothalamus
FAS	fatty acid synthase
FFA	free fatty acids
FSH	follicle-stimulating hormone
GABA	gamma-aminobutyric acid
GLUT4	type 4 glucose transporter
GnRH	gonadotrophin-releasing hormone
GR	glucocorticoid receptor
GRE	glucocorticoid-responsive element
GRα	α-subunit of the glucocorticoid receptor
HPA	hypothalamus-pituitary-adrenal
HPG	hypothalamic-pituitary-gonadal
HSL	hormone-sensitive lipase
IRS1	insulin receptor substrate 1
KISS-1R	type 1 kisspeptin receptor
LH	luteinizing hormone
LPL	lipoprotein lipase
MR	mineralocorticoid receptor
NADPH	nicotinamide adenine dinucleotide phosphate
NO	nitric oxide
NPY	neuropeptide Y
NTS	nucleus of the solitary tract
OT	oxytocin
OTr	oxytocin receptor

POA	preoptic area
POMC	proopiomelanocortin
PVN	paraventricular nucleus of hypothalamus
RFRP	RF (Arg-Phe) amide-related peptide
SCN	suprachiasmatic nucleus of the hypothalamus
SIRT1	sirtuin-1
TAG	triacylglycerol
TG	triglyceride
VIP	vasoactive intestinal peptide
VLDL	very low-density lipoproteins

Author details

Silvia Graciela Ruginsk[1]*, Ernane Torres Uchoa[2], Cristiane Mota Leite[3], Clarissa Silva Martins[4,5], Leonardo Domingues de Araujo[6], Margaret de Castro[5], Lucila Leico Kagohara Elias[6] and José Antunes Rodrigues[6]

*Address all correspondence to: sgrleitao@hotmail.com

1 Department of Physiology, Biomedical Sciences Institute, Federal University of Alfenas, Minas Gerais, Brazil

2 Department of Physiological Sciences, State University of Londrina, Parana, Brazil

3 University of North of Parana, Parana, Brazil

4 Federal University of Mato Grosso do Sul, Mato Grosso do Sul, Brazil

5 Department of Internal Medicine, Ribeirao Preto Medical School, University of Sao Paulo, Sao Paulo, Brazil

6 Department of Physiology, Ribeirao Preto Medical School, University of Sao Paulo, Sao Paulo, Brazil

References

[1] Papadimitriou A, Priftis KN. Regulation of the hypothalamic-pituitary-adrenal axis. Neuroimmunomodulation. 2009;**16**(5):265-271. DOI: 10.1159/000216184

[2] Chrousos GP, Charmandari E, Kino T. Glucocorticoid action networks—An introduction to systems biology. The Journal of Clinical Endocrinology and Metabolism. 2004;**89**(2):563-564. DOI: 10.1210/jc.2003-032026

[3] Beato M, Sánchez-Pacheco A. Interaction of steroid hormone receptors with the transcription initiation complex. Endocrine Reviews. 1996;**17**(6):587-609. DOI: 10.1210/edrv-17-6-587

[4] Uchoa ET, Aguilera G, Herman JP, Fiedler JL, Deak T, de Sousa MB. Novel aspects of glucocorticoid actions. Journal of Neuroendocrinology. 2014;**26**(9):557-572. DOI: 10.1111/jne.12157

[5] Groeneweg FL, Karst H, de Kloet ER, Joëls M. Mineralocorticoid and glucocorticoid receptors at the neuronal membrane, regulators of nongenomic corticosteroid signalling. Molecular and Cellular Endocrinology. 2012;**350**(2):299-309. DOI: 10.1016/j.mce.2011.06.020

[6] Srivastava DP, Evans PD. G-protein oestrogen receptor 1: Trials and tribulations of a membrane oestrogen receptor. Journal of Neuroendocrinology. 2013;**25**(11):1219-1230. DOI: 10.1111/jne.12071

[7] Evanson NK, Tasker JG, Hill MN, Hillard CJ, Herman JP. Fast feedback inhibition of the HPA axis by glucocorticoids is mediated by endocannabinoid signaling. Endocrinology. 2010;**151**(10):4811-4819. DOI: 10.1210/en.2010-0285

[8] Di S, Maxson MM, Franco A, Tasker JG. Glucocorticoids regulate glutamate and GABA synapse-specific retrograde transmission via divergent nongenomic signaling pathways. The Journal of Neuroscience. 2009;**29**(2):393-401. DOI: 10.1523/JNEUROSCI.4546-08.2009

[9] Nahar J, Haam J, Chen C, Jiang Z, Glatzer NR, Muglia LJ, Dohanich GP, Herman JP, Tasker JG. Rapid nongenomic glucocorticoid actions in male mouse hypothalamic neuroendocrine cells are dependent on the nuclear glucocorticoid receptor. Endocrinology. 2015;**156**(8):2831-2842. DOI: 10.1210/en.2015-1273

[10] Nader N, Chrousos GP, Kino T. Interactions of the circadian CLOCK system and the HPA axis. Trends in Endocrinology and Metabolism. 2010;**21**(5):277-286. DOI: 10.1016/j.tem.2009.12.011

[11] Nicolaides NC, Charmandari E, Chrousos GP, Kino T. Circadian endocrine rhythms: The hypothalamic-pituitary-adrenal axis and its actions. Annals of the New York Academy of Sciences. 2014;**1318**:71-80. DOI: 10.1111/nyas.12464

[12] Custodio RJ, Junior CE, Milani SL, Simões AL, de Castro M, Moreira AC. The emergence of the cortisol circadian rhythm in monozygotic and dizygotic twin infants: The twin-pair synchrony. Clinical Endocrinology. 2007;**66**(2):192-197. DOI: 10.1111/j.1365-2265.2006.02706.x

[13] Roa SLR, Martinez EZ, Martins CS, Antonini SR, de Castro M, Moreira AC. Postnatal ontogeny of the circadian expression of the adrenal clock genes and corticosterone rhythm in male rats. Endocrinology. 2017;**158**(5):1339-1346. DOI: 10.1210/en.2016-1782

[14] Reppert SM, Weaver DR. Molecular analysis of mammalian circadian rhythms. Annual Review of Physiology. 2001;**63**:647-676. DOI: 10.1146/annurev.physiol.63.1.647

[15] Kalsbeek A, Palm IF, La Fleur SE, Scheer FA, Perreau-Lenz S, Ruiter M, Kreier F, Cailotto C, Buijs RM. SCN outputs and the hypothalamic balance of life. Journal of Biological Rhythms. 2006;**21**(6):458-469. DOI: 10.1177/0748730406293854

[16] Ulrich-Lai YM, Arnhold MM, Engeland WC. Adrenal splanchnic innervations contributes to the diurnal rhythm of plasma corticosterone in rats by modulating adrenal sensitivity to ACTH. American Journal of Physiology. Regulatory, Integrative and Comparative Physiology. 2006;**290**(4):R1128-R1135. DOI: 10.1152/ajpregu.00042.2003

[17] Green Green CB, Takahashi JS, Bass J. The meter of metabolism. Cell. 2008;**134**(5):728-742. DOI: 10.1016/j.cell.2008.08.022

[18] Segall LA, Perrin JS, Walker CD, Stewart J, Amir S. Glucocorticoid rhythms control the rhythm of expression of the clock protein, Period2, in oval nucleus of the bed nucleus of the stria terminalis and central nucleus of the amygdala in rats. Neuroscience. 2006;**140**(3):753-757. DOI: 10.1016/j.neuroscience.2006.03.037

[19] Oishi K, Amagai N, Shirai H, Kadota K, Ohkura N, Ishida N. Genome-wide expression analysis reveals 100 adrenal gland-dependent circadian genes in the mouse liver. DNA Research. 2005;**12**(3):191-202. DOI: 10.1093/dnares/dsi003

[20] Le Minh N, Damiola F, Tronche F, Schütz G, Schibler U. Glucocorticoid hormones inhibit food-induced phase-shifting of peripheral circadian oscillators. The EMBO Journal. 2001;**20**(24):7128-7136. DOI: 10.1093/emboj/20.24.7128

[21] Kino T, Chrousos GP. Circadian CLOCK-mediated regulation of target-tissue sensitivity to glucocorticoids: Implications for cardiometabolic diseases. Endocrine Development. 2011;**20**:116-126. DOI: 10.1159/000321232

[22] Balsalobre A, Brown SA, Marcacci L, Tronche F, Kellendonk C, Reichardt HM, Schütz G, Schibler U. Resetting of circadian time in peripheral tissues by glucocorticoid signaling. Science. 2000;**289**(5488):2344-2347. DOI: 10.1126/science.289.5488.2344

[23] Surjit M, Ganti KP, Mukherji A, Ye T, Hua G, Metzger D, Li M, Chambon P. Widespread negative response elements mediate direct repression by agonist-liganded glucocorticoid receptor. Cell. 2011;**145**(2):224-241. DOI: 10.1016/j.cell.2011.03.027

[24] Nader N, Chrousos GP, Kino T. Circadian rhythm transcription factor CLOCK regulates the transcriptional activity of the glucocorticoid receptor by acetylating its hinge region lysine cluster: Potential physiological implications. The FASEB Journal. 2009;**23**(5):1572-1583. DOI: 10.1096/fj.08-117697

[25] Doi M, Hirayama J, Sassone-Corsi P. Circadian regulator CLOCK is a histone acetyltransferase. Cell. 2006;**125**(3):497-508. DOI: 10.1016/j.cell.2006.03.033

[26] Krieger DT. Food and water restriction shifts corticosterone, temperature, activity and brain amine periodicity. Endocrinology. 1974;**95**(5):1195-1201. DOI: 10.1210/endo-95-5-1195

[27] Leal AM, Moreira AC. Feeding and the diurnal variation of the hypothalamic-pituitary-adrenal axis and its responses to CRH and ACTH in rats. Neuroendocrinology. 1996;**64**(1):14-19. DOI: 10.1159/000127092

[28] Girotti M, Weinberg MS, Spencer RL. Differential responses of hypothalamus-pituitary-adrenal axis immediate early genes to corticosterone and circadian drive. Endocrinology. 2007;**148**(5):2542-2552. DOI: 10.1210/en.2006-1304

[29] De Araujo LD, Roa SL, Bueno AC, Coeli-Lacchini FB, Martins CS, Uchoa ET, Antunes-Rodrigues J, Elias LL, Elias PC, Moreira AC, Castro M. Restricted feeding schedules modulate in a different manner the expression of clock genes in rat hypothalamic nuclei. Frontiers in Neuroscience. 2016;**10**:567. DOI: 10.3389/fnins.2016.00567

[30] Asher G, Schibler U. Crosstalk between components of circadian and metabolic cycles in mammals. Cell Metabolism. 2011;**13**(2):125-137. DOI: 10.1016/j.cmet.2011.01.006

[31] Bogdan A, Bouchareb B, Touitou Y. Ramadan fasting alters endocrine and neuroendocrine circadian patterns. Meal-time as a synchronizer in humans? Life Sciences. 2001; **68**(14):1607-1615. DOI: 10.1016/S0024-3205(01)00966-3

[32] Ajabnoor GM, Bahijri S, Shaik NA, Borai A, Alamoudi AA, Al-Aama JY, Chrousos GP. Ramadan fasting in Saudi Arabia is associated with altered expression of CLOCK, DUSP and IL-1alpha genes, as well as changes in cardiometabolic risk factors. PLoS One. 2017;**12**(4):e0174342. DOI: 10.1371/journal.pone.0174342

[33] Nonino-Borges CB, Borges RM, Bavaresco M, Suen VM, Moreira AC, Marchini JS. Influence of meal time on salivary circadian cortisol rhythms and weight loss in obese women. Nutrition. 2007;**23**(5):385-391. DOI: 10.1016/j.nut.2007.02.007

[34] Cipolla-Neto J, Amaral FG, Afeche SC, Tan DX, Reiter RJ. Melatonin, energy metabolism, and obesity: A review. Journal of Pineal Research. 2014;**56**(4):371-381. DOI: 10.1111/jpi.12137

[35] Schwartz MW, Woods SC, Porte JRD, Seeley RJ, Baskin DG. Central nervous system control of food intake. Nature. 2000;**404**(6778):661-671. DOI: 10.1038/35007534

[36] Havel PJ. Peripheral signals conveying metabolic information to the brain: Short-term and long-term regulation of food intake and energy homeostasis. Experimental Biology and Medicine. 2001;**226**(11):963-977. PMID: 11743131

[37] Leal AM, Moreira AC. Food and the circadian activity of the hypothalamic-pituitary-adrenal axis. Brazilian Journal of Medical and Biological Research. 1997;**30**(12):1391-1405. DOI: 10.1590/S0100-879X1997001200003

[38] Honma KI, Honma S, Hiroshige T. Critical role of food amount for prefeeding corticosterone peak in rats. The American Journal of Physiology. 1983;**245**(3):R339-R344. PMID: 6614204

[39] Tataranni PA, Larson DE, Snitker S, Young JB, Flatt JP, Ravussin E. Effects of glucocorticoids on energy metabolism and food intake in humans. The American Journal of Physiology. 1996;**271**(2 Pt 1):E317-E325. DOI: 10.1152/ajpendo.1996.271.2.E317

[40] Shibli-Rahhal A, Van Bee M, Schlechte JA. Cushing's syndrome. Clinics in Dermatology. 2006;**24**(4):260-265. DOI: 10.1016/j.clindermatol.2006.04.012

[41] Karatsoreos IN, Bhagat SM, Bowles NP, Weil ZM, Pfaff DW, McEwen BS. Endocrine and physiological changes in response to chronic corticosterone: A potential model of the metabolic syndrome in mouse. Endocrinology. 2010;**151**(5):2117-2127. DOI: 10.1210/en.2009-1436

[42] Cassano AE, White JR, Penraat KA, Wilson CD, Rasmussen S, Karatsoreos IN. Anatomic, hematologic, and biochemical features of C57BL/6NCrl mice maintained on chronic oral corticosterone. Comparative Medicine. 2012;**62**(5):348-360. PMID: 23114038

[43] Nieman LK, Chanco-Turner ML. Addison's disease. Clinics in Dermatology. 2006;**24**(4):276-280. DOI: 10.1016/j.clindermatol.2006.04.006

[44] Uchoa ET, Sabino HA, Ruginsk SG, Antunes-Rodrigues J, Elias LL. Hypophagia induced by glucocorticoid deficiency is associated with an increased activation of satiety-related responses. Journal of Applied Physiology. 2009;**106**(2):596-604. DOI: 10.1152/japplphysiol.90865.2008

[45] Uchoa ET, Silva LE, de Castro M, Antunes-Rodrigues J, Elias LL. Hypothalamic oxytocin neurons modulate hypophagic effect induced by adrenalectomy. Hormones and Behavior. 2009;**56**(5):532-538. DOI: 10.1016/j.yhbeh.2009.09.007

[46] Uchoa ET, Silva LE, de Castro M, Antunes-Rodrigues J, Elias LL. Corticotrophin-releasing factor mediates hypophagia after adrenalectomy, increasing meal-related satiety responses. Hormones and Behavior. 2010;**58**(5):714-719. DOI: 10.1016/j.yhbeh.2010.07.003

[47] Uchoa ET, Silva LE, de Castro M, Antunes-Rodrigues J, Elias LL. Glucocorticoids are required for meal-induced changes in the expression of hypothalamic neuropeptides. Neuropeptides. 2012;**46**(3):119-124. DOI: 10.1016/j.npep.2012.02.002

[48] Germano CM, Castro M, Rorato R, Laguna MT, Antunes-Rodrigues J, Elias CF, Elias LL. Time course effects of adrenalectomy and food intake on cocaine- and amphetamine-regulated transcript expression in the hypothalamus. Brain Research. 2007;**1166**:55-64. DOI: 10.1016/j.brainres.2007.05.077

[49] Bruce BK, King BM, Phelps GR, Veitia MC. Effects of adrenalectomy and corticosterone administration on hypothalamic obesity in rats. The American Journal of Physiology. 1982;**243**(2):E152-E157. DOI: 10.1152/ajpendo.1982.243.2.E152

[50] Yukimura Y, Bray GA, Wolfsen AR. Some effects of adrenalectomy in the fatty rat. Endocrinology. 1978;**103**(5):1924-1928. DOI: 10.1210/endo-103-5-1924

[51] McGinnis R, Walker J, Margules D. Genetically obese (ob/ob) mice are hypersensitive to glucocorticoid stimulation of feeding but dramatically resist glucocorticoid-induced weight loss. Life Sciences. 1987;**40**(16):1561-1570. DOI: 10.1016/0024-3205(87)90121-4

[52] Uchoa ET, Zahm DS, de Carvalho Borges B, Rorato R, Antunes-Rodrigues J, Elias LL. Oxytocin projections to the nucleus of the solitary tract contribute to the increased meal-related satiety responses in primary adrenal insufficiency. Experimental Physiology. 2013;**98**(10):1495-1504. DOI: 10.1113/expphysiol.2013.073726

[53] Uchoa ET, Rorato R, Ruginsk SG, Borges Bde C, Antunes-Rodrigues J, Elias LL. Corticotrophin-releasing factor receptor 2 mediates the enhanced activation of satiety-related responses through oxytocin neurons in the paraventricular nucleus of the hypothalamus after adrenalectomy. Neuroscience Letters. 2015;**606**:123-128. DOI: 10.1016/j.neulet.2015.08.045

[54] Ibrahim MM. Subcutaneous and visceral adipose tissue: Structural and functional differences. Obesity Reviews. 2010;**11**(1):11-18. DOI: 10.1111/j.1467-789X.2009.00623.x

[55] Peckett AJ, Wright DC, Riddell MC. The effects of glucocorticoids on adipose tissue lipid metabolism. Metabolism. 2011;**60**(11):1500-1510. DOI: 10.1016/j.metabol.2011.06.012

[56] Lee MJ, Pramyothin P, Karastergiou K, Fried SK. Deconstructing the roles of glucocorticoids in adipose tissue biology and the development of central obesity. Biochimica et Biophysica Acta. 2014;**1842**(3):473-481. DOI: 10.1016/j.bbadis.2013.05.029

[57] Galitzky J, Bouloumié A. Human visceral-fat-specific glucocorticoid tuning of adipogenesis. Cell Metabolism. 2013;**18**(1):3-5. DOI: 10.1016/j.cmet.2013.06.008

[58] Spencer SJ, Tilbrook A. The glucocorticoid contribution to obesity. Stress. 2011;**4**(3):233-246. DOI: 10.3109/10253890.2010.534831

[59] Ashby P, Robinson DS. Effects of insulin, glucocorticoids and adrenaline on the activity of rat adipose-tissue lipoprotein lipids. The Biochemical Journal. 1980;**188**(1):185-192. DOI: 10.1042/bj1880185

[60] Vienberg SG, Björnholm M. Chronic glucocorticoid treatment increases de novo lipogenesis in visceral adipose tissue. Acta Physiologica (Oxford, England). 2014;**211**(2):257-259. DOI: 10.1111/apha.12283

[61] Wajchenberg BL, Giannella-Neto D, da Silva ME, Santos RF. Depot-specific hormonal characteristics of subcutaneous and visceral adipose tissue and their relation to the metabolic syndrome. Hormone and Metabolic Research. 2002;**34**(11-12):616-621. DOI: 10.1055/s-2002-38256

[62] Rebuffé-Scrive M, Brönnegard M, Nilsson A, Eldh J, Gustafsson JA, Björntorp P. Steroid hormone receptors in human adipose tissues. The Journal of Clinical Endocrinology and Metabolism. 1990;**71**(5):1215-1219. DOI: 10.1210/jcem-71-5-1215

[63] Desbriere R, Vuaroqueaux V, Achard V, Boullu-Ciocca S, Labuhn M, Dutour A, Grino M. 11beta-hydroxysteroid dehydrogenase type 1 mRNA is increased in both visceral and subcutaneous adipose tissue of obese patients. Obesity (Silver Spring). 2006;**14**(5):794-798. DOI: 10.1038/oby.2006.92

[64] Rask E, Walker BR, Söderberg S, Livingstone DE, Eliasson M, Johnson O, Andrew R, Olsson T. Tissue-specific changes in peripheral cortisol metabolism in obese women: Increased adipose 11beta-hydroxysteroid dehydrogenase type 1 activity. The Journal of Clinical Endocrinology and Metabolism. 2002;**87**(7):3330-3336. DOI: 10.1210/jcem.87.7.8661

[65] Veilleux A, Rhéaume C, Daris M, Luu-The V, Tchernof A. Omental adipose tissue type 1 11 beta-hydroxysteroid dehydrogenase oxoreductase activity, body fat distribution, and metabolic alterations in women. The Journal of Clinical Endocrinology and Metabolism. 2009;**94**(9):3550-3557. DOI: 10.1210/jc.2008-2011

[66] Masuzaki H, Paterson J, Shinyama H, Morton NM, Mullins JJ, Seckl JR, Flier JS. A transgenic model of visceral obesity and the metabolic syndrome. Science. 2001;**294**(5549): 2166-2170. DOI: 10.1126/science.1066285

[67] Tiwari A. INCB-13739, an 11beta-hydroxysteroid dehydrogenase type 1 inhibitor for the treatment of type 2 diabetes. IDrugs: The Investigational Drugs Journal. 2010;**13**(4): 266-275 20373256

[68] Arner P. Insulin resistance in type 2 diabetes: Role of fatty acids. Diabetes/Metabolism Research and Reviews. 2002;**18**(Suppl.2):S5-9, 2002. DOI: 10.1002/dmrr.254

[69] Clarkson J, d'Anglemont de Tassigny X, Moreno AS, Colledge WH, Herbison AE. Kisspeptin-GPR54 signaling is essential for preovulatory gonadotropin-releasing hormone neuron activation and the luteinizing hormone surge. The Journal of Neuroscience. 2008;**28**(35):8691-8697. DOI: 10.1523/JNEUROSCI.1775-08.2008

[70] Smith JT, Cunningham MJ, Rissman EF, Clifton DK, Steiner RA. Regulation of Kiss1 gene expression in the brain of the female mouse. Endocrinology. 2005;**146**:3686-3692. DOI: 10.1210/en.2005-0488

[71] Smith JT, Clifton DK, Steiner RA. Regulation of the neuroendocrine reproductive axis by kisspeptin-GPR54 signaling. Reproduction. 2006;**131**(4):623-630. DOI: 10.1530/rep.1.00368

[72] Piet R, de Croft S, Liu X, Herbison AE. Electrical properties of kisspeptin neurons and their regulation of GnRH neurons. Frontiers in Neuroendocrinology. 2015;**36**:15-27. DOI: 10.1016/j.yfrne.2014.05.006

[73] Pineda R, Garcia-Galiano D, Sanchez-Garrido MA, et al. Characterization of the inhibitory roles of RFRP3, the mammalian ortholog of GnIH, in the control of gonadotropin secretion in the rat: In vivo and in vitro studies. American Journal of Physiology. Endocrinology and Metabolism. 2010;**299**(1):E39-E46. DOI: 10.1152/ajpendo.00108.2010

[74] Messager S, Chatzidaki EE, Ma D, et al. Kisspeptin directly stimulates gonadotropin releasing hormone release via G protein-coupled receptor 54. Proceedings of the National Academy of Sciences of the United States of America. 2005;**102**(5):1761-1766. DOI: 10.1073/pnas.0409330102

[75] Herbison AE, Xd d T, Doran J, Colledge WH. Distribution and postnatal development of Gpr54 gene expression in mouse brain and gonadotropin-releasing hormone neurons. Endocrinology. 2010;**151**(1):312-321. DOI: 10.1210/en.2009-0552

[76] Rizwan MZ, Poling MC, Corr M, Cornes PA, Augustine RA, Quennell JH, Kauffman AS, Anderson GM. RFamide-related peptide-3 receptor gene expression in GnRH

and kisspeptin neurons and GnRH-dependent mechanism of action. Endocrinology. 2012;**153**:3770-3779. DOI: 10.1210/en.2012-1133

[77] Poling MC, Kim J, Dhamija S, Kauffman AS. Development, sex steroid regulation, and phenotypic characterization of RFamide-related peptide (Rfrp) gene expression and RFamide receptors in the mouse hypothalamus. Endocrinology. 2012;**153**:1827-1840. DOI: 10.1210/en.2011-2049

[78] Poling MC, Quennell JH, Anderson GM, Kauffman AS. Kisspeptin neurons do not directly signal to RFRP-3 neurones but RFRP-3 may directly modulate a subset of hypothalamic kisspeptin cells in mice. Journal of Neuroendocrinology. 2013;**25**:876-886. DOI: 10.1111/jne.12084

[79] Dubois SL, Acosta-Martínez M, DeJoseph MR, Wolfe A, Radovick S, Boehm U, et al. Positive, but not negative feedback actions of estradiol in adult female mice require estrogen receptor α in kisspeptin neurons. Endocrinology. 2015;**156**:1111-1120. DOI: 10.1210/en.2014-1851

[80] Molnar CS, Kallo I, Liposits Z, Hrabovszky E. Estradiol down-regulates RFamide-related peptide (RFRP) expression in the mouse hypothalamus. Endocrinology. 2011;**152**: 1684-1690. DOI: 10.1210/en.2010-1418

[81] Van der Beek EM, Horvath TL, Wiegant VM, Van den Hurk R, Buijs RM. Evidence for a direct neuronal pathway from the suprachiasmatic nucleus to the gonadotropin-releasing hormone system: Combined tracing and light and electron microscopic immunocytochemical studies. The Journal of Comparative Neurology. 1997;**384**(4):569-579. PMID: 9259490

[82] Tsukahara S. Increased Fos immunoreactivity in suprachiasmatic nucleus before luteinizing hormone surge in estrogen-treated ovariectomized female rats. Neuroendocrinology. 2006;**83**(5-6):303-312. DOI: 10.1159/000095341

[83] Smith MJ, Jiennes L, Wise PM. Localization of the VIP2 receptor protein on GnRH neurons in the female rat. Endocrinology. 2000;**141**(11):4317-4320. DOI: 10.1210/endo.141.11.7876

[84] Vida B, Deli L, Hrabovszky E, Kalamatianos T, Caraty A, Coen CW, Liposits Z, Kalló I. Evidence for suprachiasmatic vasopressin neurones innervating kisspeptin neurones in the rostral periventricular area of the mouse brain: Regulation by oestrogen. Journal of Neuroendocrinology. 2010;**22**(9):1032-1039. DOI: 10.1111/j.1365-2826.2010.02045.x

[85] Williams WP 3rd, Jarjisian SG, Mikkelsen JD, Kriegsfeld LJ. Circadian control of kisspeptin and a gated GnRH response mediate the preovulatory luteinizing hormone surge. Endocrinology 2011; 152(2):595-606. DOI: 10.1210/en.2010-0943

[86] Russo KA, La JL, Stephens SB, Poling MC, Padgaonkar NA, Jennings KJ, Piekarski DJ, Kauffman AS, Kriegsfeld LJ. Circadian control of the female reproductive Axis

through gated responsiveness of the RFRP-3 system to VIP signaling. Endocrinology. 2015;**156**:2608-2618. DOI: 10.1210/en.2014-1762

[87] Beymer M, Henningsen J, Bahougne T, Simonneaux V. The role of kisspeptin and RFRP in the circadian control of female reproduction. Molecular and Cellular Endocrinology. 2016;**438**:89-99. DOI: 10.1016/j.mce.2016.06.026

[88] Whirledge S, Cidlowski JA. A role for glucocorti-coids in stress-impaired reproduction: Beyond the hypothalamus and pituitary. Endocrinology. 2013;**154**:4450-4468. DOI: 10.1210/en.2013-1652

[89] Breen KM, Mellon PL. Influence of stress-induced intermediates on gonadotropin gene expression in gonadotrope cells. Molecular and Cellular Endocrinology. 2014;**385**:71-77. DOI: 10.1016/j.mce.2013.08.014

[90] Geraghty AC, Kaufer D. Glucocorticoid regulation of reproduction. Advances in Experimental Medicine and Biology. 2015;**872**:253-278. DOI: 10.1007/978-1-4939-2895-8_11

[91] Kamel F, Kubajak CL. Modulation of gonadotropin secretion by corticosterone: Interaction with gonadal steroids and mechanism of action. Endocrinology. 1987;**121**:561-568. DOI: 10.1210/endo-121-2-561

[92] Attardi B, Tsujii T, Friedman R, Zeng Z, Roberts JL, Dellovade TL, Pfaff DW, Chandran UR, Sullivan MW, DB DF. Glucocorticoid repression of gonadotropin-releasing hormone gene expression and secretion in morphologically distinct subpopulations of GT1-7 cells. Molecular and Cellular Endocrinology. 1997;**131**:241-255. DOI: 10.1016/S0303-7207(97)00102-0

[93] Kononen J, Hokaneimi J, Gustafsson JA, Pelto-Huikko M. Glucocorticoid receptor colocalization with pituitary hormones in the rat pituitary gland. Molecular and Cellular Endocrinology. 1993;**93**:97-103. PMID: 8319836

[94] Breen KM, Karsch FJ. New insights regarding glucocorticoids, stress and gonadotropin suppression. Frontiers in Neuroendocrinology. 2006;**27**(2):233-245. DOI: 10.1016/j.yfrne.2006.03.335

[95] Breen KM, Thackray VG, Hsu T, Mak-McCully RA, Coss D, Mellon PL. Stress levels of glucocorticoids inhibit LHbeta-subunit gene expression in gonadotrope cells. Molecular Endocrinology. 2012;**26**:1716-1731. DOI: 10.1210/me.2011-1327

[96] Kotitschke A, Sadie-Van Gijsen H, Avenant C, Fernandes S, Hapgood JP. Genomic and nongenomic cross talk between the gonadotropin-releasing hormone receptor and glucocorticoid receptor signaling pathways. Molecular Endocrinology. 2009;**23**(11):1726-1745. DOI: 10.1210/me.2008-0462

[97] Takumi K, Iijima N, Higo S, Ozawa H. Immunohistochemical analysis of the colocalization of corticotropin-releasing hormone receptor and glucocorticoid receptor in kisspeptin neurons in the hypothalamus of female rats. Neuroscience Letters. 2012;**531**(1):40-45. DOI: 10.1016/j.neulet.2012.10.010

[98] Kirby ED, Geraghty AC, Ubuka T, Bentley GE, Kaufer D. Stress increases putative gonadotropin inhibitory hormone and decreases luteinizing hormone in male rats. Proceedings of the National Academy of Sciences of the United States of America. 2009;**106**(27):11324-11329. DOI: 10.1073/pnas.0901176106

[99] Luo E, Stephens SB, Chaing S, Munaganuru N, Kauffman AS, Breen KM. Corticosterone blocks ovarian cyclicity and the LH surge via decreased kisspeptin neuron activation in female mice. Endocrinology. 2016;**157**:1187-1199. DOI: 10.1210/en.2015-1711

[100] Calisi RM, Rizzo NO, Bentley GE. Seasonal differences in hypothalamic EGR-1 and GnIH expression following capture-handling stress in house sparrows (*Passer domesticus*). General and Comparative Endocrinology. 2008;**157**:283-287. DOI: 10.1016/j.ygcen.2008.05.010

[101] Kaewwongse M, Takayanagi Y, Onaka T. Effects of RFamide-related peptide (RFRP)-1 and RFRP-3 on oxytocin release and anxiety-related behaviour in rats. Journal of Neuroendocrinology. 2010;**23**:20-27. DOI: 10.1111/j.1365-2826.2010.02077.x

[102] Soga T, Dalpatadu SL, Wong DW, Parhar IS. Neonatal dexamethasone exposure down-regulates GnRH expression through the GnIH pathway in female mice. Neuroscience. 2012;**218**:56-64. DOI: 10.1016/j.neuroscience.2012.05.023

[103] Schultz R, Isola J, Parvinen M, Honkaniemi J, Wikström AC, Gustafsson JA, Pelto-Huikko M. Localization of the glucocorticoid receptor in testis and accessory sexual organs of male rat. Molecular and Cellular Endocrinology. 1993;**95**(1-2):115-120. DOI: 10.1016/0303-7207(93)90036-J

[104] Silva EJR, Queiróz DBC, Honda L, Avellar MCW. Glucocorticoid receptor in the rat epididymis: Expression, cellular distribution and regulation by steroid hormones. Molecular and Cellular Endocrinology. 2010;**325**(1-2):64-77. DOI: 10.1016/j.mce.2010.05.013

[105] Weber MA, Groos S, Höpfl U, Spielmann M, Aumüller G, Konrad L. Glucocorticoid receptor distribution in rat testis during postnatal development and effects of dexamethasone on immature peritubular cells in vitro. Andrologia. 2000;**32**(1):23-30. DOI: 10.1111/j.1439-0272.2000.tb02861.x

[106] Penson DF, Ng C, Rajfer J, Gonzalez-Cadavid NF. Adrenal control of erectile function and nitric oxide synthase in the rat penis. Endocrinology. 1997;**138**(9):3925-3932. DOI: 10.1210/endo.138.9.5402

[107] Cumming DC, Quigley ME, Yen SS. Acute suppression of circulating testosterone levels by cortisol in men. The Journal of Clinical Endocrinology and Metabolism. 1983; **57**(3):671-673. DOI: 10.1210/jcem-57-3-671

[108] Orr T, Mann DR. Role of glucocorticoids in the stress-induced suppression of testicular steroidogenesis in adult male rats. Hormones and Behavior. 1992;**26**(3):350-363. DOI: 10.1016/0018-506X(92)90005-G

[109] Almeida SA, Petenusci SO, Anselmo-Franci JA, Rosa-e-Silva AA, Lamano-Carvalho TL. Decreased spermatogenic and androgenic testicular functions in adult rats submitted to immobilization-induced stress from prepuberty. Brazilian Journal of Medical and Biological Research. 1998;**31**(11):1443-1448. DOI: 10.1590/S0100-879X1998001100013

[110] Yazawa H, Sasagawa I, Nakada T. Apoptosis of testicular germ cells induced by exogenous glucocorticoid in rats. Human Reproduction. 2000;**15**(9):1917-1920. DOI: 10.1093/humrep/15.9.1917

[111] Bambino TH, Hsueh AJ. Direct inhibitory effect of glucocorticoids upon testicular luteinizing hormone receptor and steroidogenesis in vivo and in vitro. Endocrinology. 1981;**108**(6):2142-2148. DOI: 10.1210/endo-108-6-2142

[112] Hales DB, Payne AH. Glucocorticoid-mediated repression of P450scc mRNA and de novo synthesis in cultured Leydig cells. Endocrinology. 1989;**124**(5):2099-2104. DOI: 10.1210/endo-124-5-2099

[113] Martin LJ, Tremblay JJ. Glucocorticoids antagonize cAMP-induced star transcription in Leydig cells through the orphan nuclear receptor NR4A1. Journal of Molecular Endocrinology. 2008;**41**(3):165-175. DOI: 10.1677/JME-07-0145

[114] Xiao YC, Huang YD, Hardy DO, Li XK, Ge RS. Glucocorticoid suppresses steroidogenesis in rat progenitor Leydig cells. Journal of Andrology. 2010;**31**(4):365-371. DOI: 10.2164/jandrol.109.009019

[115] Michael AE, Pester LA, Curtis P, Shaw RW, Edwards CR, Cooke BA. Direct inhibition of ovarian steroidogenesis by cortisol and the modulatory role of 11 beta-hydroxysteroid dehydrogenase. Clinical Endocrinology. 1993;**38**:641-644. DOI: 10.1111/j.1365-2265.1993.tb02147.x

[116] Huang TJ, Shirley Li P. Dexamethasone inhibits luteinizing hormone-induced synthesis of steroidogenic acute regulatory protein in cultured rat preovulatory follicles. Biology of Reproduction. 2001;**64**(1):163-170. DOI: 10.1095/biolreprod64.1.163

[117] Yuan HJ, Han X, He N, Wang GL, Gong S, Lin J, Gao M, Tan JH. Glucocorticoids impair oocyte developmental potential by triggering apoptosis of ovarian cells via activating the Fas system. Scientific Reports. 2016;**6**:24036. DOI: 10.1038/srep24036

[118] Liu YX, Cheng YN, Miao YL, Wei DL, Zhao LH, Luo MJ, Tan JH. Psychological stress on female mice diminishes the developmental potential of oocytes: A study using the predatory stress model. PLoS One. 2012;**7**(10):e48083. DOI: 10.1371/journal.pone.0048083

6

Twenty-First Century Glucocorticoid Receptor Molecular Biology

Cheng Wang, Roel Oldenkamp,
Ronald J.W. Oellers and Colin Logie

Abstract

Glucocorticoids are central to homeostasis as a function of the circadian cycle, temporally preceding circulating adrenaline concentration circadian fluctuations. Virtually, all cell types express the glucocorticoid receptor (GR). GR is a transcription factor that activates gene expression by binding to enhancers. Intriguingly, not all cell types respond to GR stimulation in the same fashion at the molecular level. This indicates that GR activity is subject to epigenetic control. We discuss the molecular basis for epigenetic control of GR action at the genomic level, including the concept of topologically associating domains which may restrain the roaming range of distal enhancers. Furthermore, much evidence indicates that GR can repress gene expression programs. We therefore discuss current concepts of the molecular basis of GR-mediated gene expression repression, including non-genomic mechanisms that involve mRNA destabilization.

Keywords: glucocorticoid receptor, glucocorticoid response element, chromosome conformation, epigenetics, non-genomic action, RNA decay

1. Introduction

Glucocorticoids (GCs) are steroids derived from cholesterol that are mainly produced in the adrenal cortex, under the control of the hypothalamic–pituitary–adrenal axis. Due to their lipophilic nature, GCs can traverse cellular membranes and thus enter any cell. Physiologically, GCs show circadian oscillations in man, peaking at 06:00 before we wake up and then dropping until 00:00, when their levels start to rise again. Adrenaline, a catecholamine that is produced by the adrenal medulla, follows this trend with a lag of about 2 hours [1]. Ontogenetically, GC levels increase during the final weeks of human gestation and in the post-natal period. This not only stimulates gluconeogenesis, but also perinatal lung maturation [2] and many other physiological processes [3–5]. Furthermore, GCs are part of an emotion (stress, fear, and arousal) processing pathway in the brain that impacts memory and aspects of behavior that are controlled by the central nervous system [6–8].

Importantly, from a medical point of view, GCs and their synthetic analogues have strong immunosuppressive properties. Because of this, synthetic GCs belong to the top 50 World Health Organization essential medicines. Prednisone, dexamethasone, and triamcinolone are used to treat a wide range of (auto)inflammatory conditions as well as hematopoietic malignancies. The anti-inflammatory effect of GCs is due to regulation of cell survival and immune signaling molecules such as chemokines, interleukins, and cytokines such as TNFα [9, 10]. GCs are often well accepted as a long-term treatment, making them irreplaceable for medical use. Nevertheless, synthetic glucocorticoid (over)use has a number of side effects that usually involve homeostasis and tissue maintenance [11, 12]. To mitigate such side effects, a detailed understanding of the molecular mode of action of GCs is a necessity. Hence, understanding the molecular mechanisms through which GCs exert their biological function has been a highly active research field in the past century.

The glucocorticoid receptor (NR3C1, abbreviated here as GR) is a sequence-specific DNA-binding transcription factor that is expressed in virtually every human cell type. Hence, almost every tissue is potentially responsive to GCs through gene expression modulation. Since the molecular responses to GCs of given tissues are different, it is thought that epigenetic programming during cellular differentiation underlies the cell-specific GC responses [13]. Below, we will review recent developments in epigenetic research relevant to cell-specific GC response mechanisms. In the last section of this chapter, we will review recent research results that support the notion that non-genomic effects of GCs may be very important too.

2. Chromosome architecture and epigenetic control of glucocorticoid responses: DNA accessibility

Eukaryotic transcription factors (TFs) bind to regulatory DNA elements commonly called "*cis*-acting elements" to modulate the transcription rates of their target genes. *Cis*-acting elements can be located at (i) gene promoters, where mRNA transcription starts, or (ii) at enhancers, which can be located hundreds of thousands of nucleotides away from their target gene promoters, or (iii) at boundary elements that flank chromosome domains and function to restrict enhancer activity within individual topologically associated chromosome domains [13].

In order to determine the locations where TFs bind on chromosomes, a technique called chromatin immunoprecipitation (ChIP) was developed in the 1990s. ChIP is based on formaldehyde crosslinking of TFs to DNA, followed by DNA co-immunoprecipitations using antibodies directed against the TF protein [14]. Initially, PCR was used to analyze the co-immunoprecipitated DNA, using the enrichment of putative TF target sites relative to "control" chromosomal regions. Nowadays, the co-immunoprecipitated DNA fragments are prepared as DNA libraries that can be sequenced on next-generation sequencing (NGS) platforms, followed by computational mapping of the obtained reads to a reference genome [15].

Currently, more than 20 human and mouse genome-wide GR occupation profiles are available. These reveal a high degree of GR-binding variability [16]. Grøntved et al. showed that a majority (83%) of GR-DNA binding sites in mouse liver cells are liver cell-specific, while only 0.5% of events are shared between all analyzed cell-types [17]. This suggests that there is a complex and dynamic epigenetic component to GR binding that underlies the differences in GR-mediated transcriptional regulation across cell types.

The first level of epigenetic regulation is rather well defined by DNA being wrapped, or not, around histones to form nucleosomes every ~190 bp [18, 19]. Low nucleosome occupancy can be measured as DNaseI hypersensitivity, because accessible free DNA is more prone to DNaseI endonuclease cleavage than DNA wrapped around nucleosomes [20, 21].

DNA accessibility is an important indicator for GR binding. Early studies indicated that GR binding increases DNA accessibility to DNaseI [22, 23] and it was therefore concluded that GR "opens up" chromatin. Although this is true, more recent research indicates that the a majority of chromosomal GR-binding sites coincide with pre-existing hypersensitive DNA stretches, whose DNaseI accessibility profile is further modulated by GR activity, as first reported on a genome-wide level by John et al. [24–27] (**Figure 1**). Grøntved et al. indicated that 62% of glucocorticoid receptor-binding sites are occupied by the transcription factor C/EBP in mouse liver tissue and that C/EBP maintains chromatin accessibility before GC treatment [17]. Furthermore, it was shown that in HeLa cells, 88% of GR-binding sites are already occupied by the lysine acetyltransferase p300 transcription co-activator prior to GC treatment

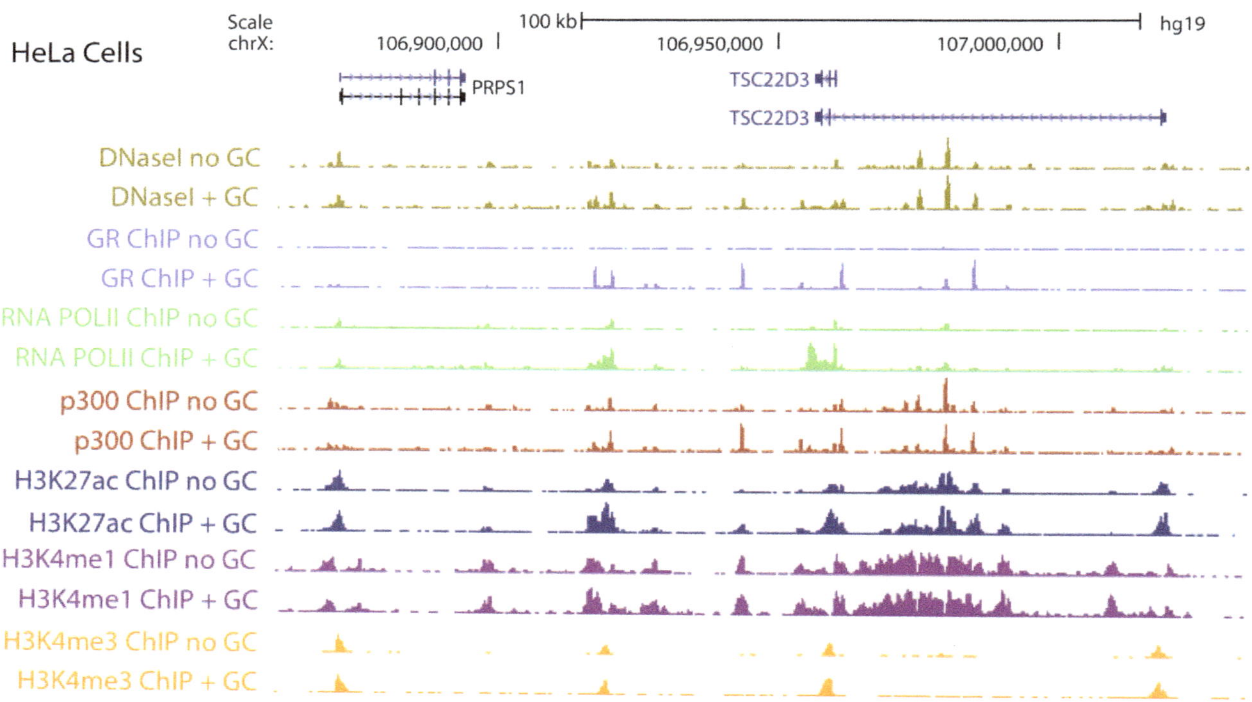

Figure 1. GR binds to GREs at several DNaseI hypersensitive locations within the *TSC22D3/GILZ* locus on human chromosome X. This can increase p300 histone acetyltransferase occupancy, H3K27ac marking, and DNaseI hypersensitivity. Notably, occupancy by RNA polymerase II is dramatically increased upon 4 hours of GC treatment, indicating transcription activation. Histone H3 lysine modifications are indicated (H3K27 acetylation, H3K4 mono-methylation, H3K4 tri-methylation). Data are from HeLa cells, Rao et al. [27].

[27, 28]. Altogether, the available evidence indicates that GR-mediated transcriptional control is dependent on other TFs that establish baseline chromatin accessibility profiles in a cell-type specific manner, as exemplified by FoxA1 [29]. However, one single pioneer TF is unlikely to be the sole key to differential use of GR response elements by different cell lineages, or by the same cell type under different conditions. Rather, combinations of DNA sequence-specific transcription factors may act together as "reciprocal pioneers" in an environmentally cued fashion [30–33].

In summary, in a given cell type, GR generally binds to a predetermined set of nucleosome free regions within enhancers that are marked by lineage determining TFs, and GR only rarely binds at sites with very low initial levels of DNA accessibility (**Figure 1**) [28, 34]. Intriguingly, GR appears to associate for rather short times with its cognate sites in vivo, with reported DNA residence times in the order of seconds [35–39]. GR binding usually results in increased histone acetylation [27] (**Figure 1**).

3. Chromosome architecture and epigenetic control of glucocorticoid responses: topologically associated domains

Over the last decade, a lot of effort was invested in mapping active *cis*-regulatory enhancer elements to susceptible promoters. This is especially relevant in GR-mediated transcriptional regulation, because the majority of GR-bound *cis*-acting DNA elements are enhancers that are located many kilobases away from the promoters of GR-responsive genes [17, 24]. An important contributor in the identification of enhancer-promoter interactions was the development of nuclear proximity-based chromosome conformation capture (3C) technology in 2002 [40]. In brief, interacting DNA regions are fixed by formaldehyde through DNA-protein-DNA crosslinks. The crosslinked chromatin is then digested using restriction enzymes and the digested ends are ligated to obtain DNA circles that harbor sequences from interacting DNA regions. In the original 3C protocol, which is considered a "one-to-one" approach, interactions between two defined genomic loci are assessed by quantitative polymerase chain reaction (RT-qPCR) using locus-specific primers. Circularized Chromatin Conformation Capture (4C), is a "one-to-all" approach that implements a second round of restriction and ligation to obtain small DNA circles which are suitable for inverse PCR amplification to identify the genome-wide DNA interactions of one defined viewpoint locus with any other chromosomal loci [41, 42]. The most recent technical development in 3C technologies is the establishment of chromosome capture followed by high-throughput sequencing (Hi-C) [43]. Crosslinked DNA is digested, labeled with biotin, and re-ligated resulting in a biotin-labeled 3C library. Ligated circles are sheared, purified, and subsequently analyzed using NGS. Hi-C is an "all-to-all" approach because it potentially identifies all possible genome-wide DNA interactions. Capture Hi-C is a further modified version of Hi-C that uses immobilized custom DNA probes and DNA hybridization to enrich for specific loci interactions present in a Hi-C library [44].

A fascinating feature of nuclear chromosome organization is its hierarchical character, containing several layers of compartmentalization. Analyses of Hi-C contact matrices confirm the existence of a first level of organization, namely the occurrence of chromosome territories [45] that were previously described in microscopy-based studies [46]. At the next level, individual chromosomes are partitioned into multi-megabase "A" and "B" compartments that have a propensity to cluster separately. "A" compartments tend to display a euchromatin profile, being gene-rich, transcriptionally active, and accessible. "B" compartments are generally gene-poor with a tendency to be more heterochromatic, transcriptionally inactive, and less accessible. Hi-C maps with improved resolution, mainly obtained through increased sequencing depth and the use of different restriction enzymes, reveal the partitioning of A and B compartments into so-called sub-Mb-sized topologically associated domains (TADs) [47]. TADs are defined by their tendency to favor internal rather than external DNA interactions. Hence, the TAD hypothesis states that TADs are flanked by left and right boundaries and that enhancers mainly interact with promoters and enhancers within their TAD, but not outside of it. It is currently thought that TADs consist of dynamic sub-Mb chromatin fiber loops that undergo continuous remodeling, among others through RNA polymerase II passage.

TADs are highly conserved between different cell lineages [48], indicating that TADs may be universal functional chromosomal units that serve as a platform within which *cis*-regulatory elements are spatially brought together with their susceptible promoter element. The basis of TAD loops is highly enriched for CCCTCF-binding factor (CTCF) [47] (**Figure 2**). CTCF

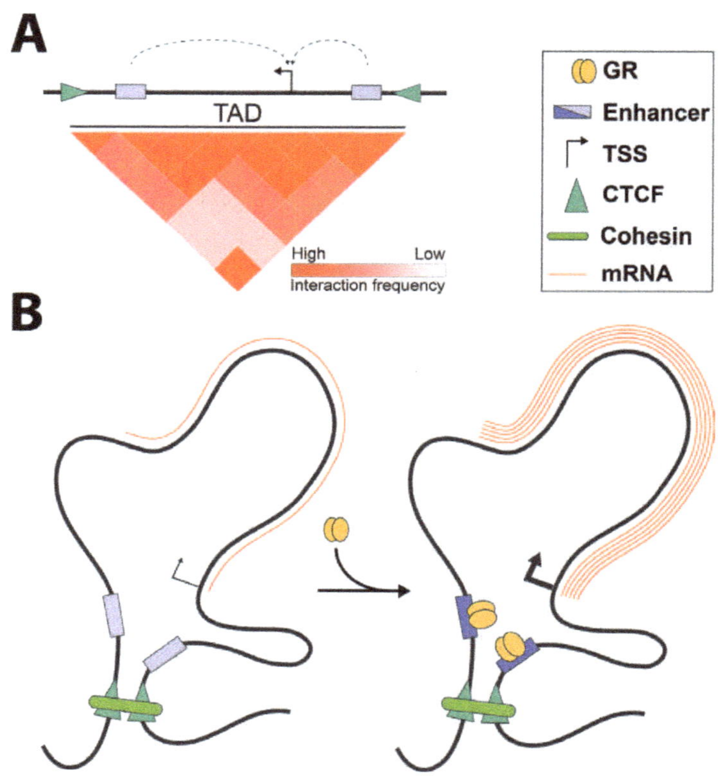

Figure 2. A model depicting long-range transactivation after glucocorticoid stimulation. (A) Linear overview of *cis*-acting element organization. Convergent CTCF motifs define TAD boundaries that restrict promoter-enhancer interactions. A schematic contact matrix of a virtual Hi-C experiment is shown as an interaction heatmap. (B) GR induces transcription through binding of a pre-configured locus without affecting its spatial chromosome architecture. Low and high levels of enhancer H3K27 acetylation are depicted by light and dark rectangles, respectively. TAD: topologically associating domain, GR: glucocorticoid receptor, and TSS: transcription start site. See also Ref. [13].

is known as a transcriptional regulator that functionally segregates chromosomal TADs by inhibiting enhancer-promoter interactions [49]. Importantly, the majority of mammalian TAD loops are flanked by a pair of convergent CTCF motifs that mark the TAD's left and right boundaries [50]. Deletion or inversion of CTCF sites can alter TAD architecture and therefore result in dysregulated enhancer-promoter interactions [51]. Moreover, CTCF depletion disrupts TAD boundaries [52] and impacts gene expression [53]. Dysregulation of CTCF is associated with improper gene regulation during development and oncogenesis [54, 55].

The cohesin complex co-localizes with CTCF when assayed by ChIP [56, 57]. Cohesin rings are composed of the core subunits SMC1, SMC3, RAD21, and STAG [58, 59]. Cohesin is most likely loaded onto its chromatid substrate by the NIPBL2/Mau2 cohesin-loading complex, which is enriched at transcription start sites (TSS) [60, 61]. Conversely, cohesin release from chromatids is facilitated by WAPL [62]. Depletion of cohesin leads to altered short-range chromatin interactions, while global TAD organization seemingly persists, suggesting that cohesin and CTCF play different mechanistic roles in TAD formation [63]. Indeed, while inhibiting cohesin loading (by inhibiting cohesin loading factors) inhibits the formation of topologically associated domains, inhibiting cohesin release by inhibiting WAPL restricts loop extension [64]. In the absence of both CTCF and WAPL, cohesin accumulates in up to 70 kilobase-long regions at the 3′-ends of active genes, in particular, if these converge on each other [60, 61]. Cohesin can be moved along chromosomes through RNA polymerase II translocation along its template in yeast and human; this indicates evolutionary conservation of the translocation of Cohesin rings during RNA polymerase II passage.

A quantitative model of "chromatin loop extrusion" was proposed that explains the dynamic features of TADs rather well [50, 65, 66]. Very recently, looping was studied in the monocytic leukemia cell line THP1 that can differentiate into macrophage-like cells. About 16,000 chromatin loops were detected in both cell types and, using stringent selection criteria, 217 were found to be "dynamic" [67]. This indicates that although loss and gain of TAD loops can occur naturally as cells adapt their gene expression landscape, it is not an obligate step in gene activation/repression. Indeed, Hi-C results obtained in parallel in eight primary human hematopoietic cell types show high correspondence [68].

In 2009, long-range interactions involving GR-bound *cis*-acting DNA sequences were identified in mouse cells using a modified 3C technique [70]. An interaction that spans 30 kb was detected between a GR-binding site in the *Lcn2* gene and the promoter of the *Ciz1* gene. This interaction may be responsible for GC-mediated *Lcn2* and *Ciz1* transcription induction in mouse mammary epithelial adenocarcinoma 3134 cells [69]. In 2011, the same research group reported that "the predominant hormone-induced changes for *Lcn2*-contacting loci can be attributed to an increased frequency of pre-existing interactions" [70]. More recently, the 4C approach and genome-wide chromatin structure analysis were applied to characterize GR-associated DNA interactions [71]. In the 3134 murine cell line, this showed that activated GR response elements can interact with a downstream enhancer of the *Tsc22d3* transcription repressor gene, whose transcription is strongly upregulated by glucocorticoids. See also **Figure 1** where human *TSC22D3* is shown. However, upon glucocorticoid receptor activation, contact intensities changed two-fold at most [71].

Theoretically, there are two types of models for transcription factor (TF)-mediated gene regulation at the level of chromatin organization and chromosome folding. In the first type, repressed loci reside in a silent and inaccessible chromatin state with a low enhancer-promoter interaction frequency. Binding of TFs to distal *cis*-regulatory elements would then enhance the accessibility of the locus for other TFs to bind the enhancers and promoters, and consequently, increased interaction between promoter and enhancer elements would alter gene expression [72, 73]. In the second type of models, the locus is dynamically pre-configured in 3D through boundary-boundary interactions controlled by CTCF and cohesin dynamics that insure that TFs can rapidly exert stimulatory or repressive effects on transcription [74] (**Figure 2**). In this model, TFs hardly affect enhancer-promoter interaction frequencies, although they do affect the histone-borne epigenetic marks such as H3K27 acetylation (see **Figure 1**). Currently, available data suggest that GR-responsive loci fit the second type of models, since dexamethasone-mediated GR activation does not greatly alter TAD structure [70, 71] (**Figure 2**).

4. GR-binding site sequences and GR-mediated transrepression

The oligomerization state and quaternary structure of GR protein on DNA is thought to influence the activity of *cis*-acting GR-binding DNA elements. Experimentally determined glucocorticoid receptor DNA-binding sites have been broadly classified as "simple," "composite" or "tethering." In the "simple" case, homodimers of GR trans-activate genes by binding to canonical GR response elements (GREs) and consequently recruit transcription co-activators [75]. In the composite DNA motif case, repression and activation are both possible outcomes. Finally, "tethering" is a DNA-binding mode whereby GR does not directly bind specific DNA sequences; instead, it is indirectly tethered to DNA by another TF via protein-protein interactions. Tethering was historically proposed to be the main mechanism of GC-induced GR-mediated transcription repression.

Canonical GREs, mineralocorticoid, progesterone, and testosterone receptor-binding sites are virtually identical, being composed of two inverted pseudo-palindromic repeats separated by a spacer sequence of three bases (GRACANNNTGTYC) [76, 112]. Spacer sequence length has been proposed to be important to maintain GR's dimerization state [77, 78]. Furthermore, it has been suggested that allosteric DNA plasticity in the GR recognition sequences influences the conformational state of GR and, thereby, its spatiotemporal regulatory character [79, 80]. However, Presman et al., shone new light on this paradigm as real-time imaging suggests that GR tetramerizes at GREs [81]. Furthermore, in another key publication, Presman et al. used GR point mutations to confirm that trans-repression and transactivation by GR are two functions that can be separated genetically, whereby loss of transactivation potential though impaired homodimerization did not always co-occur with loss of trans-repression potential [82].

The application of single-base resolution TF ChIP technology, attained by inclusion of a lambda exonuclease digestion step in the ChIP protocol (ChIP-exo), was used to reveal that many GR-bound half-sites (GRACA) coincide with recognition sequences of unrelated TFs at composite elements [83, 84]. For instance, Lim et al. revealed co-localization with liver-specific TF-binding sites, explaining part of GR's liver cell-specific binding profiles [84]. The molecular mode of regulation at composite sites still remains to be elucidated, although it was hypothesized to fit a model in which only the co-association of the involved TFs results in productive DNA binding, as seen for classical heterodimeric TFs [85, 86].

Next to its ability to bind half-sites, monomeric GR has been reported to counter the effects of other TFs through protein-protein tethering which would result in trans-repression [87, 88]. One such proposed GR-tethering partner is the activator protein 1 (AP-1) heterodimer made-up of heterodimers of bZIP TF family members. A second major proposed GR tethering partner is NF-κB, a TF that consists of heterodimers of RELA and RELB with NFKB1 and NFKB2 subunits [89–92].

For long, AP-1 and NF-κB tethering of GR to DNA were considered the dominant mechanism for GR-mediated trans-repression of transcription, through "on-DNA" repression of the GR tethering TF's transcription activation potential, as reviewed by Glass and Saijo [93]. Genomic studies showed a significant reduction of GR association upon AP-1 loss, but a majority of regulatory scenarios could neither be disentangled nor rationalized through genome-wide ChIP analyses [94]. Indeed, recent experiments indicate that the mode of GR "trans-repression" is still not fully understood. For instance, Oh et al., showed that activation of GR after LPS treatment caused similar gene repression as activation of GR before LPS treatment, and that DNA occupancy by GR was not predictive of gene expression repression, contradicting the "trans-repression by tethering" model. Rather, GR activation was found to directly induce the expression of inhibitors of NF-κB (and AP-1) and this was proposed to cause genome-wide blockade of NF-κB interaction with chromatin [95]. This suggests that protein tethering leading to DNA-bound monomeric GR trans-repression can only account for a minority of repressive events [96]. Indeed, single-molecule imaging suggests that tethering can account for only ~3% of DNA recruitment events [35].

In yet another twist of the GR tethering saga, Weikum et al. showed that GR associates with a GRE half-site that is located within an AP-1 recognition element, even in the absence of AP-1 [97]. Since AP-1 occupancy was not directly required for GR-mediated trans-repression, Weikum et al. proposed that AP-1 establishes an accessible chromatin state for subsequent GR binding to the half-sites which results in transcription repression [34]. Whether AP-1 trans-repression by GCs relies on co-repressor recruitment [98, 92] or rather on exclusion of other TFs and their co-activators is an unresolved issue at this point in time.

5. Non-genomic mechanisms of gene regulation by glucocorticoids

The classical model for GR action involves ligand-dependent release from a repressive HSP90 complex followed by genomic DNA binding and consequent transcription modulation [12, 75, 99–101]. However, over the years, non-genomic physiologically relevant GR responses have been proposed, as reviewed by Boldizsar et al. [102]. These include direct membrane binding effects of (synthetic) glucocorticoids, a putative non-GR membrane-associated receptor [103], functional interactions of GR with proteins involved in signal transduction such as kinases and phosphatases [104, 105], and mitochondrial GR translocation as a mechanism leading to T-cell apoptosis [106]. An advantage of non-genomic regulation over genomic regulation of gene expression is that non-genomic regulation can take place much faster than the transcription-translation process, which often take >20 minutes to begin to change a cell's molecular composition [107–109].

Over the past decades, it has become apparent that non-genomic mechanisms may also play vital roles in GC action, particularly in the context of immune cell regulation [108]. The mechanism we will review below concerns the apparent capacity of GR to bind to RNA.

There are reports that the growth arrest-specific 5 transcript (GAS5), which is a non-coding RNA, can sequester GR, as well as progesterone and androgen receptors, away from their genomic sites of action by acting as a "GRE decoy" [110–112]. This GAS5-dependent GC inhibitory pathway appears to also be active in some immune cells [113, 114]. Although there are no crystal structures of GR bound to RNA, such structures have been modeled [110].

On the other hand, evidence was published that GCs affect the turnover of specific mRNAs. Regulation of mRNA stability is an intricate process controlled by a complex set of interaction between phosphorylation-mediated signaling pathways like the phosphorylation of UPF1 or SMG-2, which together with *cis*-regulatory RNA elements accelerate an mRNA's decay rate [107, 115–118]. RNA *cis*-acting elements that regulate mRNA stability are usually found in their 5′ and 3′ untranslated regions (UTRs) [119, 120]. The most widely found sequences in the 3′ UTRs of unstable mRNAs belong to the adenylate-uridylate-rich elements, consisting of AUUUA ribonucleotide sequences [119]. It has been proposed that GCs can accelerate mRNA decay by inducing the transcription of genes that code for protein factors implicated in mRNA decay. One such example being the gene that codes for tristetraprolin (*TTP*, also known as *ZFP36*), which is inducible by GCs under some circumstances [121, 122]. Pro-inflammatory factor mRNAs indeed display differential half-lives through such an indirect GC-induced mechanism, an example of which is TNFα [122, 123].

Strikingly, in addition to upregulating the expression of mRNA decay factors, it would appear that GR can act directly as a ligand-dependent activator of mRNA decay. In 1999, a 5′ UTR RNA element was reported to be of particular importance for GC regulation of the expression of the MCP-1/CCL2 inflammatory chemokine [124]. In 2007, it was first reported that GR binds specifically to *CCL2* mRNA, to cause its decay [125]. In 2011, an RNA immunoprecipitation protocol was employed to define an RNA motif that recruits GR and the 5′ UTRs of *CCL2* and *CCL7* mRNAs [126]. The mechanism of GR binding to an mRNA to mediate its decay was termed "GR-mediated mRNA decay" (GMD) by Park et al. in 2015 [127]. This research group investigated how GMD occurs. They reported that GMD is a distinct mRNA decay pathway that shares factors with other forms of RNA decay [128, 129]. GMD depends on a number of proteins that have to be recruited to the mRNA. These include GR, PNRC2, UPF1, DCP1A, HRSP12, and YBX1 which then instigate rapid mRNA degradation (**Figure 3**). PNRC2 and UPF1 are known to bind to each other to bring RNA helicase activity into the complex. Another pair of factors that are known for their ability to degrade mRNA

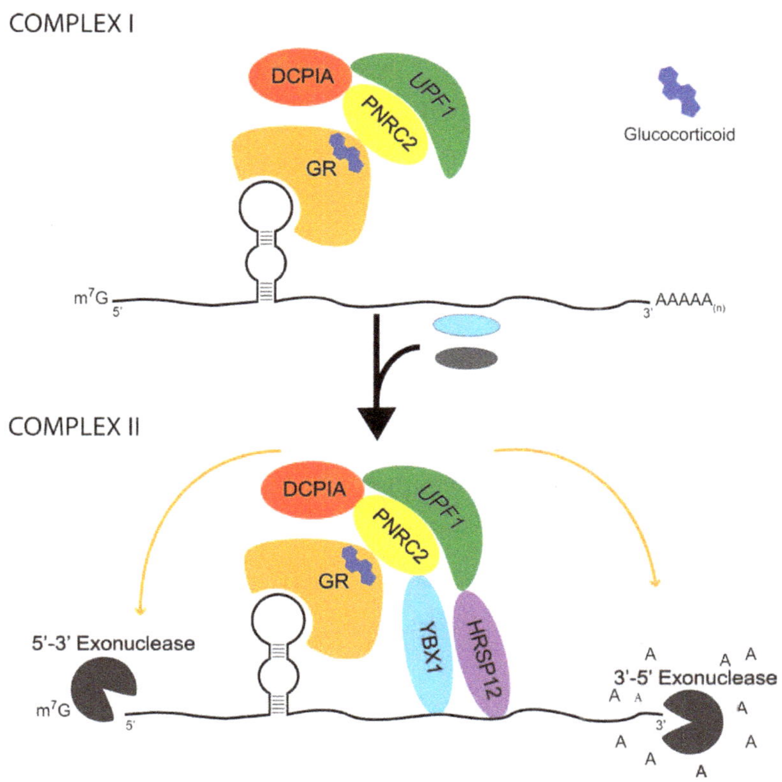

Figure 3. Model of the assembly and composition of the glucocorticoid mediated mRNA decay pathway as described by Park et al. [129]. GR with bound GC recruits PNRC2 and DCP1A together with UPF1 to the 5′ UTR of a target mRNA to form Complex I. HRSP12 and YBX1 are then recruited to form Complex II and mRNA decay is performed by exonucleases.

are DCP1A, which promotes mRNA decapping by DCP1 activity, and HRSP12, an endoribonuclease that can attack mRNA [129]. Although exciting, GMD still needs to be confirmed by unbiased approaches such as genome-wide transcriptomic comparisons of nascent RNA and steady-state RNA which have the capacity to simultaneously report mRNA transcription and decay rates [130].

6. Conclusion

Over the past decade, GR action has been studied at the molecular level in model systems using DNA accessibility assays, GR ChIP, epigenetic profiling of histone-borne epigenetic marks, transcriptome profiling, and RNA immunoprecipitation. Furthermore, chromosome conformation capture assays have been deployed to investigate the impact of GC signaling on chromosome domain topology.

In the cases where it was studied, GR was found to bind for less than a minute to its genomic targets. GR does not appear to affect the configuration of the topologically associated domains to which it binds. It therefore appears that GR binds to loci where enhancers and promoters are dynamically pre-configured in three-dimensional space. The observation that GR complies with chromosome conformation rather than influencing it offers the exciting perspective of being able to map intergenic GRE's, which are often located very far away from their target promoters, to TADs. The genes encompassed by these TADs can then be earmarked as potential GR target genes, a hypothesis that can be confirmed by monitoring their expression upon GC exposure.

Results obtained by many laboratories suggest that GR is dependent on other pioneer transcription factors to access its response elements in chromosomal DNA. Co-pioneer factor combinations appear to be cell-type-specific lineage determining TFs, largely explaining the tissue-specific responses elicited by GCs. Furthermore, much evidence indicates that GR is not only restricted to the classical inverted repeat steroid response element, but can also bind to a variety of DNA sequences that only encompass one half site. Furthermore, the concept that GR is tethered indirectly to DNA via other TFs, whose activity it would then repress "on DNA," is no longer the only model to explain trans-repression in the field. Indeed, other genomic and non-genomic interactions may explain the repression of NFKB and AP-1 target genes observed upon GC exposure.

Interestingly, GR itself appears to be subject to miRNA-mediated regulation, as recently reviewed [131].

Excitingly, following on early reports of RNA binding, it was reported multiple times that GR is also an mRNA-binding protein that induces mRNA decay. A particular target for this pathway are CCL chemokine family mRNAs that have long been known to undergo a dramatic down-regulation upon GC exposure.

Altogether, we conclude that although much effort has been invested in glucocorticoid research since the discovery in the 1940s that glucocorticoids are anti-inflammatory wonder drugs, much remains to be discovered about the molecular mechanisms of action of glucocorticoids.

Abbreviations

3C	Chromosome Conformation Capture
4C	Circularized Chromatin Conformation Capture
ChIP	Chromatin immunoprecipitation
DHS	DNaseI hypersensitive site
GC	glucocorticoid
GMD	GR-mediated mRNA decay
GR	Glucocorticoid receptor
GRE	GR response elements
Hi-C	Chromosome conformation capture with high-throughput sequencing
LPS	Lipopolysaccharides

NGS Next-generation sequencing

TAD Topologically associating domain

TF Transcription factor

TNFα Tumor necrosis factor

TSS Transcription start site

UTR mRNA untranslated region

Author details

Cheng Wang, Roel Oldenkamp, Ronald J.W. Oellers and Colin Logie*

*Address all correspondence to: c.logie@science.ru.nl

Radboud University Faculty of Science, Mathematics and Informatics, RIMLS, Nijmegen, The Netherlands

References

[1] Scheer FA et al. Impact of the human circadian system, exercise, and their interaction on cardiovascular function. Proceedings of the National Academy of Sciences of the United States of America. 2010;**107**(47):20541-20546

[2] Roberts D et al. Antenatal corticosteroids for accelerating fetal lung maturation for women at risk of preterm birth. Cochrane Database of Systematic Reviews. 2017;**3**:CD004454

[3] Liggins GC. The role of cortisol in preparing the fetus for birth. Reproduction, Fertility, and Development. 1994;**6**(2):141-150

[4] Gillies GE et al. Enduring, sexually dimorphic impact of in utero exposure to elevated levels of glucocorticoids on midbrain dopaminergic populations. Brain Sciences. 2016;**7**(1)

[5] Alcantara-Alonso V et al. Corticotropin-releasing hormone as the homeostatic rheostat of Feto-maternal Symbiosis and developmental programming in utero and neonatal life. Frontiers in Neuroendocrinology (Lausanne). 2017;**8**:161

[6] Varney NR, Alexander B, MacIndoe JH. Reversible steroid dementia in patients without steroid psychosis. The American Journal of Psychiatry. 1984;**141**(3):369-372

[7] Cahill L, McGaugh JL. Mechanisms of emotional arousal and lasting declarative memory. Trends in Neurosciences. 1998;**21**(7):294-299

[8] Hunsberger JG et al. Cellular mechanisms underlying affective resiliency: The role of glucocorticoid receptor- and mitochondrially-mediated plasticity. Brain Research. 2009;**1293**:76-84

[9] Savino W et al. Hormonal control of T-cell development in health and disease. Nature Reviews. Endocrinology. 2016;**12**(2):77-89

[10] Zen M et al. The kaleidoscope of glucorticoid effects on immune system. Autoimmunity Reviews. 2011;**10**(6):305-310

[11] Allen DB. Effects of inhaled steroids on growth, bone metabolism, and adrenal function. Advances in Pediatrics. 2006;**53**:101-110

[12] Cain DW, Cidlowski JA. Immune regulation by glucocorticoids. Nature Reviews. Immunology. 2017;**17**(4):233-247

[13] Logie C, Stunnenberg HG. Epigenetic memory: A macrophage perspective. Seminars in Immunology. 2016;**28**(4):359-367

[14] Orlando V. Mapping chromosomal proteins in vivo by formaldehyde-crosslinked-chromatin immunoprecipitation. Trends in Biochemical Sciences. 2000;**25**(3):99-104

[15] Thomas R et al. Features that define the best ChIP-seq peak calling algorithms. Briefings in Bioinformatics. 2017;**18**(3):441-450

[16] Sacta MA, Chinenov Y, Rogatsky I. Glucocorticoid signaling: An update from a genomic perspective. Annual Review of Physiology. 2016;**78**:155-180

[17] Grøntved L et al. C/EBP maintains chromatin accessibility in liver and facilitates glucocorticoid receptor recruitment to steroid response elements. The EMBO Journal, 2013. **32**(11): p. 1568-1583

[18] Valouev A et al. Determinants of nucleosome organization in primary human cells. Nature. 2011;**474**(7352):516-520

[19] Jiang C, Pugh BF. Nucleosome positioning and gene regulation: Advances through genomics. Nature Reviews. Genetics. 2009;**10**(3):161-172

[20] Gross DS, Garrard WT. Nuclease hypersensitive sites in chromatin. Annual Review of Biochemistry. 1988;**57**:159-197

[21] Dorschner MO et al. High-throughput localization of functional elements by quantitative chromatin profiling. Nature Methods. 2004;**1**(3):219-225

[22] Richard-Foy H, Hager GL. Sequence-specific positioning of nucleosomes over the steroid-inducible MMTV promoter. The EMBO Journal. 1987;**6**(8):2321-2328

[23] Reik A, Schutz G, Stewart AF. Glucocorticoids are required for establishment and maintenance of an alteration in chromatin structure: Induction leads to a reversible disruption of nucleosomes over an enhancer. The EMBO Journal. 1991;**10**(9):2569-2576

[24] John S et al. Chromatin accessibility pre-determines glucocorticoid receptor binding patterns. Nature Genetics. 2011;**43**(3):264-268

[25] Lorzadeh A et al. Nucleosome density ChIP-Seq identifies distinct chromatin modification signatures associated with MNase accessibility. Cell Reports. 2016;**17**(8):2112-2124

[26] Reddy TE et al. The hypersensitive glucocorticoid response specifically regulates period 1and expression of circadian genes. Molecular and Cellular Biology. 2012;**32**(18): 3756-3767

[27] Rao NA et al. Coactivation of GR and NFKB alters the repertoire of their binding sites and target genes. Genome Research. 2011;**21**(9):1404-1416

[28] Kuznetsova T et al. Glucocorticoid receptor and nuclear factor kappa-B affect three-dimensional chromatin organization. Genome Biology. 2015;**16**:264

[29] Eeckhoute J et al. Cell-type selective chromatin remodeling defines the active subset of FOXA1-bound enhancers. Genome Research. 2009;**19**(3):372-380

[30] Adam RC, Fuchs E. The yin and Yang of chromatin dynamics in stem cell fate selection. Trends in Genetics. 2016;**32**(2):89-100

[31] Drouin J. 60 YEARS OF POMC: Transcriptional and epigenetic regulation of POMC gene expression. Journal of Molecular Endocrinology. 2016;**56**(4):T99-T112

[32] Swinstead EE et al. Steroid receptors reprogram FoxA1 occupancy through dynamic chromatin transitions. Cell. 2016;**165**(3):593-605

[33] Zaret KS, Lerner J, Iwafuchi-Doi M. Chromatin scanning by dynamic binding of Pioneer factors. Molecular Cell. 2016;**62**(5):665-667

[34] Biddie SC et al. Transcription factor AP1 potentiates chromatin accessibility and glucocorticoid receptor binding. Molecular Cell. 2011;**43**(1):145-155

[35] Gebhardt JC et al. Single-molecule imaging of transcription factor binding to DNA in live mammalian cells. Nature Methods. 2013;**10**(5):421-426

[36] Stasevich TJ et al. Cross-validating FRAP and FCS to quantify the impact of photobleaching on in vivo binding estimates. Biophysical Journal. 2010;**99**(9):3093-3101

[37] Mikuni S, Tamura M, Kinjo M. Analysis of intranuclear binding process of glucocorticoid receptor using fluorescence correlation spectroscopy. FEBS Letters. 2007;**581**(3):389-393

[38] Morisaki T et al. Single-molecule analysis of transcription factor binding at transcription sites in live cells. Nature Communications. 2014;**5**:4456

[39] Groeneweg FL et al. Quantitation of glucocorticoid receptor DNA-binding dynamics by single-molecule microscopy and FRAP. PLoS One. 2014;**9**(3):e90532

[40] Dekker J et al. Capturing chromosome conformation. Science. 2002;**295**(5558):1306-1311

[41] Simonis M et al. Nuclear organization of active and inactive chromatin domains uncovered by chromosome conformation capture-on-chip (4C). Nature Genetics. 2006;**38**(11): 1348-1354

[42] Olivares-Chauvet P et al. Capturing pairwise and multi-way chromosomal conformations using chromosomal walks. Nature. 2016;**540**(7632):296-300

[43] van Berkum NL et al. Hi-C: A method to study the three-dimensional architecture of genomes. Journal of Visualized Experiments. 2010(39)

[44] Hughes JR et al. Analysis of hundreds of cis-regulatory landscapes at high resolution in a single, high-throughput experiment. Nature Genetics. 2014;**46**(2):205-212

[45] Lieberman-Aiden E et al. Comprehensive mapping of long-range interactions reveals folding principles of the human genome. Science. 2009;**326**(5950):289-293

[46] Bolzer A et al. Three-dimensional maps of all chromosomes in human male fibroblast nuclei and prometaphase rosettes. PLoS Biology. 2005;**3**(5):e157

[47] Dixon JR et al. Topological domains in mammalian genomes identified by analysis of chromatin interactions. Nature. 2012;**485**(7398):376-380

[48] Razin SV, Ulianov SV. Gene functioning and storage within a folded genome. Cellular & Molecular Biology Letters. 2017;**22**:18

[49] Liu M et al. Genomic discovery of potent chromatin insulators for human gene therapy. Nature Biotechnology. 2015;**33**(2):198-203

[50] Sanborn AL et al. Chromatin extrusion explains key features of loop and domain formation in wild-type and engineered genomes. Proceedings of the National Academy of Sciences of the United States of America. 2015;**112**(47):E6456-E6465

[51] Guo Y et al. CRISPR inversion of CTCF sites alters genome topology and enhancer/promoter function. Cell. 2015;**162**(4):900-910

[52] Nora EP et al. Targeted degradation of CTCF decouples local insulation of chromosome domains from genomic compartmentalization. Cell. 2017;**169**(5):930-944 e22

[53] Nikolic T et al. The DNA-binding factor Ctcf critically controls gene expression in macrophages. Cellular & Molecular Immunology. 2014;**11**(1):58-70

[54] Lettice LA et al. Enhancer-adoption as a mechanism of human developmental disease. Human Mutation. 2011;**32**(12):1492-1499

[55] Hnisz D et al. Activation of proto-oncogenes by disruption of chromosome neighborhoods. Science. 2016;**351**(6280):1454-1458

[56] Parelho V et al. Cohesins functionally associate with CTCF on mammalian chromosome arms. Cell. 2008;**132**(3):422-433

[57] Wendt KS et al. Cohesin mediates transcriptional insulation by CCCTC-binding factor. Nature. 2008;**451**(7180):796-801

[58] Gruber S, Haering CH, Nasmyth K. Chromosomal cohesin forms a ring. Cell. 2003; **112**(6):765-777

[59] Lara-Pezzi E et al. Evidence of a transcriptional co-activator function of cohesin STAG/SA/Scc3. The Journal of Biological Chemistry. 2004;**279**(8):6553-6559

[60] Lengronne A et al. Cohesin relocation from sites of chromosomal loading to places of convergent transcription. Nature. 2004;**430**(6999):573-578

[61] Busslinger GA et al. Cohesin is positioned in mammalian genomes by transcription, CTCF and Wapl. Nature. 2017;**544**(7651):503-507

[62] Kueng S et al. Wapl controls the dynamic association of cohesin with chromatin. Cell. 2006;**127**(5):955-967

[63] Zuin J et al. Cohesin and CTCF differentially affect chromatin architecture and gene expression in human cells. Proceedings of the National Academy of Sciences of the United States of America. 2014;**111**(3):996-1001

[64] Haarhuis JHI et al. The Cohesin release factor WAPL restricts chromatin loop extension. Cell. 2017;**169**(4):693-707 e14

[65] Alipour E, Marko JF. Self-organization of domain structures by DNA-loop-extruding enzymes. Nucleic Acids Research. 2012;**40**(22):11202-11212

[66] Fudenberg G et al. Formation of chromosomal domains by loop extrusion. Cell Reports. 2016;**15**(9):2038-2049

[67] Phanstiel DH et al. Static and dynamic DNA loops form AP-1-bound activation hubs during macrophage development. Molecular Cell. 2017;**67**(6):1037-1048 e6

[68] Javierre BM et al. Lineage-specific genome architecture links enhancers and non-coding disease variants to target gene promoters. Cell. 2016;**167**(5):1369-1384 e19

[69] Hakim O et al. Glucocorticoid receptor activation of the Ciz1-Lcn2 locus by long range interactions. The Journal of Biological Chemistry. 2009;**284**(10):6048-6052

[70] Hakim O et al. Diverse gene reprogramming events occur in the same spatial clusters of distal regulatory elements. Genome Research. 2011;**21**(5):697-706

[71] Stavreva DA et al. Dynamics of chromatin accessibility and long-range interactions in response to glucocorticoid pulsing. Genome Research. 2015;**25**(6):845-857

[72] Teferedegne B et al. Mechanism of action of a distal NF-kappaB-dependent enhancer. Molecular and Cellular Biology. 2006;**26**(15):5759-5770

[73] Vernimmen D et al. Long-range chromosomal interactions regulate the timing of the transition between poised and active gene expression. The EMBO Journal. 2007;**26**(8): 2041-2051

[74] Andrey G et al. A switch between topological domains underlies HoxD genes collinearity in mouse limbs. Science. 2013;**340**(6137):1234167

[75] Malovannaya A et al. Analysis of the human endogenous coregulator complexome. Cell. 2011;**145**(5):787-799

[76] Yamamoto KR. Steroid receptor regulated transcription of specific genes and gene networks. Annual Review of Genetics. 1985;**19**:209-252

[77] Luisi BF et al. Crystallographic analysis of the interaction of the glucocorticoid receptor with DNA. Nature. 1991;**352**(6335):497-505

[78] Gronemeyer H, Bourguet W. Allosteric effects govern nuclear receptor action: DNA appears as a player. Science Signaling. 2009;**2**(73):pe34

[79] Meijsing SH et al. DNA binding site sequence directs glucocorticoid receptor structure and activity. Science. 2009;**324**(5925):407-410

[80] Watson LC et al. The glucocorticoid receptor dimer interface allosterically transmits sequence-specific DNA signals. Nature Structural & Molecular Biology. 2013;**20**(7): 876-883

[81] Presman DM et al. DNA binding triggers tetramerization of the glucocorticoid receptor in live cells. Proceedings of the National Academy of Sciences of the United States of America. 2016;**113**(29):8236-8241

[82] Presman DM et al. Live cell imaging unveils multiple domain requirements for in vivo dimerization of the glucocorticoid receptor. PLoS Biology. 2014;**12**(3):e1001813

[83] Starick SR et al. ChIP-exo signal associated with DNA-binding motifs provides insight into the genomic binding of the glucocorticoid receptor and cooperating transcription factors. Genome Research. 2015;**25**(6):825-835

[84] Lim HW et al. Genomic redistribution of GR monomers and dimers mediates transcriptional response to exogenous glucocorticoid in vivo. Genome Research. 2015;**25**(6):836-844

[85] Vinson C, Acharya A, Taparowsky EJ. Deciphering B-ZIP transcription factor interactions in vitro and in vivo. Biochimica et Biophysica Acta. 2006;**1759**(1-2):4-12

[86] Cooper CD, Newman JA, Gileadi O. Recent advances in the structural molecular biology of Ets transcription factors: Interactions, interfaces and inhibition. Biochemical Society Transactions. 2014;**42**(1):130-138

[87] Karin M. New twists in gene regulation by glucocorticoid receptor: Is DNA binding dispensable? Cell. 1998;**93**(4):487-490

[88] Kassel O, Herrlich P. Crosstalk between the glucocorticoid receptor and other transcription factors: Molecular aspects. Molecular and Cellular Endocrinology. 2007;**275**(1-2): 13-29

[89] Baeuerle PA, Baltimore D. NF-kappa B: Ten years after. Cell. 1996;**87**(1):13-20

[90] De Bosscher K, Vanden Berghe W, Haegeman G. The interplay between the glucocorticoid receptor and nuclear factor-kappaB or activator protein-1: Molecular mechanisms for gene repression. Endocrine Reviews. 2003;**24**(4):488-522

[91] Hayden MS, Ghosh S. NF-kappaB, the first quarter-century: Remarkable progress and outstanding questions. Genes & Development. 2012;**26**(3):203-234

[92] Natoli G. NF-kappaB and chromatin: Ten years on the path from basic mechanisms to candidate drugs. Immunological Reviews. 2012;**246**(1):183-192

[93] Glass CK, Saijo K. Nuclear receptor transrepression pathways that regulate inflammation in macrophages and T cells. Nature Reviews. Immunology. 2010;**10**(5):365-376

[94] Uhlenhaut NH et al. Insights into negative regulation by the glucocorticoid receptor from genome-wide profiling of inflammatory cistromes. Molecular Cell. 2013;**49**(1):158-171

[95] Oh KS et al. Anti-inflammatory chromatinscape suggests alternative mechanisms of glucocorticoid receptor action. Immunity. 2017;**47**(2):298-309 e5

[96] Kadiyala V et al. Cistrome-based cooperation between airway epithelial glucocorticoid receptor and NF-kappaB orchestrates anti-inflammatory effects. The Journal of Biological Chemistry. 2016;**291**(24):12673-12687

[97] Weikum ER et al. Tethering not required: The glucocorticoid receptor binds directly to activator protein-1 recognition motifs to repress inflammatory genes. Nucleic Acids Research. 2017;**45**(14):8596-8608

[98] Chinenov Y et al. Role of transcriptional coregulator GRIP1 in the anti-inflammatory actions of glucocorticoids. Proceedings of the National Academy of Sciences of the United States of America. 2012;**109**(29):11776-11781

[99] Logie C, Stewart AF. Ligand-regulated site-specific recombination. Proceedings of the National Academy of Sciences of the United States of America. 1995;**92**(13):5940-5944

[100] Inayoshi Y et al. Repression of GR-mediated expression of the tryptophan oxygenase gene by the SWI/SNF complex during liver development. Journal of Biochemistry. 2005;**138**(4):457-465

[101] Muratcioglu S et al. Structural modeling of GR interactions with the SWI/SNF chromatin remodeling complex and C/EBP. Biophysical Journal. 2015;**109**(6):1227-1239

[102] Boldizsar F et al. Emerging pathways of non-genomic glucocorticoid (GC) signalling in T cells. Immunobiology. 2010;**215**(7):521-526

[103] Lowenberg M et al. Novel insights into mechanisms of glucocorticoid action and the development of new glucocorticoid receptor ligands. Steroids. 2008;**73**(9-10):1025-1029

[104] Buttgereit F, Scheffold A. Rapid glucocorticoid effects on immune cells. Steroids. 2002;**67**(6):529-534

[105] Beck IM et al. Crosstalk in inflammation: The interplay of glucocorticoid receptor-based mechanisms and kinases and phosphatases. Endocrine Reviews. 2009;**30**(7):830-882

[106] Sionov RV et al. Role of mitochondrial glucocorticoid receptor in glucocorticoid-induced apoptosis. The Journal of Experimental Medicine. 2006;**203**(1):189-201

[107] Stellato C. Post-transcriptional and nongenomic effects of glucocorticoids. Proceedings of the American Thoracic Society. 2004;**1**(3):255-263

[108] Cruz-Topete D, Cidlowski JA. One hormone, two actions: Anti- and pro-inflammatory effects of glucocorticoids. Neuroimmunomodulation. 2015;**22**(1-2):20-32

[109] Battich N, Stoeger T, Pelkmans L. Control of transcript variability in single mammalian cells. Cell. 2015;**163**(7):1596-1610

[110] Kino T et al. Noncoding RNA gas5 is a growth arrest- and starvation-associated repressor of the glucocorticoid receptor. Science Signaling. 2010;**3**(107):ra8

[111] Tani H, Torimura M, Akimitsu N. The RNA degradation pathway regulates the function of GAS5 a non-coding RNA in mammalian cells. PLoS One. 2013;**8**(1):e55684

[112] Strahle U et al. Glucocorticoid- and progesterone-specific effects are determined by differential expression of the respective hormone receptors. Nature. 1989;**339**(6226): 629-632

[113] Mayama T, Marr AK, Kino T. Differential expression of glucocorticoid receptor noncoding RNA repressor Gas5 in autoimmune and inflammatory diseases. Hormone and Metabolic Research. 2016;**48**(8):550-557

[114] Lucafo M et al. Role of the long non-coding RNA growth arrest-specific 5 in glucocorticoid response in children with inflammatory bowel disease. Basic & Clinical Pharmacology & Toxicology. 2017

[115] Page MF et al. SMG-2 is a phosphorylated protein required for mRNA surveillance in *Caenorhabditis elegans* and related to Upf1p of yeast. Molecular and Cellular Biology. 1999;**19**(9):5943-5951

[116] Bhattacharya A et al. Characterization of the biochemical properties of the human Upf1 gene product that is involved in nonsense-mediated mRNA decay. RNA. 2000;**6**(9): 1226-1235

[117] Shyu AB, Wilkinson MF. The double lives of shuttling mRNA binding proteins. Cell. 2000;**102**(2):135-138

[118] Anderson P, Kedersha N. RNA granules: Post-transcriptional and epigenetic modulators of gene expression. Nature Reviews. Molecular Cell Biology. 2009;**10**(6):430-436

[119] Chen CY, Shyu AB. AU-rich elements: Characterization and importance in mRNA degradation. Trends in Biochemical Sciences. 1995;**20**(11):465-470

[120] Chen CY et al. Nucleolin and YB-1 are required for JNK-mediated interleukin-2 mRNA stabilization during T-cell activation. Genes & Development. 2000;**14**(10):1236-1248

[121] Anderson P. Post-transcriptional control of cytokine production. Nature Immunology. 2008;**9**(4):353-359

[122] Ishmael FT et al. Role of the RNA-binding protein tristetraprolin in glucocorticoid-mediated gene regulation. Journal of Immunology. 2008;**180**(12):8342-8353

[123] Kratochvill F et al. Tristetraprolin limits inflammatory cytokine production in tumor-associated macrophages in an mRNA decay-independent manner. Cancer Research. 2015;**75**(15):3054-3064

[124] Poon M, Liu B, Taubman MB. Identification of a novel dexamethasone-sensitive RNA-destabilizing region on rat monocyte chemoattractant protein 1 mRNA. Molecular and Cellular Biology. 1999;**19**(10):6471-6478

[125] Dhawan L et al. A novel role for the glucocorticoid receptor in the regulation of monocyte chemoattractant protein-1 mRNA stability. The Journal of Biological Chemistry. 2007;**282**(14):10146-10152

[126] Ishmael FT et al. The human glucocorticoid receptor as an RNA-binding protein: Global analysis of glucocorticoid receptor-associated transcripts and identification of a target RNA motif. Journal of Immunology. 2011;**186**(2):1189-1198

[127] Cho H et al. Glucocorticoid receptor interacts with PNRC2 in a ligand-dependent manner to recruit UPF1 for rapid mRNA degradation. Proceedings of the National Academy of Sciences of the United States of America. 2015;**112**(13):E1540-E1549

[128] Park OH, Do E, Kim YK. A new function of glucocorticoid receptor: Regulation of mRNA stability. BMB Reports. 2015;**48**(7):367-368

[129] Park OH et al. Identification and molecular characterization of cellular factors required for glucocorticoid receptor-mediated mRNA decay. Genes & Development. 2016;**30**(18):2093-2105

[130] Rabani M et al. High-resolution sequencing and modeling identifies distinct dynamic RNA regulatory strategies. Cell. 2014;**159**(7):1698-1710

[131] Wang H et al. The effects of microRNAs on glucocorticoid responsiveness. Journal of Cancer Research and Clinical Oncology. 2017;**143**(6):1005-1011

7

66 Years of Corticosteroids in Dentistry: And We are Still at a Cross Road?

Wei Cheong Ngeow, Daniel Lim and Nurhalim Ahmad

Abstract

Most of the corticosteroids prescribed in dentistry are for topical applications or short-term usage, rarely for its systemic effects or for long-term consumption, as in the treatment of some medical conditions. Among the various specialties in dentistry, oral and maxillofacial surgery, oral medicine and endodontics are the more frequent users of corticosteroids. Corticosteroids are used in oral and maxillofacial procedures to reduce associated post-operative inflammation. The most researched outcome on the use of corticosteroids in oral and maxillofacial surgery revolves around their impact to reduce post-operative pain, swelling and trismus. Topical corticosteroids, on the other hand, are effective in treating various oral mucosal lesions including oral ulcerations and oral presentations of auto-immune diseases. Corticosteroids are also used as part of the treatment of temporomandibular joint disorders. Intracanal placement of corticosteroids is used in endodontic treatment. This chapter reviews the use of corticosteroids in the three specialties of dentistry as mentioned.

Keywords: corticosteroids, dentistry, oral and maxillofacial surgery, oral medicine, endodontology

1. Introduction

Corticosteroids is one well-known anti-inflammatory group of drugs that is listed in the Dental' Practitioners' Formulary. Among the various specialties in dentistry, oral medicine, oral and maxillofacial surgery and endodontics are the more frequent users of corticosteroids. Most of the corticosteroids prescribed in dentistry are for topical applications or short-term usage, rarely for its systemic effects or for long-term consumption, as in the treatment of some medical conditions. Five years ago, a chapter entitled "The role of Corticosteroids in today's Oral and

Maxillofacial Surgery" [1] has been published in the book "Glucocorticoids—New Recognition of Our Familiar Friend". The objective of this chapter is therefore to complement the previous publication as well as providing an update on the use of corticosteroids in dentistry, instead of merely oral and maxillofacial surgery.

Although corticosteroids were already used in the field of medicine since 1944, it was not until 1951 that they were introduced to dentistry. Then, Strean published a paper which represented the first scientific approach to the general use of corticosteroids in dentistry [2]. Strean and Horton [3] and Spies et al. [4] were the first to use (hydro)cortisone for the treatment of oral diseases related to local causes and oral manifestations of inflammatory systemic disease. Back then, corticosteroids were prescribed as topical medicament as well as systemic medication, depending on the oral manifestations of systemic diseases. Topical corticosteroids have proven to be effective in treating various oral mucosal lesions including oral ulcerations and oral presentations of auto-immune diseases. In oral medicine, injection of corticosteroids is part of the treatment of temporomandibular joint degeneration.

Corticosteroids are used in oral and maxillofacial surgical procedures to reduce associated post-operative inflammation. The suggestion of their use for managing post-operative sequelae of dentoalveolar surgery began as an editorial by Kenny in 1954 [5]. Following this, Ross and White performed a clinical trial comparing oral hydrocortisone against placebo in a double-blind study involving third molar surgeries that confirmed the former's efficacy [6]. The most researched outcome on the use of corticosteroids in oral surgery revolves around their effect in reducing post-operative pain, swelling and trismus. Over the last 6 decades, the use of corticosteroids for third molar surgery had been studied extensively in different formulations, dosings, routes and sites of administration [7]. These corticosteroids include dexamethasone (per-oral/p.o.), dexamethasone acetate (intramuscular), dexamethasone sodium phosphate (intravenous and intramuscular), methylprednisolone (p.o.), methylprednisolone acetate and methylprednisolone sodium succinate (both intravenous and intramuscular) [8]. In recent years, a twin-mix combination of 2% lignocaine with 1:200,000 adrenaline and 4 mg dexamethasone was even given as an inferior alveolar nerve block [9]. A recent review concluded that there are benefits that can be derived from the short-term use of corticosteroids in reducing these inflammatory sequelae, with no side effects observed when given using the methods listed above [7]. However, the use of corticosteroids for periodontal and implant surgeries has not been investigated. The other use of corticosteroids in oral surgery is as medication for various cranial nerve disorders and application/injections for the treatment of facial scars [10]. It is a standard medication for Bell's palsy [11], with prednisolone coupled with acyclovir being the most popular choice. The recommended dose is prednisolone 60–80 mg daily during first 5 days with dose tapering over next 5 days [12]. It is a drug within a cocktail with NSAIDs given to patients suffering from traumatic trigeminal nerve injuries [13]. One study even reported their beneficial effect on lingual and inferior alveolar nerve hypersensitivity following third molar surgery [14]. More controversial use of corticosteroids is related to their administration to patients with maxillofacial space infection. Low et al. recently reported that corticosteroids are useful as adjunct treatment for such cases [15]. Their patients experienced significant clinical improvement with reduction of pain, swelling and trismus, and shortening hospital stay to an average of 3.5 days, in addition to omission of surgical intervention in 50% of cases.

Lastly, corticosteroids are used as exposed pulp lining and intracanal medicament in endodontic therapy. This chapter reviews the use of corticosteroids in the three specialties of dentistry as mentioned. It shall answer the routinely asked impression: are dental surgeons and dental specialists still at a cross road in deciding whether corticosteroids should be routinely used in clinical dentistry?

2. Corticosteroids in oral and maxillofacial surgery

Corticosteroids are used mainly by oral and maxillofacial surgeons to reduce the post-operative sequelae (pain, swelling and trismus) of dentoalveolar surgery, orthognathic surgery, facial fractures and reconstructive surgery [16, 17]. Post-operative nausea and vomiting have been reported to be less in patients who were given corticosteroids when these surgeries were done under general anaesthesia [18]. In addition, corticosteroids have been proven to improve interpalpebral width as well as reducing post-operative pain after surgical repair of orbital blowout fractures [19, 20]. Local steroid injection of the tongue base had proven to reduce the incidence and severity of post-palatoplasty upper airway obstruction in children undergoing cleft palate surgery [21]. A questionnaire survey in North America reported that close to half of oral and maxillofacial surgeons stated that they use short-term, high-dose perioperative corticosteroids to control post-operative oedema [22]. Only 20% of oral and maxillofacial surgeons claimed that they never use it for dentoalveolar surgery [23]. In comparison, corticosteroids are less preferred for dentoalveolar surgeries by surgeons in at least one European country [16]. Their popularity for dentoalveolar surgeries elsewhere has not been established.

The group of corticosteroids of interest is the glucocorticoids (dexamethasone and betamethasone, and prednisolone and methylprednisolone), because of their anti-inflammatory activities with little or no effect on fluid and electrolyte balance [7]. Their effect has been well studied using the third molar surgery model over the past 6 decades (**Table 1**). In a study that reviewed the reported outcome of corticosteroids over the last 10 years (2006–2015), Ngeow and Lim [7] reviewed 34 studies that administered corticosteroids via different routes which included intravenous, intramuscular (masseter, deltoid or gluteus), submucosal, endoalveolar and oral administrations. They found that benefits could be derived from the short-term use of corticosteroids with regards to pain, swelling and trismus control following third molar surgery, with no side effects observed. However, there were two limitations to their study, namely restriction to studies performed only throughout the last decade, and exclusion of studies that compared corticosteroids with other drugs, intervention or treatment, except when the corticosteroid was administered with an adjuvant therapy related to third molar surgery, namely an antibiotic.

Some 10 years ago, a systematic review and meta-analysis by Markiewicz et al. [24] reported that perioperative administration of corticosteroids produced a mild to moderate reduction in swelling and improvement of trismus after third molar surgery. More recently, another three meta-analyses specifically reported on the effect of dexamethasone in third molar surgery. Two reviewed the effect of submucosal injection of dexamethasone [25, 26], while the third reviewed the preemptive effect of dexamethasone [27]. The findings of two meta-analyses on submucosal injection are different. Chen et al. reported that submucosal injection of dexamethasone

Authors (year)	Corticosteroids studied	Summary outcomes			
		Swelling	Pain	Trismus	Others
Ross and White (1958) [6]	Hydrocortisone 40 mg (multiple doses)	Reduced	No difference	Reduced	—
Ware et al. (1963) [51]	Dexamethasone 9 mg or 13.5 mg (multiple doses)	No difference	—	No difference	—
Lineberg (1965) [29]	Dexamethasone 9 mg (multiple doses)	Reduced	—	Reduced	—
Nathanson and Seifert (1964) [52]	Betamethasone 0.6 mg; multiple tablets (multiple doses)	Reduced	Reduced	Reduced	Reduced ecchymosis
Hooley and Francis (1969) [53]	Betamethasone 1.2 g (multiple doses)	Reduced	Reduced	Reduced	Increased dry socket (4%)
Messer and Keller (1975) [54]	Dexamethasone 4 mg (single dose)	Reduced	Reduced	Reduced	—
Caci and Gluck (1976) [55]	Prednisolone 5 mg (multiple doses)	No difference	Reduced	Reduced	Comparison against papase; reduced ecchymosis
Huffman (1977) [56]	Methylprednisolone sodium succinate 40 mg or 125 mg (single dose)	Reduced	—	—	—
Edilby et al. (1982) [57]	Dexamethasone 4 mg and 8 mg (Two doses)	No difference	No difference	No difference	—
Skjelbred and Løkken (1982) [58]	Betamethasone 9 mg (single dose)	Reduced	Reduced	Reduced	Given preoperative
Skjelbred and Løkken (1982) [59]	Betamethasone 9 mg (single dose)	Reduced	Reduced	—	Give post-operative
Skjelbred and Løkken (1983) [60]	Methylprednisolone succinate 40 mg (single dose)	Reduced	—	—	—
Bystedt and Nordenram (1985) [61]	Methylprednisolone 12 mg followed by 4 mg (multiple doses)	No difference	No difference	No difference	—
ElHaq et al. (1985) [62]	Dexamethasone 10 mg (two doses)	Reduced	—	Reduced	Comparison against ulatrasound, which is equally as effective
Pedersen (1985) [63]	Betamethasone 4 mg (single dose)	Reduced	Reduced	Reduced	

Authors (year)	Corticosteroids studied	Summary outcomes			
		Swelling	Pain	Trismus	Others
Sisk and Bonnington (1985) [64]	Methylprednisolone 125 mg (single dose)	No difference	Reduced	No difference	Comparison against flurbiprofen or placebo
Beirne and Hollander (1986) [65]	Methylprednisolone 125 mg (single dose)	Reduced	Reduced	No difference	—
Olstad and Skjelbred (1986) [66]	Methylprednisolone (multiple tapering doses)	Reduced	Reduced	—	—
Holland (1987) [67]	Methylprednisolone 40 mg (single dose)	Reduced	Reduced	—	—
Troullos et al. (1990) [68]	Methylprednisolone 125 mg (single dose)	Reduced	Reduced	Reduced	Less effective pain control than flurbiprofen or ibuprofen
Neupert et al. (1992) [69]	Dexamethasone 4 mg (single dose)	No difference	No difference	Reduced	—
Baxendale et al. (1993) [70]	Dexamethasone 8 mg (single dose)	Reduced	Reduced	No difference	—
Hyrkäs et al. (1993) [71]	Methylprednisolone 40 mg (single dose)	—	Reduced	No difference	Increased efficacy in pain control in combination with diclofenac sodium
Milles and Desjardins (1993) [72]	Methylprednisolone 16 mg and 20 mg (two doses)	Reduced	—	No difference	—
Schmelzeisen and Frölich (1993) [73]	Dexamethasone 6 mg (two doses)	Reduced	Reduced	Reduced	—
Schultze-Mosgau et al. (1995) [74]	Methylprednisolone 32 mg (single dose)	Reduced	Reduced	—	Co-administered with ibuprofen
Esen et al. (1999) [75]	Methylprednisolone 125 mg (single dose)	Reduced	Reduced	Reduced	—
Dionne et al. (2003) [76]	Dexamethasone 4 mg (two doses)	—	Reduced	—	Synergistic pain relief with ketorolac
Üstün et al. (2003) [77]	Methylprednisolone 1.5 mg/kg or 3 mg/kg (single dose)	No difference	No difference	No difference	Comparison of two different doses of corticosteroids
Bamgbose et al. (2005) [78]	Dexamethasone 8 mg and 4 mg (two doses)	Reduced	Reduced	No difference	Co-administered with diclofenac sodium

Authors (year)	Corticosteroids studied	Summary outcomes			
		Swelling	Pain	Trismus	Others
López-Carriches et al. (2005) [79]	Methylprednisolone 40 mg (single dose)	—	No difference	—	Comparison with diclofenac
Moore et al. (2005) [80]	Dexamethasone 10 mg (single dose)	—	Reduced	Reduced	Synergistic effect with rofecoxib
Tiwana et al. (2005) [81]	Dexamethasone 8 mg or methylprednisolone 40 mg (single dose)	No difference	No difference	No difference	Improved sleep and decreased nausea
Buyukkurt et al. (2006) [82]	Prednisolone 25 mg (single dose)	Reduced	Reduced	Reduced	Synergistic effect with diclofenac
Graziani et al. (2006) [83]	Dexamethasone 4 mg or 10 mg (single dose)	Reduced	Reduced	Reduced	—
López-Carriches et al. (2006) [84]	Methylprednisolone 40 mg (single dose)	Reduced	—	No difference	Comparison with diclofenac
Mico Llorens et al. 2006 [85]	Methylprednisolone 40 mg (single dose)	Reduced	No difference	Reduced	
Ordulu et al. (2006) [86]	Methylprednisolone 1.5 mg/kg (single dose)	No difference	No difference	Reduced	Comparison with tube drainage
Grossi et al. (2007) [87]	Dexamethasone 4 mg or 8 mg (single dose)				
Filho et al. (2008) [88]	Dexamethasone 4 mg or 8 mg (single dose)	Reduced	No difference	Reduced	No difference between two dosages
Zandi et al. (2008) [89]	Dexamethasone 8 mg (single dose) followed by methylprednisolone 5 mg (multiple doses)	Reduced	Reduced	Reduced	Comparison against rubber drain, which reduced pain and trismus
Vegas-Bustamante et al. (2008) [90]	Methylprednisolone 40 mg (single dose)	Reduced	Reduced	Reduced	
Chopra et al. (2009) [91]	Betamethasone 0.5 mg (single dose)	Reduced	Reduced	Reduced	Comparison against paracetamol, serratiopeptidase, ibuprofen
Gataa and Nemat (2009) [92]	Methylprednisolone 10 mg (single dose)	Reduced	Reduced	Reduced	Oral route more effective than submucosal route in controlling pain and trismus
Tiigimae-Saar et al. (2010) [93]	Prednisolone 30 mg (single dose)	Reduced	Reduced	Reduced	

Authors (year)	Corticosteroids studied	Summary outcomes			
		Swelling	Pain	Trismus	Others
Kang et al. (2010) [94]	Prednisolone 10 mg or 20 mg (single dose)				No difference between the two dosages. Dose need to be more than 20 mg to be effective
Majid and Mahmood (2011) [95]	Dexamethsone 4 mg (single dose)	Reduced	Reduced	Reduced	No difference between intramuscular and submucosal routes
Majid (2011) [96]	Dexamethasone 4 mg (single dose)	Reduced	Reduced	Reduced	No difference between intramuscular and submucosal routes. Improved QoL
Deo and Shetty (2011) [97]	Dexamethasone 8 mg (single dose)	Reduced	Reduced	Reduced	—
Antunes et al. (2011) [98]	Dexamethasone 8 mg (single dose)	Reduced	Reduced	Reduced	No difference between submucosal and intramuscular (masseter) routes
Kaur et al. (2011) [99]	Methylprednisolone 40 mg (single dose)	Reduced	Reduced	Reduced	—
Mushtaq et al. (2011) [100]	Dexamethasone 4 mg (single dose)	Reduced	Reduced	Reduced	—
Boonsiriseth et al. (2012) [101]	Dexamethasone 8 mg (single dose)	Reduced	Reduced	Reduced	No difference between oral and intramuscular (deltoid) routes
Klongnoi et al. (2012) [102]	Dexamethasone 8 mg (single dose)	Reduced	Reduced	No difference	
Loganathan and Srinivasan (2012) [103]	Methylprednisolone 40 mg (single dose) or dexamethasone 4 mg (single dose)	Reduced	Reduced	Reduced	No difference between the two drugs
Murugesan et al. (2012) [104]	Dexamethasone 1 mg (multiple doses)	Reduced	Reduced	No difference	Comparison with serratiopeptidase
Panwar (2012) [105]	Prednisolone 5 mg (single dose)	Reduced	Reduced	Reduced	—
Acham et al. (2013) [106]	Methylprednisolone 60–80 mg based on body weight (single dose)	Reduced	Reduced	Reduced	—
Arakeri et al. (2013) [107]	Dexamethasone 8 mg (single dose)	Reduced	Reduced	—	Comparison with aprotinin (a serine protease inhibitor)
Bauer et al. (2013) [108]	Dexamethasone 8 mg (single dose)	—	Reduced	—	Synergistic effect with ibuprofen

Authors (year)	Corticosteroids studied	Summary outcomes			
		Swelling	Pain	Trismus	Others
Bortoluzzi et al. (2013) [109]	Dexamethasone 8 mg (single dose)	No difference	No difference	No difference	Dexamethasone was combined with amoxicillin or placebo
Channar et al. (2013) [110]	Dexamethasone 8 mg (two doses)	No difference	—	No difference	—
Chaurand-Lara and Facio-Umaña (2013) [111]	Methylprednisolone 20 mg (single dose)	Reduced	Reduced	—	—
Christensen et al. (2013) [112]	Methylprednisolone 16 mg (two doses)	Reduced	Reduced	—	Co-administered with bupivacaine or lignocaine
Flores et al. (2013) [113]	Betamethasone 11.4 mg (single dose)	Reduced	—	Reduced	Comparison with oral deflazacort
Majid and Mahmood (2013) [114]	Dexamethasone 4 mg (single dose) IM deltoid, IV, submucosal, endoalveolar, divided doses of 4× 1 mg)	Reduced	Reduced	Reduced	Improved quality of life
Mehra et al. (2013) [115]	Dexamethasone 8 mg (single dose)	Reduced	Reduced	Reduced	Synergistic effect with ibuprofen
Nair et al. (2013) [116]	Dexamethasone 4 mg (single dose)	Reduced	No difference	No difference	—
Warraich et al. (2013) [117]	Dexamethasone 4 mg (single dose)	Reduced	Reduced	Reduced	—
Agostinho et al. (2014) [118]	Dexamethasone 4 mg or 12 mg (single dose)	Reduced	Reduced	Reduced	No difference between two dosages
Bhargava et al. (2014) [9]	Dexamethasone 4 mg (single dose)	Reduced	Reduced	Reduced	—
Ehsan (2014) [119]	Dexamethasone 4 mg (single dose)	Reduced	—	Reduced	—
Kaur et al. (2014) [120]	Methylprednisolone (single dose)	Reduced	Reduced	Reduced	Studied the synergistic effects with ibuprofen
Marques et al. (2014) [121]	Betamethasone 12 mg (single dose)	No difference	No difference	No difference	
Noboa et al. (2014) [122]	Dexamethasone 4 mg (single dose)	Reduced	Reduced	Reduced	Submucosal injection is as effective as oral intake
Shaikh et al. (2014) [123]	Dexamethasone 8 mg (two doses)	Reduced	—	Reduced	—

Authors (year)	Corticosteroids studied	Summary outcomes			
		Swelling	Pain	Trismus	Others
Ashraf et al. (2014) [124]	Methylprednisolone 125 mg (single dose)	Reduced	Reduced	Reduced	No difference between submucosal and intramuscular (gluteus) routes
Kocer et al. (2014) [125]	Methylprednisolone 20 mg (single dose)	Reduced	Not studied	Reduced	No difference in reducing trismus. IM masseter better in reducing swelling
Selvaraj et al. (2014) [126]	Methylpredniolone 40 mg (single dose)	Reduced	Reduced	Reduced	No difference between the masseter and gluteus intramuscular routes
Vyas et al. (2014) [127]	Methylprednisolone 40 mg (single dose)	Reduced	Reduced	Reduced	IM masseter more effective
Alcantara et al. (2014) [128]	Dexamethasone 8 mg (single dose) or Methylprednisolone 40 mg (single dose)	Reduced	Reduced	Reduced	Dexamethasone better in reducing swelling and trismus but no difference in reducing pain
Darawade et al. (2014) [129]	Dexamethasone 8 mg (single dose) or methylprednisolone 40 mg (single dose)	Reduced	Reduced	Reduced	Dexamethasone better in reducing swelling and trismus but no difference in reducing pain
Chappi et al. (2015) [130]	Methylprednisolone 5 m (multiple doses)	No difference	Reduced	No difference	Comparison against serratiopeptidase
Chaudhary et al. (2015) [131]	Dexamethasone 4 mg or 8 mg (single dose)	Reduced	Reduced	Reduced	—
Gopalakrishnan et al. (2015) [132]	Dexamethasone 4 mg (single dose)	Reduced	Reduced	Reduced	Submucosal more effective than intramuscular (deltoid) route
Sabhlok et al. (2015) [133]	Dexamethasone 4 mg (multiple dose) or dexamethasone 4 mg (single dose)	No difference	No difference	Reduced	Continuous oral medication is more effective than single IM
Zerener et al. (2015) [134]	Dexamethasone 4 mg (single dose) or triamcinolone acetonide 4 mg (single dose)	Reduced	Reduced	Reduced	No difference between the two drugs
Dereci et al. (2016) [135]	Dexamethasone 8 mg (single dose)	Reduced	—	—	—
Paiva-Oliveira et al. (2016) [136]	Dexamethasone 8 mg (single dose)	No difference	No difference	Reduced	Comparison with ketorolac tromethamine
Quadri et al. (2016) [137]	Dexamethasone 4 mg (single dose)	Reduced	Reduced	Reduced	—
Saravanan et al. (2016) [138]	Dexamethasone 4 mg/2 ml (single dose)	Reduced	Reduced	Reduced	SC is more effective than IM

Authors (year)	Corticosteroids studied	Summary outcomes			
		Swelling	Pain	Trismus	Others
Al-Dajani et al. (2017) [139]	Dexamethasone 0.1 mg/kg (single dose)	Reduced	Reduced	Reduced	
Al-Shamiri et al. (2017) [140]	Dexamethasone 8 mg (single dose)	Reduced	Reduced	Reduced	
Barbalho et al. (2017) [141]	Dexamethasone 8 mg (single dose)	Reduced	No difference	No difference	Co-administered with nimesulide 100 mg
Chugh et al. (2017) [142]	Dexamethasone 8 mg (single dose) or methylprednisolone 40 mg (single dose)	No difference	Reduced	Reduced	Dexamethasone more efficacious than methylprednisolone
Gozali et al. (2017) [143]	Dexamethasone 8 mg (single dose)	—	Reduced	—	—
Khalida et al. (2017) [144]	Dexamethasone 4 mg (single dose)	Reduced	—	Reduced	—
Lim and Ngeow (2017) [145]	Dexamethasone 4 mg or methylprednisolone 40 mg (single dose)	Reduced	Reduced	Reduced	—
Lima et al. (2017) [146]	Dexamethasone	Reduced	Reduced	Reduced	Comparison with diclofenac sodium
Lima et al. (2017) [147]	Dexamethasone 8 mg (single dose)	Reduced	Reduced	No difference	Comparison with diclofenac sodium
Mojsa et al. (2017) [148]	Dexamethasone 4 mg (single dose)	Reduced	Reduced	Reduced	Post-operative superior to preoperative in pain control
Rocha-Neto et al. (2017) [149]	Dexamethasone 8 mg (single dose)	No difference	Reduced	Reduced	Preoperative superior to post-operative in swelling reduction
Selimović et al. (2017) [150]	Methylprednisolone 32 mg (single dose)	—	—	Reduced	Co-administered with meloxicam
Syed et al. (2017) [151]	Dexamethasone 4 mg (single dose)	Reduced	Reduced	Reduced	—

Table 1. Summary of outcome of various researches related to the use of corticosteroids in oral and maxillofacial surgery, using impacted third molar surgery model.

reduced not only early and late oedema but also early trismus [25], while Moraschini et al. reported that submucosal dexamethasone was effective in reducing pain and swelling, but not trismus [26]. The last meta-analysis looking solely on preemptive dexamethasone against other oral anti-inflammatories found that it is more effective than methylprednisolone for reducing swelling and trismus. However, the authors found insufficient evidence to conclude that dexamethasone is better than other nonsteroidal anti-inflammatories or methylprednisolone as a preemptive analgesic [27]. In term of mode of administration, it has been suggested that systemic administration of corticosteroids is more effective [8].

Table 1 summarises all relevant studies on the use of corticosteroids using the third molar surgical model throughout the last 61 years. It shows a change in the trend of corticosteroid prescription, with low-dose single dose being favoured in the last two decades instead of the multiple or high-doses popular in the 1970s till 1990s. However, not many studies have look into the effect of corticosteroids in other oral surgical procedures. One reason for this limitation is the lack of opportunity to perform standardisation that is needed with other oral surgery/dentoalveolar surgical procedures. Mead et al. and Linenburg were among the few researchers who were able to conduct tests on patients undergoing different types of oral surgical procedure, including third molar surgery [28, 29]. Mead et al. administered oral triamcinolone postoperatively to 96 patients who had undergone varied oral surgical procedures and reported that it was superior to placebo in reducing oedema, pain and trismus [28].

In contrast, Linenburg studied the effect of dexamethasone on patients undergoing treatment of cellulitis and trismus due to an infectious process [29]. He reported a higher percentage of patients treated with corticosteroids being cured of cellulitis and trismus after 4 days than conventional treatment of hospitalisation, antibiotics, drainage and heat application. Linenburg also conducted a trial on 12 patients undergoing a full-mouth or a maxillary alveoloplasty and found that oedema and trismus last longer in patients without dexamethasone. A double-blinded comparison was performed on 50 patients undergoing both removal of bilaterally impacted third molars and full-mouth or maxillary alveoloplasty, and again he found that oedema and trismus last longer in patients without dexamethasone [29].

Not many randomised trials have been undertaken to study the effects of corticosteroids in oral and maxillofacial surgery. With regards to pain and swelling, its effect in traumatology has been studied once only in two separate RCTs; one on patients with blow out fracture [20] and the other on those with mandibular fracture [30]. In the observer-blinded study on the effect of dexamethasone 30 mg in blowout fracture surgery, Kormi et al. concluded that dexamethasone decreased post-operative pain and recommended it as a preemptive analgesic. In comparison, Dongol et al. reported that submucosal administration of dexamethasone after open reduction and internal fixation for mandibular fractures was effective in reducing post-operative swelling and pain. However, they did not observe any significant difference in mouth opening or difficulty in mandibular function [30].

Systemic corticosteroids are used to prevent post-surgical facial oedema, enhance patient comfort and prevent potential upper airway compromise in orthognathic surgery. Several trials even hinted a neuroregenerative effect on inferior alveolar nerve affected by orthognathic surgery [31]. Seo et al. reported that corticosteroids have the potential to accelerate the recovery of sensory impairment and it is desirable to start treatment later than 1 week post-operatively. For the record, the first recommendation for using corticosteroids in orthognathic surgery was made by Guernsey and DeChamplain [32] who reviewed complications affecting 22 patients who underwent sagittal ramisection. They suggested that post-operative swelling could be controlled by a regimen of dexamethasone used perioperatively. They described the diminution of post-operative oedema empirically but did not explain how they arrived at their recommended regime of corticosteroids. A study undertaken by Munro et al. [33] 2 years later however, failed to support this recommendation. There are, however, several trials that later confirmed the reduction of swelling in orthognathic patients [17, 34]. Most of them have been meta-analysed and/or underwent systematic review by several authors throughout the last 7 years [35]. Among others, Schaberg et al. reported that perioperative methylprednisolone (1 mg/kg) was effective in patients who underwent either a Le Fort I osteotomy or a transoral vertical osteotomy, as compared to control patients who were not given this medication [36]. Similarly, Weber and Griffin reported a reduction of swelling when dexamethasone was given perioperatively in patients undergoing bilateral sagittal split osteotomy (BSSO) [37]. This finding has been confirmed by other authors [34] who recently reported that the most effective dose of dexamethasone for bilateral sagittal split osteotomy was 16 mg given preoperatively.

Widar et al. although reported that betamethasone (single dose or multiple repeated dose up to 16 mg) reduces swelling, it does not reduce neurosensory disturbances over time in patients undergoing bilateral sagittal split osteotomy [17]. Similar findings have been reported by Mensink et al. and Pourdanesh et al. [38, 39]. Similar impact on the neurosensory disturbances after zygomatic complex fracture has been reported recently by Haapanen et al. [40]. Because of the limited number of studies that listed the benefit of administration of corticosteroids in orthognathic surgery, there is still a need for more robust evidence to support their use [41].

Although many studies and systematic reviews found that corticosteroids are beneficial in controlling various post-operative sequelae, there are some who discouraged their use because of the fear of several potential adverse side effects [42]. A most recent systemic review and meta-analysis on the perioperative use of corticosteroids in orthognathic surgery although confirmed that they reduced facial oedema, found that adverse effects were inconsistently screened and reported [37]. The least severe adverse effect is the development of steroid induced acne in some female orthognathic surgery patients [43]. Other more severe complications include adrenal suppression [44], acute psychiatric reactions such as psychosis or inappropriate euphoria [42], a higher infection rate and decreased healing potential.

There are several recent studies that reported conflicting adverse effects with regards to disturbance in surgical wound healing, especially in major oral and maxillofacial surgeries. Thorén et al. in a retrospective study reported that the rate of disturbance in surgical wound healing for patients who had received perioperative steroids was more than twice (6.0%) the corresponding rate for patients who did not receive steroids (2.8%), although this difference was not statistically significant. They reported that intraoral surgical approach was a significant predictor to this adverse effect [45]. Snäll et al. in contrast, did not observe similar problem in operative treatment of mandibular fractures, although they found that older age was a significant predictor of impaired healing [46]. However, in another study on open reduction and fixation of zygomatic complex fractures, Snäll et al. reported increased disturbance in surgical wound healing and did not recommend the administration of corticosteroids for such surgery [47].

Other serious complications associated with the administration of corticosteroids are acute gastrointestinal reactions (abdominal pain, haematemesis, and/or maelena), hyperglycemia, superinfection and septicaemia [48] and avascular necrosis of the femoral head [49]. It has been reported that common regimes used in orthognathic surgery involve a total dose of 1830 mg of methylprednisolone over a 30-hour period, a dosage similar to some short-term, high-dose regimens described in orthopaedic case reports of avascular necrosis of the femoral head [49]. Hence, there is a potential risk for this group for patients to develop avascular necrosis. Fortunately, Precious et al., found no evidence that this has occurred in the only study that reviewed the need of total hip replacement in 1276 orthognathic patients. They concluded that the use of systemic corticosteroids for short duration in orthognathic surgery is unlikely related to AVN of the femoral head and the attendant need for total hip replacement [50].

3. Corticosteroids in oral medicine

3.1. Recurrent aphthous ulcer

Recurrent apthous ulcers top the list of the commonest oral mucosal lesions encountered by any dental practitioners. Generally, this condition is self-limiting and resolves within 2–3 weeks with the exception of major recurrent aphthous ulcer [162]. Despite it being self-limiting, the pain and the frequency of recurrence can be very devastating to the patients. Corticosteroid is one of the available treatment options for recurrent aphthous ulcers.

The use of topical corticosteroids can be advocated when topical anesthetic, antiseptics and anti-inflammatory agents are no longer effective in relieving the discomfort caused by these ulcers. It was suggested to begin with less potent drug such as triamcinolone and moving gradually to more potent corticosteroids like clobetasol [163]. These corticosteroids come in the form of mouthwashes, ointments, creams and adhesive pastes.

Triamcinolone acetonide 0.1% is the commonly used concentration although it can actually be used at concentration ranging from 0.05 to 0.5%, and is usually applied 3–4 times a day [164]. For maximum effect of the drug, it should be in contact with the ulcer for as long as possible. Therefore, it is advisable to refrain from any oral intake within 20 minutes after application or touching the affected area [164]. Fluocinolone acetonide and clobetasol require lower concentrations of 0.025–0.05% since they are potent corticosteroid. These drugs are usually applied 4–5 times a day [164]. Al-Na'amah et al. in 2009 studied the use of dexamethasone 0.1% by comparing it to triamcinolone acetonide 0.1% and found that both drugs are effective in the treatment of recurrent aphthous ulcers [159].

On the other hand, systemic corticosteroids are rarely required in the treatment of recurrent aphthous ulcers except for cases that are not responsive to topical medications [165]. Oral prednisone with starting dose of 25 mg/day is recommended [165]. This is then followed by tapering of the dosage during a period of 2 months. The tapering regime as reported by Femiano et al. in 2003 and 2010 (**Table 2**) had been shown to be effective in the treatment and prevention of recurrence of aphthous ulcer [161].

3.2. Oral lichen planus

Table 3 shows that topical corticosteroids are reasonably effective in the treatment of oral lichen planus. The use of more potent corticosteroids was associated with more improvement following therapy. However, incidence of oral candidiasis also increased in proportion

Authors (year)	Corticosteroids	Outcomes			
		Pain reduction	Ulcer size reduction	Duration of ulcer	Recurrence
Topical					
Yeoman (1978) [152]	Betamethasone valerate 1 puff QID (max 16 puff/24 hours)	Reduced	–	Reduced	–
Pimlott (1983) [153]	0.05% fluocinonide ointment + orabase	Reduced	–	Reduced	Less
Lo Muzio et al. (2001) [154]	0.05% clobetasol ointment	Reduced	–	–	–
Rhodus and Bereuter (1998) [155]	Kenalog-in-Orabase, TDS	Reduced	–	Reduced	–
Teixeira et al. (1999) [156]	0.1% mometasone furoate lotion QID	Reduced	–	Reduced	–
Rodriguez (2007) [157]	0.05% clobetasol propionate oral paste QID × 5 days	Reduced	Faster	–	–
Al-Na'amah et al. (2009) [158]	Dexamucobase; 0.1% dexamethasone QID	Reduced	Faster	Reduced	–
Al-Na'amah et al. (2009) [158]	Kenalog; 0.1% triamcinolone acetonide QID	Reduced	Fast	Reduced	–
Fani et al. (2012) [159]	0.1% triamcinolone acetonide ointment TDS	Significantly better therapeutic effect in triamcinolone group			
Systemic					
Femiano et al. (2003) [160]	Prednisone 25 mg OD × 1 week, 20 mg OD × 2 weeks, 15 mg OD × 2 weeks, 10 mg OD × 2 weeks, 5 mg OD × 1 week	Reduced	–	Reduced	Less
Femiano et al. (2010) [161]	Prednisone 25 mg OD × 15 days, 12.5 mg OD × 15 days, 6.25 mg OD × 15 days, 6.25 mg EOD × 15 days	Reduced.	–	Reduced	Less

Table 2. Topical and systemic corticosteroids used in the treatment of recurrent aphthous ulcer.

Corticosteroid	Author (year)	Results (%)		
		Complete response	Partial response	No response
Hydrocortisone hemisuccinate	Holbrook et al. (1988) [165]	48	37	15
Betamethasone sodium phosphate	Hegarty et al. (2002) [166]	0	73	27
Betamethasone valerate 0.1 mg	Cawson (1968) [167]	43	23	34
Triamcinolone acetonide 0.1%	Thongprasom et al. (1992) [168]	42	Not mentioned	Not mentioned
Fluocinolone acetonide 0.1%	Thongprasom et al. (1992) [168]	68	Not mentioned	Not mentioned
Fluocinonide 0.05%	Lozada and Silverman (1980) [169]	52	48	0
	Voute et al. (1993) [170]	20	60	20
	Carbone et al. (1999) [171]	25	65	10
Fluticasone propionate 0.05%	Hegarty et al. (2002) [166]	0	80	20
Clobetasol propionate 0.05%	Lozada-Nur et al. (1991) [172]	56	22	22
	Sardella et al. (1988) [173]	57	21.5	21.5
	Carbone et al. (1999) [170]	75	25	0
	Gonzales-Moles et al. (2002) [174]	93	0	7

Table 3. Topical corticosteroids used in the treatment of oral lichen planus.

to the potency of corticosteroids used [169, 171]. Carbone et al. in 2003 reported that the use of topical corticosteroid can be as effective or even more effective than systemic corticosteroids in the treatment of oral lichen planus [175]. On the other hand, the use of systemic corticosteroids should be restricted to acute exacerbations or multiple lesions. Topical regime can be prescribed in combination of systemic regime to reduce side effects of systemic corticosteroids [176]. The commonly used systemic corticosteroid is prednisone which is usually prescribed within the range of 40–80 mg/day to achieve clinical response. To avoid adverse effects of this drug, it is best to prescribe the lowest dose for the shortest duration possible. To achieve this, prednisone can either be given for a brief period of 5–7 days and stop abruptly or the dose can be tapered down by 5–10 mg/day gradually over a period of 2–4 weeks [177].

Intralesional injection is another alternative for administrating corticosteroids in the treatment of oral lichen planus. Hydrocortisone, dexamethasone, betamethasone, triamcinolone acetonide and methylprednisolone have been used for intralesion injection. This method is however, painful and causes localised mucosal atrophy. Intralesional injection is also not feasible in cases of multiple widespread lesions [176, 178].

3.3. Pemphigus vulgaris and mucous membrane pemphigoid

Corticosteroids have become the mainstay of treatment for pemphigus ever since the first case series reported by Ryan in 1971 [179]. Despite being the gold standard in the treatment of pemphigus, the use of corticosteroids is still mulled by many physicians due to the adverse effects of long-term treatment and difficulty in ascertaining the best regimen [180]. Due to the high mortality rate of this condition, studies conducted were just comparing various groups of drugs used, different dosages and modes of administration rather than purely investigating the efficacy of a particular drug. Most of the articles published were mainly case reports and case series [181].

More than three-quarter of the patients with pemphigus vulgaris presented with oral lesions. And these lesions are the presenting signs of half of the patients diagnosed with pemphigus vulgaris [182]. As in the treatment of oral lesions in pemphigus vulgaris, oral lesions secondary to mucous membrane pemphigoid are also treated with moderate to high potency topical corticosteroids (fluocinonide 0.05%, clobetasol 0.05%), applied 2–3 times per day. The frequency of application can be tapered gradually with improvement of symptoms [182]. Bear in mind that as a result of prolonged topical corticosteroids use, infection such as candidiasis and reactivation herpes simplex virus can occur. Combination of other drugs such as dapsone, tetracycline and nicotinamide is recommended.

As for systemic corticosteroids, an initial dose of 0.5–1 mg/kg/day of prednisone plus adjuvant immunosuppressants is recommended. This dose is continued until all existing lesions have healed and no development of new lesions is noticed clinically. Once this is achieved, tapering of the dose can be performed [182]. The ultimate aim in the treatment strategy is to minimise the dose of systemic corticosteroids while controlling the disease with immunosuppressants.

In patient with severe pemphigus vulgaris, corticosteroid pulse therapy can be administered to induce remission. In this therapy, a very high-dose of corticosteroid (500–1000 mg methylprednisolone or 100–200 mg dexamethasone given in divided dose on 3 consecutive days) is given in a short period of time in combination immunosuppressants and maintenance dose of corticosteroids [183].

3.4. Bell's palsy

With an unclear knowledge of the aetiology of Bell's palsy, it poses a great challenge in coming up with an optimal treatment of the condition. To achieve a good outcome, corticosteroid needs to be given within 72 hours of onset of facial palsy. Berg et al. in 2012 found that prednisolone given within 72 hours of onset of palsy significantly improve outcome in mild to moderate palsy but not in severe palsy. The regime used was prednisolone 60 mg/day for 5 days, followed by 10 mg/day for another 5 days [184]. Using the same regimen, another study found that prednisolone significantly achieve complete recovery in mild to severe palsy and less synkinesis observed in mild and moderate palsy. However, no significant reduction of synkinesis in severe cases was reported [185]. Murthy and Saxena in 2011 suggested two corticosteroid regimens for the treatment of Bell's palsy which were either prednisolone 60 mg/day for 5 days followed by 10 mg/day for another 5 days or prednisolone 25 mg twice a day for 10 days [186]. The American Academy of Otolaryngology-Head and Neck Surgery recommended a 10-day course of oral steroids with at least 5 days at a high-dose (either prednisolone 50 mg for 10 days or prednisone 60 mg for 5 days with a 5-day taper) initiated within 72 hours of symptom onset [187].

Conflicting results were reported in different studies on the benefit of combining anti viral therapy with corticosteroid to achieve better outcome. Minnerop et al. reported that combination of famciclovir and prednisone was superior to prednisone alone in cases of severe Bell's palsy [188]. Combining antiviral therapy with prednisone increase the recovery rate slightly but not significantly compared to prednisone monotherapy [189]. On the other hand, valacyclovir was found to have no additional effect to prednisolone in sequelae of Bell's palsy [869] and the addition of acyclovir to prednisolone did not significantly improve recovery from Bell's palsy [190]. Despite conflicting results from various studies, Madhok et al. in their Cochrane review in 2016 concurred with current evidences that corticosteroids showed significant benefit in the treatment of Bell's palsy [191].

3.5. Temporomandibular joint

In year 1953, Horten reported the use of intraarticular injection of steroids into the temporomandibular joint (TMJ) space. Being the first to perform this procedure in the TMJ, he was then inspired by Hollander and colleagues' work where they injected hydrocortisone into other arthritic joints [192]. Kopp et al. in 1985 injected betamethasone into the TMJ space in a group of patients with TMJ pain and dysfunction, showed that betamethasone was effective in reducing joint pain up to 4 weeks [193]. About 6 years later, Kopp and colleagues performed intraarticular injection using methylprednisolone which showed similar promising results up to 4 weeks [194]. Bjørnland et al. injected betamethasone into the TMJ space of patients with osteoarthritis and myofascial pain 10 years ago. Although betamethasone managed to reduce joint pain, sodium hyaluronate which was given in the other study group was found to be more effective [195]. Another promising use of corticosteroids is for the management of disc displacement without reduction. Samiee et al. found that combined intraarticular injection of local anaesthetic and corticosteroids improved mouth opening [196].

Using computed tomography (CT) scan, Møystad et al. evaluated the bony changes in osteoarthritic TMJ following intraarticular injection of sodium hyaluronate and corticosteroid (betamethasone). The number of cases that showed disease progression, regression and no changes were almost equal [197]. This finding raised the question on the effectiveness of corticosteroids as intraarticular injection. Another study by Bouloux et al. recently again showed no added effect of using corticosteroids or another agent, hyaluronic acid in arthrocentesis [198]. In cases of juvenile idiopathic arthritis, a study by Resnick et al. showed that although intraarticular corticosteroid (triamcinolone hexacetonide) injection did reduce TMJ sinovitis pain, its efficacy for long-term inflammation and joint destruction control needs further studies.

4. Corticosteroids in endodontology

The first intracanal medication using corticosteroids was reported by Wolfsohn in 1954. In that study, he showed that hydrocortisone was effective in reducing severe secondary inflammatory reactions in the apical periodontal tissue following endodontic treatment [208]. Other authors who also used corticosteroids as intracanal medication, as listed in **Table 4**, reported beneficial outcome in the post-operative or post-instrumentation pain. Besides reducing pain, Thong et al. reported that the use of corticosteroid-antibiotic and calcium hydroxide significantly inhibited periodontal ligament inflammation and inflammatory root resorption [209]. A well-known intracanal medication, Ledermix®, is corticosteroid-antibiotic compound which consists of 1% triamcinolone acetonide and 3.2% demeclocycline hydrochloride in a polyethylene glycol base. The function of antibiotic in that paste is to compensate for the possible corticosteroid-induced immunosuppessing effect [210]. Despite being an effective intracanal medication, Ledermix® was found to cause discolouration of the teeth especially when it is placed above the cementoenamel junction. Therefore, to avoid this Ledermix® should be placed below the gingival margin [211].

Similar to the use of corticosteroids in third molar surgery, local injection of corticosteroids have been found to reduce post treatment pain. Kaufman et al. evaluated the effect of intraligamental injection of corticosteroids on post treatment pain. They found that intraligamental injection of methylprednisolone significantly decreased post treatment pain [202]. Nobuhara et al. in their histological study found that local infiltration of dexamethasone significantly reduced inflammation of the periapical tissue [212].

Author (year)	**Corticosteroids**	**Outcome**
		Post treatment pain
Intracanal		
Rogers et al. (1999) [199]	Dexamethasone 0.4 mg (intracanal) and ketorolac tromethamine 3 mg (intracanal)	Reduced
Negm (2001) [200]	Kenacomb (antibiotics and triamcinolone acetonide 0.1%)	Reduced
Ehrmann et al. (2003) [201]	Ledermix (1% triamcinolone acetonide, 3.2% demeclocycline)	Reduced
Local (injection)		
Kaufman et al. (1994) [202]	4–8 mg methylprednisolone (intraligamental injection)	Reduced
Systemic		
Stewart and Chilton (1958) [203]	Metreton (2.5 mg prednisone, 2 mg chlopheniramine) TDS × 2 days, penicillin 250 mg TDS × 3 days	Reduced
Stewart (1962) [204]	Dexamethasone 0.75 mg BD × 2 days	Reduced
Krasner and Jackson (1986) [205]	Dexamethasone 0.75 mg × 7 tablets, 3 tablets immediately after procedure, one tablet every 3 hours	Reduced
Glassman et al. (1989) [206]	Dexamethsone 4 mg × 3 tablets, one tablet taken immediately after procedure, one tablet every 4 hours	Reduced
Liesinger et al. (1993) [207]	Dexamethasone 0.07–0.09 mg/kg (intramuscular injection)	Reduced

Table 4. Studies on usage of corticosteroids via various routes of administration.

From the studies shown in **Table 4**, it is obvious that they confirmed the favourable result of systemic administration of corticosteroids in alleviating post treatment pain. In all the studies, corticosteroids were only given for a very short period. Therefore, the possibility of adverse effects arising from short-term corticosteroids is very unlikely [7].

5. Conclusion

The uses of corticosteroids are very well established in the field of oral medicine and endodontology. On the other hand, in the field of oral and maxillofacial surgery, despite being consistently effective in controlling post-surgical oedema, corticosteroids provide rather less consistent outcome in pain control as well as trismus reduction. Its impact on wound healing is varied.

Author details

Wei Cheong Ngeow*, Daniel Lim and Nurhalim Ahmad

*Address all correspondence to: ngeowy@um.edu.my

Faculty of Dentistry, University of Malaya, Kuala Lumpur, Malaysia

References

[1] Zandi M. The role of corticosteroids in today's oral and maxillofacial surgery. In: Qian X, editor. Glucocorticoids—New Recognition of Our Familiar Friend. InTech; 2012. DOI: 10.5772/48655. Available from: https://www.intechopen.com/books/glucocorticoids-new-recognition-of-our-familiar-friend/the-role-of-corticosteroids-in-today-s-oral-and-maxillofacial-surgery

[2] Strean LP. The possible role of cortisone in dentistry. New York Journal of Dentistry. 1951; **22**:102-104

[3] Strean LP, Horton C. Hydrocortisone in dental practice. Dental Digest. 1954;**59**:8-16

[4] Spies TD, Dreizen S, Stone RE, Garcia-Lopez G, Lopez-Toca R, Reboredo A. A clinical appraisal of ACTH and cortisone as therapeutic agents in dental medicine. Oral Surgery, Oral Medicine, and Oral Pathology. 1952;**5**:25-40

[5] Kenny FA. Editorial & clinical observation. Journal of Oral Surgery. 1954;**12**:314

[6] Ross R, White CP. Evaluation of hydrocortisone in prevention of postoperative complications after oral surgery: A preliminary report. Journal of Oral Surgery. 1958;**16**:220-226

[7] Ngeow WC, Lim D. Do corticosteroids still have a role in the management of third molar surgery? Advances in Therapy. 2016;**33**:1105-1139. DOI: 10.1007/s12325-016-0357-y

[8] Alexander R, Throndson R. A review of perioperative corticosteroid use in dentoalveolar surgery. Oral Surgery, Oral Medicine, Oral Pathology, Oral Radiology, and Endodontics. 2000;**90**:406-415. DOI: 10.1067/moe.2000.109778

[9] Bhargava D, Sreekumar K, Deshpande A. Effects of intra-space injection of twin mix versus intraoral-submucosal, intramuscular, intravenous and per-oral administration of dexamethasone on post-operative sequelae after mandibular impacted third molar surgery: A preliminary clinical comparative study. Oral and Maxillofacial Surgery. 2014;**18**:293-296. DOI: 10.1007/s10006-013-0412-7

[10] Carroll W, Patel K. Steroids and fluorouracil for keloids and hypertrophic scars. JAMA Facial Plastic Surgery. 2015;**17**:77-79. DOI: 10.1001/jamafacial.2014.1355

[11] Lagalla G, Logullo F, Di Bella P, Provinciali L, Ceravolo MG. Influence of early high-dose steroid treatment on Bell's palsy evolution. Neurological Sciences. 2002;**23**:107-112. DOI: 10.1007/s100720200035

[12] Baker PR. Diagnosis and management of Bell's palsy. Oral and Maxillofacial Surgery Clinics of North America. 2000;**12**:303-308

[13] Greenstein G, Carpentieri JR, Cavallaro J. Nerve damage related to implant dentistry: Incidence, diagnosis, and management. The Compendium of Continuing Education in Dentistry. 2015;**36**:652-659

[14] Barron RP, Benoliel R, Zeltser R, Eljay E, Nahlieli O, Gracely RH. Effect of dexamethasone and dipyrone on lingual and inferior alveolar nerve hypersensitivity following third molar extractions: Preliminary report. Journal of Orofacial Pain. 2014;**18**:62-68

[15] Low LF, Audimulam H, Lim HW, Selvaraju K, Balasundram S. Steroids in maxillofacial space infection: A retrospective cohort study. Open Journal of Stomatology. 2017;**7**:397-407. DOI: 10.4236/ojst.2017.79034

[16] Kormi E, Snäll J, Törnwall J, Thorén H. A survey of the use of perioperative glucocorticoids in oral and maxillofacial surgery. Journal of Oral and Maxillofacial Surgery. 2016;**74**:1548-1551. DOI: 10.1016/j.joms.2016.02.027

[17] Widar F, Kashani H, Alsén B, Dahlin C, Rasmusson L. The effects of steroids in preventing facial oedema, pain, and neurosensory disturbances after bilateral sagittal split osteotomy: A randomized controlled trial. International Journal of Oral and Maxillofacial Surgery. 2015;**44**:252-258. DOI: 10.1016/j.ijom.2014.08.002

[18] Baxendale BR, Vater M, Lavery KM. Dexamethasone reduces pain and swelling following extraction of third molar teeth. Anaesthesia. 1993;**48**:961-964

[19] Flood TR, McManners J, el-Attar A, Moos KF. Randomized prospective study of the influence of steroids on postoperative eye-opening after exploration of the orbital floor. The British Journal of Oral & Maxillofacial Surgery. 1999;**37**:312-315

[20] Kormi E, Snäll J, Koivusalo AM, Suominen AL, Thorén H, Törnwall J. Analgesic effect of perioperative systemic dexamethasone on blowout fracture surgery. Journal of Oral and Maxillofacial Surgery. 2017;**75**:1232-1237. DOI: 10.1016/j/joms.2016.09.026

[21] Abdel-Aziz M, Ahmed A, Naguib N, Abdel-Khalik MI. The effect of steroid injection of the tongue base on reducing postoperative airway obstruction in cleft palate repair. International Journal of Oral and Maxillofacial Surgery. 2012;**41**:612-615. DOI: 10.1016/j.ijom.2012.01.013

[22] Assimes T, Lessard ML. The use of perioperative corticosteroids in craniomaxillofacial surgery. Plastic and Reconstructive Surgery. 1999;**103**:313-321

[23] Moore PA, Nahouraii HS, Zovko JG, Wisniewski SR. Dental therapeutic practice patterns I the U.S. II. Analgesics, corticosteroids, and antibiotics. General Dentistry. 2006;**54**:201-207

[24] Markiewicz MR, Brady MF, Ding EL, Dodson TB. Corticostreoids reduce postoperative morbidity after third molar surgery: A systematic review and meta-analysis. Journal of Oral and Maxillofacial Surgery. 2008;**66**:1881-1894. DOI: 10.1016/j.joms.2008.04.022

[25] Chen Q, Chen J, Hu B, Feng G, Song J. Submucosal injection of dexamethasone reduces postoperative discomfort after third-molar extraction: A systemic review and meta-analysis. Journal of the American Dental Association. 2017;**148**:81-91. DOI: 10.1016/j.adaj.2016.09.014

[26] Moraschini V, Hidalgo R, Porto Barboza E. Effect of submucosal injection of dexamethasone after third molar surgery: A meta-analysis of randomized controlled trials. International Journal of Oral and Maxillofacial Surgery. 2016;**45**:232-240. DOI: 10.1016/j.ijom.2015.09.008

[27] Falci SGM, Lima TC, Martins CC, Santos CRRD, Pinheiro MLP. Preemptive effect of dexamethasone in third-molar surgery: A meta-analysis. Anesthesia Progress. 2017;**64**:136-143. DOI: 10.2344/anpr-64-05-08

[28] Mead SV, Lynch DF, Mead SC, Wolkowicz J. Triamcinolone given orally to control postoperative reactions to oral surgery. Journal of Oral Surgery. 1964;**22**:484-487

[29] Linenberg W. The clinical evaluation of dexamethasone in oral surgery. Oral Surgery, Oral Medicine, and Oral Pathology. 1965;**20**:6-28

[30] Dongol A, Jaisani MR, Pradhan L, Dulal S, Sagtani A. A randomized clinical trial of the effects of submucosal dexamethasone after surgery for mandibular fractures. Journal of Oral and Maxillofacial Surgery. 2015;**73**:1124-1132. DOI: 10.1016/j.joms.2014.12.042

[31] Seo K, Tanaka Y, Terumitsu M, Someya G. Efficacy of steroid treatment for sensory impairment after orthognathic surgery. Journal of Oral and Maxillofacial Surgery. 2004;**62**:1193-1197

[32] Guernsey LH, DeChamplain RW. Sequelae of complications of the intraoral sagittal oseotomy in the mandibular rami. Oral Surgery. 1971;**32**:176-192

[33] Munro IR, Boyd JB, Wainwright DJ. Effect of steroids in maxillofacial surgery. Annals of Plastic Surgery. 1986;**17**:440-444

[34] Abukawa H, Ogawa T, Kono M, Koizumi T, Kawase-Koga Y, Chikazu D. Intravenous dexamethasone administration before orthognathic surgery reduces the postoperative edema

fo the masseter muscle: A randomized controlled trial. Journal of Oral and Maxillofacial Surgery. 2017;**75**:1257-1262. DOI: 10.1016/j.joms.2016.12.048

[35] Jean S, Dionne PL, Bouchard C, Giasson L, Turgeon AF. Perioperative systemic corticosteroids in orthognathic surgery: A systematic review and meta-analysis. Journal of Oral and Maxillofacial Surgery. DOI: 10.1016/j.joms.2017.06.014

[36] Schaberg SJ, Stuller CB, Edwards SM. Effect of methylprednisolone on swelling after orthognathic surgery. Journal of Oral and Maxillofacial Surgery. 1984;**42**:356-361

[37] Weber CR, Griffin JM. Evaluation of dexamethasone for reducing postoperative edema and inflammatory response after orthognathic surgery. Journal of Oral and Maxillofacial Surgery. 1994;**52**:35-39

[38] Mensink G, Zweers A, Wolterbeek R, Dicker GG, Groot RH, van Merkesteyn RJ. Neurosensory disturbances one year after bilateral sagittal split osteotomy of the mandibula performed with separators: A multi-centre prospective study. Journal of Cranio-Maxillo-Facial Surgery. 2012;**40**:763-767. DOI: 10.1016/j.jcms.2012.02.003

[39] Pourdanesh F, Khayampour A, Jamalian A. Therapeutic effects of local application of dexamethasone during bilateral sagittal split ramus osteotomy surgery. Journal of Oral and Maxillofacial Surgery. 2014;**72**:1391-1394. DOI: 10.1016/j.joms.2013.12.025

[40] Haapanen A, Thorén H, Apajalahti S, Suominen AL, Snäll J. Does dexamethasone facilitate neurosensory function regeneration after zygomatic fracture? A randomized controlled trial. Journal of Oral and Maxillofacial Surgery. DOI: 10.1016/j.joms.2017.08.009

[41] Chegini S, Dhariwal DK. Review of evidence for the use of steroids in orthognathic surgery. The British Journal of Oral & Maxillofacial Surgery. 2012;**50**:97-101. DOI: 10.1016/j.bjoms.2010.11.019

[42] Galen DM, Beck M, Buchbinder D. Steroid psychosis after orthognathic surgery: A case report. Journal of Oral and Maxillofacial Surgery. 1997;**55**:294-297

[43] Precious DS, Hoffman CD, Miller R. Steroid acne after orthognathic surgery. Oral Surgery, Oral Medicine, Oral Pathology and Oral Radiology. 1992;**74**:279-281

[44] Cawson RA, James J. Adrenal crisis in a dental patient having systemic corticosteroid. The British Journal of Oral Surgery. 1973;**10**:305-309

[45] Thorén H, Snäll J, Kormi E, Numminen L, Fäh R, Iizuka T, Lindqvist C, Törnwall J. Does perioperative glucocorticosteroid treatment correlate with disturbance in surgical wound healing after treatment of facial fractures? A retrospective study. Journal of Oral and Maxillofacial Surgery. 2009;**67**:1884-1888. DOI: 10.1016/j.joms.2009.04.089

[46] Snäll J, Kormi E, Lindqvist C, Suominen AL, Mesimäki K, Törnwall J, Thorén H. Impairment of wound healing after operative treatment of mandibular fractures, and the influence of dexamethasone. The British Journal of Oral & Maxillofacial Surgery. 2013;**51**:808-812. DOI: 10.1016/j.bjoms.2013.08.015

[47] Snäll J, Kormi E, Koivusalo AM, Lindqvist C, Suominen AL, Törnwall J, Thorén H. Effects of perioperatively administered dexamethasone on surgical wound healing in patients undergoing surgery for zygomatic fracture: A prospective study. Oral Surgery, Oral Medicine, Oral Pathology, Oral Radiology. 2014;**117**:685-659. DOI: 10.1016/j.oooo.2014.02.033

[48] Boston Collaborative Drug Surveillance Program: Acute adverse reactions to prednisone in relation to dosage. Clinical Pharmacology and Therapeutics. 1972;**13**:694-698

[49] Anderson JM, Helm R. Multiple joint osteonecrosis following short-term steroid therapy: Case report. The Journal of Bone and Joint Surgery. American Volume. 1982;**64**:139-141

[50] Precious D, Armstrong J, Morrison A, Field C. The incidence of total hip replacement in orthognathic surgery patients receiving short-term steroid therapy. Journal of Oral and Maxillofacial Surgery. 1992;**50**:956-957

[51] Ware WH, Campbell JC, Taylor RC. Effect of a steroid on postoperative swelling and trismus. Dental Progress. 1963;**3**:116-120

[52] Nathanson NR, Seifert DM. Betamethasone in dentistry. A clinical report. Oral Surgery, Oral Medicine, Oral Pathology and Oral Radiology. 1964;**18**:715-721

[53] Hooley JR, Francis FH. Betamethasone in traumatic oral surgery. Journal of Oral Surgery. 1969;**27**:398-403

[54] Messer EJ, Keller JJ. The use of intraoral dexamethasone after extraction of mandibular third molars. Oral Surgery, Oral Medicine, and Oral Pathology. 1975;**40**:594-598

[55] Caci F, Gluck GM. Double-blind study of prednisolone and papase as inhibitors of complications after oral surgery. Journal of the American Dental Association (Chicago, IL). 1976;**93**:325-328

[56] Huffman GG. Use of methylprednisolone sodium succinate to reduce post-operative edema after removal of impacted third molars. Journal of Oral Surgery. 1977;**35**:198-199

[57] Edilby GI, Canniff JP, Harris M. A double-blind placebo-controlled trial of the effect of dexamethasone on postoperative swelling. Journal of Dental Research. 1982;**61**:556

[58] Skjelbred P, Løkken P. Post-operative pain and inflammatory reaction reduced by injection of a corticosteroid: A controlled trial in bilateral oral surgery. European Journal of Clinical Pharmacology. 1982;**21**:391-396

[59] Skjelbred P, Løkken P. Reduction of pain and swelling by a corticosteroid injected 3 hours after surgery. European Journal of Clinical Pharmacology. 1982;**23**:141-146

[60] Skjelbred P, Lokken P. Effects of naloxone on post-operative pain and steroid-induced analgesia. British Journal of Clinical Pharmacology. 1983;**15**:221-226

[61] Bystedt H, Nordenram A. Effect of methylprednisolone on complications after removal of impacted mandibular third molars. Swedish Dental Journal. 1985;**9**:65-69

[62] ElHag M, Coghlan K, Christmas P, Harvey W, Harris M. The anti-inflammatory effects of dexamethasone and therapeutic ultrasound in oral surgery. The British Journal of Oral & Maxillofacial Surgery. 1985;**23**:17-23

[63] Pederson A. Decadronphosphate in the relief of complaints after third molar surgery. International Journal of Oral and Maxillofacial Surgery. 1985;**14**:235-240

[64] Sisk A, Bonnington GJ. Evaluation of methylprednisolone and flurbiprofen for inhibition of postoperative inflammatory response. Oral Surgery, Oral Medicine, and Oral Pathology. 1985;**60**:137-145

[65] Beirne OR, Hollander BH. The effect of methylprednisolone on pain trismus and swelling after removal of third molars. Oral Surgery, Oral Medicine, and Oral Pathology. 1986;**61**: 134-138

[66] Olstad OA, Skjelbred P. Comparison of the analgesic effect of a corticosteroid and paracetamol in patients with pain after oral surgery. British Journal of Clinical Pharmacology. 1986;**22**:437-442

[67] Holland CS. The influence of methylprednisolone on post-operative swelling following oral surgery. The British Journal of Oral & Maxillofacial Surgery. 1987;**25**:293-299

[68] Troullos ES, Hargreaves KM, Butler DP, Dionne RA. Comparison of nonsteroidal anti-inflammatory drugs, ibuprofen and flurbiprofen, with methylprednisolone and placebo for acute pain, swelling, and trismus. Journal of Oral and Maxillofacial Surgery. 1990;**48**: 945-952

[69] Neupert EA, Lee JW, Philput CB, Gordon JR. Evaluation of dexamethasone for reduction of postsurgical sequelae of third molar removal. Journal of Oral and Maxillofacial Surgery. 1992;**50**:1177-1182

[70] Baxendale BR, Vater M, Lavery KM. Dexamethasone reduces pain and swelling following extraction of third molar teeth. Anesthesia. 1993;**48**:961-964

[71] Hyrkäs T, Ylipaavalniemi P, Oikarinen VJ, Paakkari I. A comparison of diclofenac with and without single-dose intravenous steroid to prevent postoperative pain after third molar removal. Journal of Oral and Maxillofacial Surgery. 1993;**51**:634-636

[72] Milles M, Desjardins PJ. Reduction of postoperative facial swelling by low-dose methylprednisolone: An experimental study. Journal of Oral and Maxillofacial Surgery. 1993;**51**: 987-991

[73] Schmelzeisen R, Frölich JC. Prevention of postoperative swelling and pain by dexamethasone after operative removal of impacted third molar teeth. European Journal of Clinical Pharmacology. 1993;**44**:275-277

[74] Schultze-Mosgau S, Schmelseizen R, Frölich JC, Schmele H. Use of ibuprofen and methylprednisolone for the prevention of pain and swelling after removal of impacted third molars. Journal of Oral and Maxillofacial Surgery. 1995;**53**:2-7

[75] Esen E, Tasar F, Akhan O. Determination of the antiinflammatory effects of methylprednisolone on the sequelae of third molar surgery. Journal of Oral and Maxillofacial Surgery. 1999;**57**:1201-1206

[76] Dionne RA, Gordon SM, Rowan J, Kent A, Brahim JS. Dexamethasone suppresses peripheral prostanoid levels without analgesia in a clinical model of acute inflammation. Journal of Oral and Maxillofacial Surgery. 2003;**61**:997-1003

[77] Ustün Y, Erdogan O, Esen E, Karsli ED. Comparison of the effects of 2 doses of methylprednisolone on pain, swelling, and trismus after third molar surgery. Oral Surgery, Oral Medicine, Oral Pathology, Oral Radiology, and Endodontics. 2003;**96**:535-539. DOI: 10.1016/s1079210403004645

[78] Bamgbose BO, Akinwande JA, Adeyomo WL, Ladeinde AL, Arotiba GT, Ogunlewe MO. Effects of co-administered dexamethasone and diclofenac potassium on pain, swelling and trismus following third molar surgery. Head & Face Medicine. 2005;**7**:1-11. DOI: 10.1186/1746-160X-1-11

[79] López-Carriches C, Martínez-González JM, Donado-Rodríguez M. Analgesic efficacy of diclofenac versus methylprednisolone in the control of postoperative pain after surgical removal of lower third molars. Medicina Oral, Patología Oral y Cirugía Bucal. 2005;**10**:432-439

[80] Moore PA, Brar P, Smiga ER, Costello BJ. Preemptive rofecoxib and dexamethasone for prevention of pain and trismus following third molar surgery. Oral Surgery, Oral Medicine, Oral Pathology, Oral Radiology, and Endodontics. 2005;**99**:1-7. DOI: 10.1016/j.tripleo.2004.08.028

[81] Tiwana PS, Foy SP, Shugars DA, Marciani RD, Conrad SM, Phillips C, White RP. The impact of intravenous corticosteroids with third molar surgery in patients at high risk for delayed health-related quality of life and clinical recovery. Journal of Oral and Maxillofacial Surgery. 2005;**63**:55-62

[82] Buyukkurt MC, Gungormus M, Kaya O. The effect of a single dose prednisolone with and without diclofenac on pain, trismus, and swelling after removal of mandibular third molars. Journal of Oral and Maxillofacial Surgery. 2006;**64**:1761-1766. DOI: 10.1016/j.joms.2005.11.107

[83] Graziani F, D'Aiuto F, Arduino PG, Tonelli M, Gabriele M. Perioperative dexamethasone reduces post-surgical sequelae of wisdom tooth removal. A split-mouth randomized double-masked clinical trial. International Journal of Oral and Maxillofacial Surgery. 2006;**35**:241-246. DOI: 10.1016/j.joms.2005.07.010

[84] López-Carriches C, Martínez-González JM, Donado-Rodríguez M. The use of methylprednisolone versus diclofenac in the treatment of inflammation and trismus after surgical removal of lower third molars. Medicina Oral, Patología Oral y Cirugía Bucal. 2006;**11**:E440-E445

[85] Micó-Llorens JM, Satorres-Nieto M, Gargallo-Albiol J, Arnabat-Domínquez J, Berini-Aytés L, Gay-Escoda C. Efficacy of methylprednisolone in controlling complications after impacted lower third molar surgical extraction. European Journal of Clinical Pharmacology. 2006;**62**:693-698. DOI: 10.1007/s00228-006-0164-5

[86] Ordulu M, Aktas I, Yalcin S, Azak AN, Evlioglu G, Disci R, Emes Y. Comparative study of the effect of tube drainage versus methylprednisolone after third molar surgery. Oral Surgery, Oral Medicine, Oral Pathology, Oral Radiology, and Endodontics. 2006;**101**:e96-e100. DOI: 10.1016/j.tripleo.2005.09.002

[87] Grossi GB, Maiorana C, Garramone RA, Borgonovo A, Beretta M, Farronato D, Santoro F. Effect of submucosal injection of dexamethasone on postoperative discomfort after third molar surgery: A prospective study. Journal of Oral and Maxillofacial Surgery. 2007; **65**:2218-2226. DOI: 10.1016/j.joms.2006.11.036

[88] Filho JRL, Maurette PE, Allais M, Cotinho M, Fernandes C. Clinical comparative study of the effectiveness of two dosages of dexamethasone to control post-operative swelling, trismus and pain after the surgical extraction of mandibular impacted third molars. Medicina Oral, Patología Oral y Cirugía Bucal. 2008;**13**:E129-E132

[89] Zandi M. Comparison of corticosteroids and rubber drain for reduction of sequelae after third molar surgery. Oral and Maxillofacial Surgery. 2008;**12**:29-33. DOI: 10.1007/s10006-008-0096-6

[90] Vegas-Bustamante E, Micó-Llorens J, Gargallo-Albiol J, Satorres-Nieto M, Berini-Aytes L, Gay-Escoda C. Efficacy of methylprednisolone injected into the masseter muscle following the surgical extraction of impacted lower third molars. International Journal of Oral and Maxillofacial Surgery. 2008;**37**:260-263. DOI: 10.1016/j/ijom.2007.07.018

[91] Chopra D, Rehan HS, Mehra P, Kakkar AK. A randomized, double-blind, placebo-controlled study comparing the efficacy and safety of paracetamol, serratiopeptidase, ibuprofen and betamethasone using the dental impaction pain model. International Journal of Oral and Maxillofacial Surgery. 2009;**38**:350-355. DOI: 10.1016/j.ijom.2008.12.013

[92] Gataa IS, Nemat AH. Evaluation of the effectiveness of two methods using methylprednisolone on post-operative sequelae following lower third molar surgery. Kufa Medical Journal. 2009;**12**:257-266

[93] Tiigimae-Saar J, Leibur E, Tamme T. The effect of prednisolone on reduction of complaints after impacted third molar removal. Stomatologija. 2010;**12**:17-22

[94] Kang S-H, Choi Y-S, Byun I-Y, Kim M-K. Effect of preoperative prednisolone on clinical post-operative symptoms after surgical extractions of mandibular third molars. Australian Dental Journal. 2010;**55**:462-467. DOI: 10.111/j.1834-7819.2010.01271.x

[95] Majid OW, Mahmood WK. Effect of submucosal and intramuscular dexamethasone on post-operative sequelae after third molar surgery: Comparative study. The British Journal of Oral & Maxillofacial Surgery. 2011;**49**:647-652. DOI: 10.1016/j.bjoms.2010.09.021

[96] Majid OW. Submucosal dexamethasone injection improves quality of life measures after third molar surgery: A comparative study. Journal of Oral and Maxillofacial Surgery. 2011;**69**:2289-2297. DOI: 10.1016/j.joms.2011.01.037

[97] Deo SP, Shetty P. Effect of submucosal injection of dexamethasone on post-operative sequelae of third molar surgery. Journal of Nepal Medical Association. 2011;**51**:71-77

[98] Antunes AA, Avelar RL, Neto ECM, Frota R, Dias E. Effect of two routes of administration of dexamethasone on pain, edema, and trismus in impacted lower third molar surgery. Oral and Maxillofacial Surgery. 2011;**15**:217-223. DOI: 10.1007/s10006-011-0290-9

[99] Kaur J, Sandhu S, Kaur T, Bhullar RS, Sandhu Y, Singh P. Effect of methylprednisolone on postoperative pain, swelling and trismus following the surgical removal of bilateral impacted mandibular third molars. IJCDC. 2011;**1**:36-42

[100] Mushtaq M, Khan AH, Hussain A. Effect of dexamethasone on swelling, pain and trismus following third molar surgery. Gomal Journal of Medical Sciences. 2011;**9**:74-77

[101] Boonsiriseth K, Klongnoi B, Sirintawat N, Saengsirinavin C, Wongsirichat N. Comparative study of the effect of dexamethasone injection and consumption in lower third molar surgery. International Journal of Oral and Maxillofacial Surgery. 2012;**41**:244-247. DOI: 10.1016/j.ijom.2011.12.011

[102] Klongnoi B, Kaewpradub P, Boonsiriseth K, Wongsirichat N. Effect of single dose preoperative intramuscular dexamethasone injection on lower impacted third molar surgery. International Journal of Oral and Maxillofacial Surgery. 2012;**41**:376-379. DOI: 10.1016/j.ijom.2011.12.014

[103] Loganathan S, Srinivasan H. A comparative evaluation of methylprednisolone and dexamethasone injection into the masseter muscle in surgical removal of impacted lower third molars. International Journal of Current Research and Review. 2012;**4**:133-136

[104] Murugesan K, Sreekumar K, Sabapathy B. Comparison of the roles of serratiopeptidase and dexamethasone in the control of inflammation and trismus following impacted third molar surgery. Indian Journal of Dental Research. 2012;**23**:709-713

[105] Panwar SK. The role of oral prednisolone on swelling, trismus and pain after removal of impacted mandibular third molar. JMST. 2012;**1**:44-52

[106] Acham S, Klampfl A, Truschnegg A, Kirmeier R, Sandner-Kiesling A, Jakse N. Beneficial effect of methylprednisolone after mandibular third molar surgery: A randomized, double-blind, placebo-controlled split-mouth trial. Clinical Oral Investigations. 2013;**17**:1693-1700. DOI: 10.1007/s00784-012-0867-1

[107] Arakeri G, Raj KK, Shivakumar HR, Jayade B. A randomized clinical trial to compare efficacy of submucosal aprotinin injection and intravenous dexamethasone in reducing pain and swelling after third molar surgery: A prospective study. Journal of Maxillofacial and Oral Surgery. 2013;**12**:73-79

[108] Bauer HC, Duarte FL, Horliana AC, Torta-mano IP, Perez FE, Simone JL, Jorge WA. Assessment of preemptive analgesia with ibuprofen coadministered or not with dexamethasone in third molar surgery: A randomized double-blind controlled clinical trial. Oral and Maxillofacial Surgery. 2013;**17**:165-171. DOI: 10.1007/s10006-012-0360-7

[109] Bortoluzzi MC, Capella DL, Barbieri T, Plagiarini M, Cavalier T, Manfro R. A single dose of amoxicillin and dexamethasone for prevention of post-operative complications in third molar surgery: A randomized, double-blind, placebo controlled clinical trial. Journal of Clinical Medicine Research. 2013;**5**:26-33. DOI: 10.4021/jocmr1160w

[110] Channar KA, Kumar N, Ul Hassan Q, Memon AB. Dexamethasone in control of post-operative sequelae after extraction of mandibular impacted third molars. Medical Channel. 2013;**19**:63-66

[111] Chaurand-Lara J, JA F-U. Methylprednisolone injection following the surgical extraction of impacted lower third molars: A split-mouth study. Open Journal of Stomatology. 2013;**3**:192-196. DOI: 10.4236/ojst.2013.32033

[112] Christensen J, Matzen LH, Vaeth M, Wenzel A, Schou S. Efficiency of bupivacaine versus lidocaine and methylprednisolone versus placebo to reduce postoperative pain and swelling after surgical removal of mandibular third molars: A randomized, double-blinded, crossover clinical trial. Journal of Oral and Maxillofacial Surgery. 2013;**71**:1490-1499. DOI: 10.1016/j.joms.2013.05.001

[113] Flores RJM, Aguilar OSH, Ochoa ZMG. Betamethasone (sodium phosphate + acetate) prevents inflammation and trismus in retained lower third-molar surgery. Glucocorticoids in third-molar surgery. Revista ADM. 2013;**70**:190-196

[114] Majid OW, Mahmood WK. Use of dexamethasone to minimise post-operative sequelae after third molar surgery: Comparison of five different routes of administration. Oral Surgery. 2013;**6**:200-208. DOI: 10.1111/ors.12049

[115] Mehra P, Reebye U, Nadershah M, Cottrell D. Efficacy of anti-inflammatory drugs in third molar surgery: A randomized clinical trial. International Journal of Oral and Maxillofacial Surgery. 2013;**42**:835-842. DOI: 10.1016/j/ijom.2013.02.017

[116] Nair RB, Rahman NMM, Ummar M, Hafiz KAA, Isaac JK, Sameer KM. Effect of submucosal injection of dexamethasone on post-operative discomfort after third molar surgery: A prospective study. The Journal of Contemporary Dental Practice. 2013;**14**:401-404

[117] Warraich R, Faisal M, Rana M, Shaheen A, Gellrich N-C, Rana M. Evaluation of post-operative discomfort following third molar surgery using submucosal dexamethasone—A randomized observer blind prospective study. Oral Surgery, Oral Medicine, Oral Pathology, Oral Radiology. 2013;**116**:16-22. DOI: 10.1016/j.oooo.2012.12.007

[118] Agostinho CN, da Silva VC, Maia Filho EM, Cruz ML, Bastos EG. The efficacy of 2 different doses of dexamethasone to control post-operative swelling, trismus and pain after third molar extractions. General Dentistry 2014;**62**:e1–e5.

[119] Ehsan A, Bukhairi SGA, Ashar AM, Junaid M. Effects of pre-operative submucosal dexamethasone injection on the post-operative swelling and trismus following surgical extraction of mandibular third molar. Journal of the College of Physicians and Surgeons–Pakistan. 2014;**24**:489-492

[120] Kaur N, Misurya R, Narula R, Kumar M, Neelkamal N. Comparison of the clinical efficacy of methylprednisolone with ibuprofen and ibuprofen alone on the postoperative sequelae of surgical removal of impacted third molar. Indian Journal of Pain. 2014;**28**:105-110

[121] Marques J, Pié-Sánchez J, Figueiredo R, Valmaseda-Castellón E, Gay-Escoda C. Effect of the local administration of betamethasone on pain, swelling and trismus after impacted lower third molar extraction. A randomized, tripleblinded, controlled trial. Medicina Oral, Patología Oral y Cirugía Bucal. 2014;**19**:e49-e54. DOI: 10.4317/medoral.19280

[122] Noboa MM, Ramacciato JC, Teixeira RG, Vicentini CB, Groppo FC, Lopes Motta RH. Evaluation of effects of two dexamethasone formulations in impacted third molar surgeries. Rev Dor São Paulo. 2014;**15**:163-168. DOI: 10.5935/1806-0013.20140036

[123] Shaikh MI, Khatoon S, Rajput F, Shah SYA. Impacted mandibular third molar surgery; the role of dexamethasone in postoperative swelling and trismus. Professional Medizinhistorisches Journal. 2014;**21**:1272-1278

[124] Ashraf J, Yaqoob A, Yaqoob G, Ahad M, Rasheed N, Yaqoob M. Evaluation and comparison of locally infiltrated methylprednisolone and intramuscularly injected methylprednisolone in controlling the post-operative sequelae of impacted mandibular third molar extraction—In vivo study. IJRID. 2014;**4**:98-116

[125] Koçer G, Yuce E, Tuzuner Oncul A, Dereci O, Koskan O. Effect of the route of administration of methylprednisolone on edema and trismus in impacted lower third molar surgery. International Journal of Oral and Maxillofacial Surgery. 2014;**43**:639-643. DOI: 10.1016/j.ijom.2013.11.005

[126] Selvaraj L, Rao SH, Lankupalli AS. Comparison of efficacy of methylprednisolone injection into masseter muscle versus gluteal muscle for surgical removal of impacted lower third molar. Journal of Maxillofacial and Oral Surgery. 2014;**13**:495-498. DOI: 10.1007/s12663-013-0562-z

[127] Vyas N, Agarwal S, Shah N, Patel D, Aapaliya P. Effect of single dose intramuscular methylprednisolone injection into the masseter muscle on the surgical extraction of impacted lower third molars: A randomized controlled trial. Kathmandu University Medical Journal. 2014;**12**:4-8

[128] Alcântara CEP, Faici SGM, Oliveria-Ferreira F, Santos CRR, Pinheiro MLP. Pre-emptive effect of dexamethasone and methylprednisolone on pain, swelling, and trismus after third molar surgery: A split-mouth randomized triple-blind clinical trial. International Journal of Oral and Maxillofacial Surgery. 2014;**43**:93-98. DOI: 10.1016/j.ijom.2013.05.016

[129] Darwade DA, Kumar S, Mehta R, Sharma AR, Reddy GS. Search of a better option: Dexamethasone versus methylprednisolone in third molar impaction surgery. Journal of International Oral Health. 2014;**6**:14-17

[130] Chappi DM, Suresh KV, Patil MR, Desai R, Tauro DP, Shiva Bharani KNS, Parkar MI, Babaji HV. Comparison of clinical efficacy of methylprednisolone and serratiopeptidase for reduction of postoperative sequelae after lower third molar surgery. Journal of Clinical and Experimental Dentistry. 2015;**7**:e197-e202. DOI: 10.4317/jced.51868

[131] Chaudhary PD, Rastogi S, Gupta P, Niranjanaprasad Indra B, Thomas R, Choudhury R. Pre-emptive effect of dexamethasone injection and consumption on post-operative swelling, pain and trismus after third molar surgery. A prospective, double blind and randomized study. Journal of Oral Biology and Craniofacial Research. 2015;**5**:21-27. DOI: 10.1016/j.jobcr.2015.02.001

[132] Gopalakrishnan V, Darekar HS, Sahoo NK. Effectiveness of submucosal v/s intramuscular dexamethasone in mandibular third molar surgeries. IJMSCI. 2015;**2**:648-655

[133] Sabhlok S, Kenjale P, Mony D, Khatri I, Kumar P. Randomized controlled trial to evaluate the efficacy of oral dexamethasone and intramuscular dexamethasone in mandibular third molar surgeries. Journal of Clinical and Diagnostic Research. 2015;**9**:ZC48-ZC51. DOI: 10.7860/JCDR/2015/13930.6813

[134] Zerener T, Aydintug YS, Sencimen M, Bayar GR, Yazici M, Altug HA, Misir AF, Acikel C. Clinical comparison of submucosal injection of dexamethasone and triamcinolone acetonide on post-operative discomfort after third molar surgery. Quintessence International. 2015;**46**:317-326. DOI: 10.3290/j.qi.a33281

[135] Dereci O, Tuzuner-Oncul AM, Kocer G, Yuce E, Askar M, Ozturk A. Efficacy of immediate postoperative intramasseteric dexamethasone injection on postoperative swelling after mandibular impacted third molar surgery: A preliminary split-mouth study. The Journal of the Pakistan Medical Association. 2016;**66**:320-323

[136] Paiva-Oliveira JG, Bastos PR, Cury Pontes ER, da Silva JC, Delgado JA, Oshiro-Filho NT. Comparison of the anti-inflammatory effect of dexamethasone and ketorolac in the extractions of third molars. Oral and Maxillofacial Surgery. 2016;**20**:123-133. DOI: 10.1007/s10006-015-0533-2

[137] Quadri A, Imran M, Quadri S. Comparative clinical evaluation of submucosal and intramuscular dexamethasone in reducing post operative sequelae following impacted mandibular third molar surgery. IJSS Journal of Surgery. 2016;**2**:84-87. DOI: 10.17354/SUR/2016/61

[138] Saravanan K, Kannan R, John RR, Nantha Kumar C. A single pre operative dose of sub mucosal dexamethasone is effective in improving post operative quality of life in the surgical management of impacted third molars: A comparative randomised prospective study. Journal of Maxillofacial and Oral Surgery. 2016;**15**:67-71. DOI: 10.1007/s12663-015-0795-0

[139] Al-Dajani M. Can preoperative intramuscular single-dose dexamethasone improve patient-centered outcomes following third molar surgery? Journal of Oral and Maxillofacial Surgery. 2017;**75**:1616-1626. DOI: 10.1016/j.joms.2017.03.037

[140] Al-Shamiri HM, Shawky M, Hassanein N. Comparative assessment of preoperative versus postoperative dexamethasone on postoperative complications following lower third molar surgical extraction. International Journal of Dentistry. 2017;**2017**:1350375. DOI: 10.1155/2017/1350375

[141] Barbalho JC, Vasconcellos RJ, de Morais HH, Santos LA, Almeida RA, Rêbelo HL, Lucena EE, de Araújo SQ. Effects of co-administered dexamethasone and nimesulide on pain, swelling, and trismus following third molar surgery: A randomized, triple-blind, controlled trial. International Journal of Oral and Maxillofacial Surgery. 2017;**46**:236-242. DOI: 10.1016/j.ijom.2016.10.011

[142] Chugh A, Singh S, Mittal Y, Chugh V. Submucosal injection of dexamethasone and methylprednisolone for the control of postoperative sequalae after third molar surgery: Randomized controlled trial. International Journal of Oral and Maxillofacial Surgery. 2017. DOI: 10.1016/j.ijom.2017.07.009.

[143] Gozali P, Boonsiriseth K, Kiattavornchareon S, Khanijou M, Wongsirichat N. Decreased post-operative pain using sublingual injection of dexamethasone (8mg) in lower third molar surgery. Journal of Dental Anesthesia and Pain Medicine. 2017 Mar;**17**:47-53. DOI: 10.17245/jdapm.2017.17.1.47

[144] Khalida B, Fazal M, Muntaha ST, Khan K. Effect of submucosal injection of dexamethasone on post-operative swelling and trismus following impacted mandibular third molar surgery. Pakistan Oral & Dental Journal. 2017;**37**:231-234

[145] Lim D, Ngeow WC. A comparative study on the efficacy of submucosal injection of dexamethasone versus methylprednisolone in reducing postoperative sequelae after third molar surgery. Journal of Oral and Maxillofacial Surgery. 2017;**75**:2278-2286. DOI: 10.1016/j.joms.2017.05.033

[146] Lima CAA, Favarinj VT, Torres AM, da Silva RA, Sato FRL. Oral dexamethasone decreases postoperative pain, swelling, and trismus more than diclofenac following third molar removal: A randomized controlled clinical trial. Oral and Maxillofacial Surgery. DOI: 10.1007/s10006-017-0635-0

[147] Lima TC, Bagordakis E, Falci SGM, Dos Santos CRR, Pinheiro MLP. Pre-Emptive effect of dexamethasone and diclofenac sodium associated with codeine on pain, wwelling, and trismus after third molar surgery: A split-mouth, randomized, triple-blind, controlled clinical trial. Journal of Oral and Maxillofacial Surgery. DOI: 10.1016/j.joms.2017.06.012

[148] Mojsa IM, Pokrowiecki R, Lipczynski K, Czerwonka D, Szczeklik K, Zaleska M. Effect of submucosal dexamethasone injection on postoperative pain, oedema, and trismus following mandibular third molar surgery: A prospective, randomized, double-blind clinical trial. International Journal of Oral and Maxillofacial Surgery. 2017;**46**:524-530. DOI: 10.1016/j.ijom.2016.11.006

[149] Rocha-Neto AM, Nogueira EF, Borba PM, Laureano-Filho JR, Vasconcelos BC. Application of dexamethasone in the masseter muscle during the surgical removal of lower third molars. The Journal of Craniofacial Surgery. 2017;**28**:e43-e47. DOI: 10.1097/SCS.0000000000003188.

[150] Selimović E, Ibrahimagić-Šeper L, Šišić I, Sivić S, Huseinagić S. Prevention of trismus with different pharmacological therapies after surgical extraction of impacted mandibular third molar. Medicinski Glasnik (Zenica). 2017;**14**:145-151. DOI: 10.17392/871-16

[151] Syed KB, AlQahtani FH, Mohammad AH, Abdullah IM, Qahtani HS, Hameed MS. Assessment of pain, swelling and trismus following impacted third molar surgery using injection dexamethasone submucosally: A prospective, randomized, crossover clinical study. Journal of International Oral Health. 2017;**9**:116-121. DOI: 10.4103/jioh.jioh_65_17

[152] Yeoman CM, Greenspan JS, Harding SM. Recurrent oral ulceration. A double-blind comparison of treatment with betamethasone valerate aerosol and placebo. British Dental Journal. 1978;**144**:114-116

[153] Pimlott SJ, Walker DM. A controlled clinical trial of the efficacy of topically applied fluocinonide in the treatment of recurrent aphthous ulceration. British Dental Journal. 1983;**154**:174-177

[154] Lo Muzio L, della Valle A, Mignogna MD, Pannone G, Bucci P, Bucci E, Sciubba J. The treatment of oral aphthous ulceration or erosive lichen planus with topical clobetasol propionate in three preparations: A clinical and pilot study on 54 patients. Journal of Oral Pathology & Medicine. 2001;**30**:611-617

[155] Rhodus NL, Bereuter J. An evaluation of a chemical cautery agent and an anti-inflammatory ointment for thr treatment of recurrent aphthous stomatitis: A pilot study. Quintessence International. 1998;**29**:769-773

[156] Teixeira F, Mosqueda-Taylor A, Montano S, Dominguea-Soto L. Treatment of recurrent oral ulcers with mometasone furoate lotion. Postgraduate Medical Journal. 1999;**75**:574. DOI: 10.1136/pgmj.75.887.574a

[157] Rodriguez M, Rubio JA, Sanchez R. Effectiveness of two oral pastes for the treatment of recurrent aphthous stomatitis. Oral Diseases. 2007;**13**:490-494. DOI: 10.1111/j.1601-0825.2006.01327.x

[158] Al-Na'mah ZM, Carson R, Thanoon IAJ. Dexamucobase: A novel treatment for oral aphthous ulceration. Quintessence International. 2009;**40**:399-404

[159] Fani MM, Ebrahimi H, Pourshahidi S, Aflaki E, Shafiee Sarvestani S. Comparing the effect of phenytoin syrup and triamcinolone acetonide ointment on aphthous ulcers in patients with Bechet's syndrome. Iranian Red Crescent Medical Journal. 2012;**14**:75-79

[160] Femiano F, Gombos F, Scully C. Recurrent aphthous stomatitis unresponsive to topical corticosteroids: A study of the comparative therapeutic effects of systemic prednisone

and systemic sulodexide. International Journal of Dermatology. 2003;**42**:394-397. DOI: 10.1046/j.1365-4362.2003.01853.x

[161] Femiano F, Buonaiuto C, Gombos F, Lanza A, Cirillo N. Pilot study on recurrent aphthous stomatitis (RAS): A randomized placebo-controlled trial for the comparative therapeutic effects of systemic prednisone and systemic montelukast in subjects unresponsive to topical therapy. Oral Surgery, Oral Medicine, Oral Pathology, Oral Radiology, and Endodontics. 2020;**109**:402-407. DOI: 10.1016/j.tripleo.2009.10.024

[162] Ship JA. Recurrent aphthous stomatitis: An update. Oral Surgery, Oral Medicine, and Oral Pathology. 1996;**81**:141-147

[163] Belenguer-Guallar I, Jiménez-Soriano Y, Claramunt-Lozano A. Treatment of recurrent aphthous stomatitis. A literature review. Journal of Clinical and Experimental Dentistry. 2014;**6**:e168-e174. DOI: 10.4317/jced.51401

[164] Brocklehurst P, Tickle M, Glenny AM, Lewis MA, Pemberton MN, Taylor J, Walsh T, Riley P, Yates JM. Systemic interventions for recurrent aphthous stomatitis (mouth ulcers). Cochrane Database of Systematic Reviews. 2012;**9**:CD005411. DOI: 10.1002/14651858.CD005411.pub2

[165] Holbrook WP, Kristmundsdottir T, Loftsson T. Aqueous hydrocortisone mouthwash solution: Clinical evaluation. Acta Odontologica Scandinavica. 1998;**56**:157-160

[166] Hegarty MA, Hodgson AT, Lewsey DJ, Porter RS. Fluticasone propionate spray and betamethasone sodium phosphate mouthrinse: A randomized crossover study for the treatment of symptomatic oral lichen planus. Journal of the American Academy of Dermatology. 2002;**47**:271-279

[167] Cawson RA. Treatment of oral lichen planus with betamethasone. British Medical Journal. 1968;**1**:86-89

[168] Thongprasom K, Luangjarmekorn L, Sererat T, Taweesap W. Relative efficacy of fluocinolone acetonide compared with triamcinolone acetonide in treatment of oral lichen planus. Journal of Oral Pathology & Medicine. 1992;**21**:456-458

[169] Lozada F, Silverman S Jr. Topically applied fluocinonide in an adhesive base in the treatment of oral vesiculoerosive diseases. Archives of Dermatology 1980;**116**:898-901.

[170] Voute AB, Schulten EA, Langendijk PN, Kostense PJ, van der Waal I. Fluocinonide in an adhesive base for treatment of oral lichen planus. A double-blind, placebo-controlled clinical study. Oral Surgery, Oral Medicine, Oral Pathology, Oral Radiology, and Endodontology. 1993;**75**:181-185

[171] Carbone M, Conrotto D, Carrozzo M, Broccoletti R, Gandolfo S, Scully C. Topical corticosteroids in association with miconazole and chlorhexidine in the long-term management of atrophic-erosive oral lichen planus: A placebo-controlled and comparative study between clobetasol and fluocinonide. Oral Diseases. 1999;**5**:44-49

[172] Lozada-Nur F, Huang MZ, Zhou GA. Open preliminary clinical trial of clobetasol propionate ointment in adhesive paste for treatment of chronic oral vesiculoerosive diseases. Oral Surgery, Oral Medicine, Oral Pathology, Oral Radiology, and Endodontics. 1991;**71**:283-287

[173] Sardella A, Demarosi F, Oltolina A, Rimondini L, Carrassi A. Efficacy of topical mesalazine compared with clobetasol propionate in treatment of symptomatic oral lichen planus. Oral Diseases. 1998;**4**:255-259

[174] Gonzalez-Moles MA, Morales P, Rodriguez-Archilla A, Isabel IR, Gonzalez-Moles S. Treatment of severe chronic oral erosive lesions with clobetasol propionate in aqueous solution. Oral Surgery, Oral Medicine, Oral Pathology, Oral Radiology, and Endodontics. 2002;**93**:264-270

[175] Carbone M, Goss E, Carrozzo M, Castellano S, Conrotto D, Broccoletti R, Gandolfo S. Systemic and topical corticosteroid treatment of oral lichen planus: A comparative study with long-term follow-up. Journal of Oral Pathology & Medicine. 2003;**32**:323-329

[176] Lodi G, Scully C, Carrozzo M, Griffiths M, Sugerman PB, Thongprasom K. Current controversies in oral lichen planus: Report of an international consensus meeting. Part 2. Clinical management and malignant transformation. Oral Surgery, Oral Medicine, Oral Pathology, Oral Radiology, and Endodontics. 2005;**100**:164-178. DOI: 10.1016/j.tripleo.2004.06.077

[177] Eisen D, Carrozzo M, Bagan Sebastian J-V, Thongprasom K. Oral lichen planus: Clinical features and management. Oral Diseases. 2005;**11**:338-349. DOI: 10.1111/j.1601-0825.2005.01142.x

[178] Liu C, Xie B, Yang Y, Lin D, Wand C, Lin M, Ge L, Zhou H. Efficacy of intralesional betamethasone for erosive oral lichen planus and evaluation of recurrence: A randomized controlled trial. Oral Surgery, Oral Medicine, Oral Pathology, Oral Radiology. 2013;**116**:584-590. DOI: 10.1016/j.oooo.2013.07.023

[179] Ryan JG. Pemphigus. A 20-year survey of experience with 70 cases. Archives of Dermatology. 1971;**104**:14-20

[180] Zhao CY, Murrell DF. Pemphigus vulgaris: An evidence-based treatment update. Drugs. 2015;**75**:271-284. DOI: 10.1007/s40265-015-0353-6

[181] Cholera M, Chainai-Wu N. Management of pemphigus. Advances in Therapy. 2016;**33**: 910-958. DOI: 10.1007/s12325-016-0343-4

[182] Knudson RM, Kalaaji AN, Bruce AJ. The management of mucous membrane pemphigoid and pemphigus. Dermatologic Therapy. 2010;**23**:268-280. DOI: 10.1111/j.1529-8019.2010.01323.x

[183] Mentink LF, Mackenzie MW, Toth GG, Laseur M, Lambert FP, Veeger NJ, Cianchini G, Pavlovic MD, Jonkman MF. Randomized controlled trial of adjuvant oral dexamethasone pulse therapy in pemphigus vulgaris. Archives of Dermatology. 2006;**142**:570-576. DOI: 10.1001/archderm.142.5.570

[184] Berg T, Bylund N, Marsk E, Jonsson L, Kanerva M, Hultcrantz M, Engström M. The effect of prednisolone on sequelae in Bell's palsy. Archives of Otolaryngology – Head & Neck Surgery. 2012;**138**:445-449. DOI: 10.1001/archoto.2012.513

[185] Axelsson S, Berg T, Jonsson L, Engström M, Kanerva M, Stjernquist-Desatnik A. Bell's palsy—The effect of prednisolone and/or valaciclovir versus placebo in relation to baseline severity in a randomised controlled trial. Clinical Otolaryngology. 2012;**37**:283-290. DOI: 10.1111/j.1749-4486.2012.02526.x

[186] Murthy JMK, Saxena AB. Bell's palsy: Treatment guidelines. Annals of Indian Academy of Neurology. 2011;**14**(Suppl 1):S70-S72. DOI: 10.4103/0972-2327.83092

[187] Baugh RF, Basura GJ, Ishii LE, Schwartz SR, Drumheller CM, Burkholder R, Deckard NA, et al. Clinical practice guideline: Bell's palsy. Otolaryngology and Head and Neck Surgery. 2013;**149**(Suppl 3):S1-S27. DOI: 10.1177/0194599813505967

[188] Minnerop M, Herbst M, Fimmers R, Matz B, Klockgether T. Wüllner. Bell's palsy. Combined treatment of famciclovir and prednisone is superior to prednisone alone. Journal of Neurology. 2008;**255**:1726-1730. DOI: 10.1007/s00415-008-0008-6

[189] Numthavaj P, Thakkinstian A, Dejthevaporn C, Attia J. Corticosteroid and antiviral therapy for Bell's palsy: A network meta-analysis. BMC Neurology. 2011;**11**:1. DOI: 10.1186/1471-2377-11-1

[190] Al-Hamadani HA, Abdul-Ameer AJ, Abed AN, Hamzah MT. Bell's palsy: Evaluation of clinical response to medical treatment. Iraqi Journal of Medical Sciences. 2013;**11**:84-88

[191] Madhok VB, Gagyor I, Daly F, Somasundara D, Sullivan M, Gammie F, Sullivan F. Corticosteroids for Bell's palsy (idiopathic facial paralysis). Cochrane Database of Systematic Reviews. 2016;**7**:CD001942. DOI: 10.1002/14651858.CD001942.pub5

[192] Horten CP. The treatment of arthritic temporomandibular joints by intra-articular injection of hydrocortisone. Oral Surgery. 1953;**6**:826-829

[193] Kopp S, Wenneberg B, Haraldson T, Carlsson GE. The short-term effect of intra-articular injections of sodium hyaluronate and corticosteroid on temporomandibular joint pain and dysfunction. Journal of Oral and Maxillofacial Surgery. 1985;**43**:429-435

[194] Kopp S, Akerman S, Nilner M. Short-term effects of intra-articular sodium hyaluronate, glucocorticoid, and saline injections on rheumatoid arthritis. Journal of Craniomandibular Disorders. 1991;**5**:231-238

[195] Bjørnland T, Gjaerum AA, Møystad A. Osteoarthritis of the temporomandibular joint: An evaluation of the effects and complications of corticosteroid injection compared with injection with sodium hyaluronate. Journal of Oral Rehabilitation. 2007;**34**:583-589. DOI: 10.1111/j.365-2842.2007.01759.x

[196] Samiee A, Sabzerou D, Edalatpajouh F, Clark GT, Ram S. Temporomandibular joint injection with corticosteroid and local anesthetic for limited mouth opening. Journal of Oral Science. 2011;**53**:321-325

[197] Møystad A, Mork-Knutsen BB, Bjørnland T. Injection of sodium hyaluronate compared to a corticosteroid in the treatment of patients with temporomandibular joint osteoarthritis: A CT evaluation. Oral Surgery, Oral Medicine, Oral Pathology, Oral Radiology, and Endodontics. 2008;**105**:e53-e60. DOI: 10.1016/j.tripleo.2007.08.024

[198] Bouloux GF, Chou J, Krishnan D, Aghaloo T, Kahenasa N, Smith JA, Giannakopoulus H. Is hyaluronic acid or corticosteroid superior to lactated ringer solution in the short term for improving function and quality of life after arthrocentesis? Part 2. Journal of Oral and Maxillofacial Surgery. 2017;**75**:63-72. DOI: 10.1016/j.joms.2016.08.008

[199] Rogers MJ, Johnson BR, Remeikis NA, BeGole EA. Comparison of effect of intracanal use of ketorolac tromethamine and dexamethasone with oral ibuprofen on post treatment endodontic pain. Journal of Endodontia. 1999;**25**:381-384. DOI: 10.1016/S0099-2399(06)81176-3

[200] Negm MM. Intracanal use of a corticosteroid-antibiotic compound for the management of post treatment endodontic pain. Oral Surgery, Oral Medicine, Oral Pathology, Oral Radiology, and Endodontics. 2001;**92**:435-439. DOI: 10.1067/moe.2001.115975

[201] Ehrmann EH, Messer HH, Adams GG. The relationship of intracanal medicaments to postoperative pain in endodontics. International Endodontic Journal. 2003;**36**:868-875

[202] Kaufman E, Heling I, Rotstein I, Friedman S, Sion A, Moz C, Stabholtz A. Intraligamentary injection of slow-release methylprednisolone for the prevention of pain after endodontic treatment. Oral Surgery, Oral Medicine, and Oral Pathology. 1994;**77**:651-654

[203] Stewart GG, Chilton NW. Role of antihistamines and corticosteroids in endodontic practice. Oral Surgery, Oral Medicine, and Oral Pathology. 1958;**11**:433-440

[204] Stewart G. Combined use of an antibiotic and a corticosteroid for postoperative sequelae in endodontic practice. The Journal of Dental Medicine. 1962;**17**:142-146

[205] Krasner P, Jackson E. Management of posttreatment endodontic pain with oral dexamethasone: A double-blind study. Oral Surgery, Oral Medicine, and Oral Pathology. 1986;**62**:187-190

[206] Glassman G, Krasner P, Morse DR, Rankow H, Lang J, Furst ML. A prospective randomized double-blind trial on efficacy of dexamethasone for endodontic interappointment pain in teeth with asymptomatic inflamed pulps. Oral Surgery, Oral Medicine, and Oral Pathology. 1989;**67**:96-100

[207] Liesinger A, Marshall FJ, Marshall JG. Effect of variable doses of dexamethasone on post treatment endodontic pain. Journal of Endodontia. 1993;**19**:35-39

[208] Wolfson BC. The role of hydrocortisone in the control of apical periodontitis. Oral Surgery, Oral Medicine, and Oral Pathology. 1954;**7**:314-321

[209] Thong YL, Messer HH, Siar CH, Saw LH. Periodontal response to two intracanal medicaments in replanted monkey incisors. Dental Traumatology. 2001;**17**:254-259

[210] Abbott PV. Medicaments: Aids to success in endodontics. Part 1. A review of literature. Australian Dental Journal. 1990;**35**:438-448

[211] Kim ST, Abbott PV, McGinley P. The effects of Ledermix paste on discolouration of mature teeth. International Endodontic Journal. 2000;**33**:227-232

[212] Nobuhara WK, Carnes DL, Giles JA. Anti-inflammatory effects of dexamethasone on periapical tissues following endodontic over-instrumentation. Journal of Endodontia. 1993;**19**:501-507

8

Corticosteroids and their Use in Respiratory Disorders

Ibrahim A. Janahi, Abdul Rehman and Noor Ul-Ain Baloch

Abstract

Corticosteroids are adrenal hormones that play important physiologic roles including modulation of glucose metabolism, protein catabolism, alteration of calcium metabolism, regulation of bone turnover, suppression of immune system, and down-regulation of the inflammatory cascade. Because of their diverse effects, corticosteroids have been used therapeutically for treating a wide variety of auto-immune, rheumatologic, inflammatory, neoplastic and infectious diseases. In the field of pulmonology, corticosteroids have been used for the treatment of reactive airway diseases (such as asthma and allergic bronchopulmonary aspergillosis), chronic obstructive pulmonary disease, sarcoidosis, collagen vascular diseases (such as vasculitic disorders), eosinophilic pneumonitis, idiopathic interstitial pneumonias and infectious disorders (such as laryngotracheobronchitis). Different formulations of corticosteroids are commercially available including tablets, intravenous injections, intramuscular formulations and inhaled preparations. Long-term use of corticosteroids is often limited by their adverse effects, which include abnormal fat deposition, weight gain, diabetes mellitus, cataracts, glaucoma, osteoporosis, osteonecrosis, elevated risk of fractures, increased susceptibility to infections, proximal myopathy, depression, psychosis, adrenal atrophy with risk of Addisonian crisis, abdominal striae, acne vulgaris, delayed wound healing, easy bruising, electrolyte abnormalities and increased risk of peptic ulcer disease. As our understanding of corticosteroids advances, we may be able to identify individuals at higher risk of experiencing adverse effects.

Keywords: corticosteroids, glucocorticoids, respiratory diseases, airway disorders, asthma, chronic obstructive pulmonary disease, pneumonia, sarcoidosis

1. Introduction to corticosteroids

Corticosteroids are steroid hormones produced by the adrenal gland. Adrenal glands constitute the endocrine system of the body and are a pair of pyramidal shaped glands located just above the kidneys on either side of the body. Because of their location, they are also known as suprarenal glands and are perfused by suprarenal arteries, which arise on either side from renal arteries [1]. These endocrine glands are important as they secrete a number of hormones into the blood, which play a vital role in maintaining homeostasis. With respect to the structure of the adrenal glands, they consist of an outer cortex and inner medulla. The adrenal medulla secretes catecholamines (epinephrine and norepinephrine), which are stress hormones and are mediators of the sympathetic autonomic nervous system [2]. The adrenal cortex itself comprises of three layers viz. zona glomerulosa, zona fasciculata and zona reticularis. These three layers are responsible for secreting mineralocorticoids, glucocorticoids, and adrenal androgens (sex hormones) respectively [3]. As the name suggests, mineralocorticoids are responsible for maintenance of fluid and mineral (electrolyte) balance; the chief mineralocorticoid is aldosterone. Glucocorticoids are involved in regulating glucose metabolism (glycolysis and gluconeogenesis) and storage (glycogenesis and glycogenolysis); the prototype glucocorticoid is cortisol. The primary adrenal androgen is dehydroepiandrosterone and possesses virilizing properties. Cortisol and other related hormones (such as 11-deoxycortisol and corticosterone) are collectively referred to as corticosteroids [4].

2. Physiologic effects

Corticosteroids play important physiologic roles in the human body and are referred to as "stress hormones" as they prepare the body during periods of physiologic stress. One of the most important actions of corticosteroids is their ability to up-regulate glucose synthesis [5]. Glycogen is the principal storage form of glucose in humans and is stored in various organs of the body, especially the liver. Glycogen is a multibranched polysaccharide and its structure consists of a core protein (glycogenin), which gives off multiple branches composed of glucose monomers [6]. Glycogen is produced by a biochemical pathway known as glycogenesis, which occurs chiefly in the liver. Glycogen is broken down during periods of fasting to provide a supply of glucose monomers. Glucose monomers can be utilized by all cells of the body through the processes of glycolysis. Pyruvate produced during glycolysis can then produce acetyl-CoA which can enter the Krebs cycle. Oxidation of glucose (in conjunction with the electron transport chain) produces adenosine 1,4,5-triphosphate (ATP), which is the energy currency of the cell. Stress hormones (such as catecholamines) generally up-regulate gluconeogenesis and glycogenolysis to induce hyperglycemia, which helps in fulfilling energy demands of various cells of the body [7]. Corticosteroids also induce fasting hyperglycemia by up-regulating gluconeogenesis; this is achieved by increasing expression of several key enzymes involved in gluconeogenesis including phosphoenol pyruvate-carboxykinase, fructose-1,6-bisphosphatase and glucose-6-phosphatase [8]. Cortisol and other corticosteroids are unique in that they up-regulate gluconeogenesis while inhibiting glycogenolysis. This seemingly contradictory effect of corticosteroids is important in intrauterine life when release of cortisol from the fetal adrenal gland helps in building glycogen stores in the fetal liver to prepare for delivery.

Protein metabolism is also affected by corticosteroids. Increased catabolism of proteins to amino acids provides a supply of alanine, which can be converted to glucose by the process of gluconeogenesis. Cahill cycle (glucose-alanine cycle) refers to a series of chemical reactions in which amino groups and carbon skeletons from muscles are transported to the liver in the form of alanine, which are subsequently converted to glucose [9]. An essential enzyme for Cahill cycle is alanine aminotransferase (ALT), which is present in both muscles and liver. Alanine aminotransferase (also known as serum glutamate-pyruvate transaminase [SGPT]) is responsible for transferring an amino group from alanine to α-ketoglutarate, which results in the production of pyruvate and glutamate [10]. Pyridoxal phosphate is a co-factor for this reaction and is formed from pyridoxine (vitamin B_6). As corticosteroids up-regulate protein catabolism, they induce a state of negative nitrogen balance in the body, which is important during periods of starvation.

Corticosteroids have important effects on bone turnover and affect bone mass. Bone is a type of connective tissue composed of osteocytes, osteoblasts and osteoclasts [11]. Osteoclasts are derivatives of the reticuloendothelial system and are responsible for bone resorption. Osteoblasts are mesenchymal origin cells and are responsible for giving rise to osteocytes—the mature cells that make up bones. Osteoclasts and their progenitors express a receptor on their surface for nuclear factor-κB (NFκB) commonly referred to as RANK. Ligand for RANK (known as RANKL) is expressed on the surface of osteoblasts and RANK–RANKL interaction is necessary for the differentiation and formation of osteoclasts [12]. Osteoprotegerin (OPG) is a cytokine receptor that is secreted by stromal cells and osteoblasts, which acts as a decoy receptor for RANKL. Secretion of OPG is one of the mechanisms by which the body prevents excessive resorption of bones. Due to this reason, OPG is sometimes also referred to as "osteoclastogenesis inhibitory factor." Corticosteroids can affect bone turnover by inhibiting the secretion of OPG and increasing RANK–RANKL interaction, which leads to enhanced formation of osteoclasts. By tipping the balance in favor of osteoclasts, corticosteroids favor bone resorption and loss of mineral bone mass [13]. Calcium homeostasis in the body is tightly regulated by a number of hormones including parathyroid hormone (PTH), calcitonin and other hormones. Under physiologic conditions, serum calcium level is not drastically affected by corticosteroids. However, in pathologic states including Cushing's syndrome and Addison's disease, hypocalcemia and hypercalcemia (respectively) may be occasionally seen.

Vascular tone is also affected by corticosteroids, which has important implications during states of physiologic stress. Under resting conditions, cortisol and other corticosteroids are not necessary for maintaining vascular tone. However, during periods of stress, corticosteroids have a "permissive effect" for catecholamines and help in maintaining the vascular tone [14]. In patients with severe deficiency of glucocorticoids (such as Addison's disease), catecholamines are ineffective in increasing the blood pressure; this may manifest clinically as overt or orthostatic hypotension. This is especially important for patients with severe sepsis (or septic shock), myxedema coma, pituitary apoplexy and other diseases. Presence of stress hormones (including thyroid hormones and corticosteroids) is necessary for the optimal action of catecholamines, which helps in the maintenance of vascular tone and blood pressure [15]. This in turn maintains adequate perfusion of vital organs and allows the body to cope with physiologic stress.

Fluid status of the body is principally controlled by steroid hormones. Mineralocorticoids (such as aldosterone) are primarily responsible for maintaining the fluid and salt balance in the body. Renin is a hormone secreted by the juxtaglomerular apparatus of nephrons, which is responsible for cleaving angiotensinogen to angiotensin I. Angiotensinogen is produced in the liver and is a precursor to angiotensin I, which is produced in the circulation by action of renin. Angiotensin

I is then converted to angiotensin II in the pulmonary microvasculature through the action of dipeptidyl peptidase (commonly referred to as angiotensin converting enzyme [ACE]) [16]. Angiotensin II has at least four important effects in the body: (a) stimulation of aldosterone synthesis and secretion; (b) increasing thirst; (c) vasoconstriction; and (d) enhancing activity of sodium (Na^+)-hydrogen (H^+) exchanger in the proximal convoluted tubule of nephrons. The overall impact of angiotensin II is to retain salt and water with expansion of the effective circulating volume [17]. Aldosterone leads to further expansion of the extracellular fluid by increasing reabsorption of sodium (Na^+) and chloride (Cl^-) in the distal convoluted tubule of nephrons. At the same time, aldosterone increases tubular secretion of potassium (K^+) and loss of hydrogen (H^+) ions in the urine, which can potentially induce hypokalemia and metabolic alkalosis respectively. The overall effect of the renin–angiotensin–aldosterone system (RAAS) is to retain salt and water, thereby expanding the effective circulating volume and blood pressure. Although corticosteroids possess mainly glucocorticoid effects, they do have weak mineralocorticoid effects at physiologic concentrations. In disease states, and when used therapeutically, corticosteroids can have substantial mineralocorticoid activity with clinically significant effects on the body [18].

A number of other effects are also possessed by corticosteroids, which are not evident in physiologic states; however, in disease states, these actions can result in protean manifestations. Corticosteroids are necessary for optimal functioning of the body and excess or deficiency of these hormones can manifest as Cushing's syndrome or Addison's disease respectively. Cushing syndrome is most commonly iatrogenic and results from exogenous use of steroids, although it can also result from cortisol or adrenocorticotrophic hormone (ACTH)-secreting tumors (such as pituitary adenoma, adrenal adenoma or carcinoma, small cell carcinoma of lung, etc.) [19]. Common features of this disease include obesity, buffalo lump (lipodystrophy), moon facies, purple abdominal striae, easy bruising, depression, psychosis, cataracts, glaucoma, hypertension, hypokalemia and hypocalcemia. On the other hand, Addison's disease can be caused by auto-immune destruction of the adrenal gland (in developed countries) or infiltration of the adrenal gland by infections such as tuberculosis (in developing countries). Hypocortisolism manifests as weakness, fatigue, weight loss, hyperpigmentation of skin (due to increased release of ACTH from the pituitary gland), hyponatremia, hyperkalemia, orthostatic or resting hypotension, hypercalcemia, basophilia and/or eosinophilia [20]. Treatment of these diseases is directed at restoring the balance of steroid hormones back to normal. In the case of Cushing syndrome, the underlying cause is addressed (e.g. removal of primary tumor); rarely, bilateral adrenalectomy with exogenous replacement of steroids may be required. In Addison's disease, replacement of steroid hormones is generally needed for life. These two diseases exemplify the importance of corticosteroids and the deleterious consequences of their excess or deficiency on the human body.

3. Mechanism of action

From a therapeutic standpoint, corticosteroids have been exploited most for their anti-inflammatory and immunosuppressive effects [21]. While these properties of corticosteroids are not evident during physiologic states, they are clinically important in the treatment of numerous diseases including auto-immune diseases, neoplastic diseases, inflammatory disorders, rheumatologic conditions and infectious diseases (in conjunction with other drugs).

Inflammation is the response of the body to any noxious stimulus with an aim to eliminate the noxious stimulus and start the process of tissue repair. Inflammatory response of the body involves leukocytes, chemical mediators and vascular changes. Acute inflammation begins with a series of vascular changes that increases blood flow to the inflamed tissue. Chemical mediators of inflammation, such as histamine and serotonin, cause arteriolar vasodilation and venous vasoconstriction. This in turn promotes the exudation of fluid from the intravascular compartment to the interstitial space [22]. Leukocytes are then recruited to the area of inflammation through the expression of selectins on endothelium and integrins on leukocytes. Selectins are responsible for weak binding of leukocytes to the endothelium, which results in "rolling" of leukocytes along the endothelium. On the other hand, integrins are responsible for high-affinity binding of leukocytes ("adhesion") to the endothelium with pavementing of the endothelium with leukocytes. Through the interaction of various cell surface molecules, such as platelet–endothelial cell adhesion molecule-1 (PECAM-1), leukocytes migrate through the microvasculature into the interstitium [23]. Neutrophils, monocytes and macrophages can phagocytose microbes and other offending agents by binding to their pathogen-associated molecular patterns (PAMPs) using pattern recognition receptors (PRRs). Following phagocytosis, microbes are trapped inside vacuoles called "phagosomes," which are then fused with lysosomes to form phagolysosomes. Microbes and dead cells are thus degraded through the action of hydrolytic enzymes present inside lysosomes. Neutrophils and macrophages can also generate free radicals through the action of enzymes, which can damage different micro-organisms and offending agents [24].

A number of chemical mediators play a crucial role in the process of inflammation. These include biogenic amines, prostaglandins, leukotrienes, lipoxins, cytokines, chemokines, complement proteins, bradykinin, nitric oxide and other molecules [25]. Histamine and serotonin are biogenic amines and mediate vascular changes implicated in acute inflammation; histamine also causes bronchoconstriction. Prostaglandins are eicosanoids and have a variety of actions in the body. PGE_2 is the mediator of pain, $PGF_{2\alpha}$ causes increased vascular permeability, PGI_2 (prostacyclin) causes vasodilation and thromboxane A_2 causes platelet aggregation and vasoconstriction. Leukotrienes are derivatives of arachidonic acid and mediate bronchoconstriction. Lipoxins are lipid-derived autacoids that have a modulatory effect on the overall process of inflammation [26]. Bradykinin is a product of the kinin cascade and is derived by the action of kallikrein on high-molecular weight kininogen. This molecule irritates bronchiolar smooth muscle and mediates cough and vasodilation. Nitric oxide is released from endothelium and causes vasodilation. Complement cascade plays an important role in inflammation and is a part of the humoral immune system. Some complement proteins act as opsonins and anaphylatoxins. C5a, a complement protein, also causes chemotaxis of leukocytes to the area of inflammation. Cytokines are a group of small protein molecules that play various roles in the body including chemotaxis of leukocytes (chemokines), communication between leukocytes (interleukins), mounting fever (pyrogens) and so on [27]. All these chemical mediators play a crucial role in mounting an inflammatory response and pharmacologic interruption of their actions can blunt or modulate the inflammatory response.

Phospholipase A_2 is an enzyme that is responsible for the synthesis of arachidonic acid from phospholipids present in cell membranes of various cells. Arachidonic acid is an important lipophilic compound that serves as the precursor for the synthesis of prostaglandins, thromboxane A_2, leukotrienes and lipoxins (**Figure 1**). Cyclooxygenase is an enzyme that is responsible

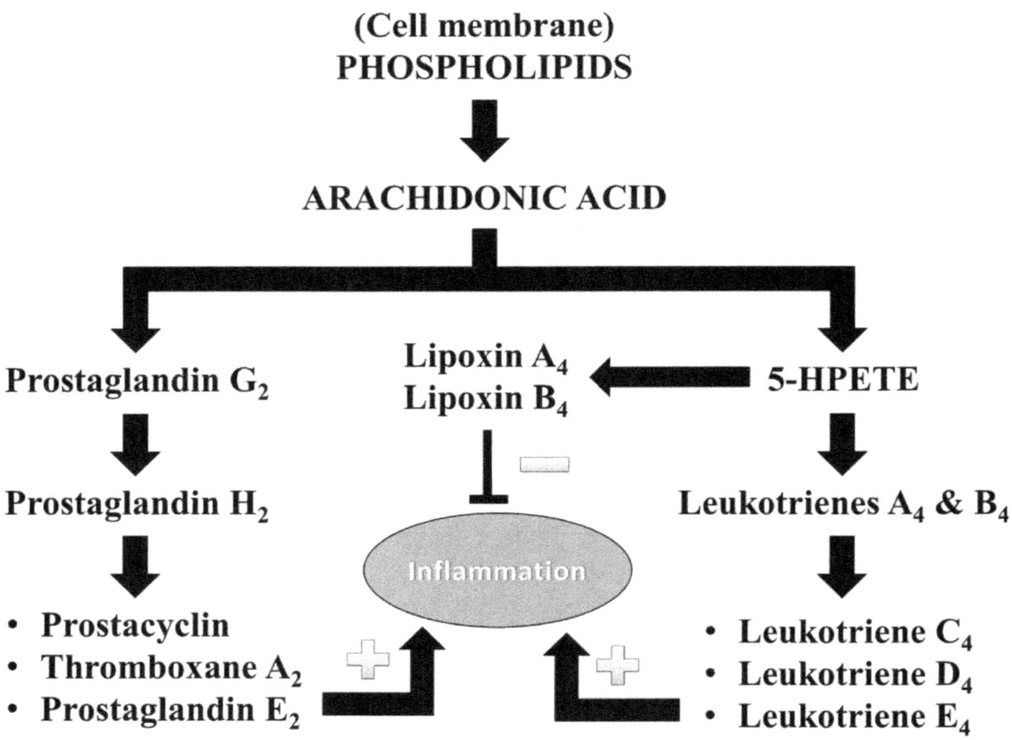

Figure 1. Arachidonic acid metabolism with cyclooxygenase and lipoxygenase pathways. *HPETE* = hydroperoxyeicosatetraenoic acid.

for the formation of prostaglandins from arachidonic acid. Non-steroidal anti-inflammatory drugs (NSAIDs) and acetaminophen exert their anti-inflammatory effects by inhibiting cyclooxygenase and preventing formation of prostaglandins and thromboxane [28]. Arachidonic acid can also be acted upon by 12-lipoxygenase that results in the formation of lipoxins A_4 and B_4, both of which modulate inflammation by inhibiting neutrophil adhesion and chemotaxis. Another enzyme, 5-lipoxygenase, is involved in the synthesis of leukotrienes from arachidonic acid. Leukotrienes C_4, D_4 and E_4 induce bronchospasm, vasoconstriction and increased vascular permeability. Synthesis of arachidonic acid is inhibited by corticosteroids and this effect of corticosteroids is exploited therapeutically for treating inflammatory disorders [29].

The anti-inflammatory effects of corticosteroids are chiefly achieved by altering the synthesis of chemical mediators of inflammation. When commercially available corticosteroids are administered therapeutically, these molecules are readily absorbed and penetrate into various cells of the body due to their highly lipophilic nature. Glucocorticoids enter the cytosol of cells and bind to the glucocorticoid receptor. The glucocorticoid–receptor complex can repress the expression of pro-inflammatory genes by preventing translocation of certain transcription factors (especially NFκB) from the cytosol into the nucleus [30]. Moreover, the glucocorticoid–receptor complex can translocate into the nucleus and up-regulate transcription of anti-inflammatory genes by binding to "zing fingers" of glucocorticoid-response elements (GRE). Glucocorticoids inhibit translocation of NFκB by inducing the expression of IκBα inhibitory protein, which sequesters NFκB in the cytosol and prevents transcription of pro-inflammatory genes [31]. This is in turn inhibits the expression of pro-inflammatory genes and results in a blunted inflammatory response.

One of the most important effects of glucocorticoids is the modulation of gene expression of enzymes involved in the metabolism of arachidonic acid. Most notably, glucocorticoids reduce the expression of the enzyme phospholipase A_2, which is responsible for the formation of arachidonic acid [32]. By inhibiting the formation of arachidonic acid, synthesis of prostaglandins, lipoxins, leukotrienes and thromboxane is inhibited. Since arachidonic acid metabolites mediate several key steps in the process of inflammation, their inhibition results in a blunted inflammatory response. Consequently, margination, chemotaxis and phagocytosis by phagocytes are inhibited by corticosteroids, which manifests as an overall anti-inflammatory effect. Additionally, through inhibition of the NFκB pathway, inflammatory cells begin to produce anti-inflammatory cytokines, which down-regulate the overall immune and inflammatory response. This has important therapeutic implications for the treatment of many diseases in which chronic inflammation lies at the core of their pathogenesis [33].

4. Formulations

Different formulations of corticosteroids are commercially available and have been used in a variety of diseases. Tablets, intravenous formulations and intramuscular preparations are available for systemic use. Systemic formulations are generally more efficacious as compared to other formulations (such as inhaled or topical steroids). However, this greater efficacy comes at the cost of increased adverse effects, which may be substantial in some cases [34]. Oral formulations are available for various corticosteroids with the most popular ones being prednisolone, methylprednisolone, hydrocortisone, and dexamethasone. Given the lipophilic nature of steroids, adequate absorption of steroids is achieved in most patients as they readily cross cell membranes of enterocytes [35]. Oral formulations are convenient for patients who require chronic use of steroids, such as lung transplant recipients. Tablets are the most commonly used oral formulation of corticosteroids. Prednisone syrup and dexamethasone oral solution or elixirs are also available, which may be useful for pediatric patients and those with feeding tubes. Conversion from one systemic steroid to another requires knowledge of equipotent dosages, which are provided in **Table 1**. Frequency of dosage is determined by the half-life and duration of action for individual corticosteroids; for instance, hydrocortisone lasts for 8–12 hours whereas dexamethasone may last for 36–72 hours [36].

Parenteral systemic formulations of steroids are also available and have a number of important uses. Intramuscular preparations of steroids, such as methylprednisolone or triamcinolone acetonide, are often used to provide a delayed release of steroids over a prolonged period of time with a relatively steady plasma concentration. Intravenous methylprednisolone and hydrocortisone are often used in patients with life-threatening or organ-threatening inflammatory conditions. Very high doses of steroids can be given intravenously (termed 'pulse therapy'), which have been postulated to have physicochemical effects on plasmalemma of various cells, which may modulate the function of transmembrane proteins [37]. Steroid therapy has also been employed via many other parenteral routes of administration. Intralesional triamcinolone acetonide injections have been used for the treatment of several dermatologic disorders, such as keloids, alopecia areata, granuloma annulare, lichen planus and psoriasis.

Steroids	Dexamethasone	Methylprednisolone	Prednisone	Hydrocortisone	Fludrocortisone
Glucocorticoid effect*	0.75 mg	4 mg	5 mg	20 mg	-
Mineralocorticoid effect*	-	-	50 mg	20 mg	100 mcg
Duration of action	36–72 hours (long)	12–36 hours (intermediate)	12–36 hours (intermediate)	8–12 hours (short)	12–36 hours (intermediate)

*Fludrocortisone has no glucocorticoid effect, while dexamethasone and methylprednisolone have negligible mineralocorticoid effects

Table 1. Comparison of equivalent doses of various steroids.

Gout and other inflammatory joint disorders have been treated with intra-articular injections of steroids. In the field of oncology, intrathecal administration of hydrocortisone along with chemotherapeutic drugs has been used for the treatment of leukemia [38].

Inhaled preparations of corticosteroids come in the form of nebulizer solutions, metered-dose inhalers or dry powder inhalers. Inhaled formulations are useful for the treatment of various airway disorders as these preparations exert their maximal effects locally with minimal systemic absorption. Consequently, the risk of systemic adverse effects is reduced, although oral thrush, dysphonia and systemic adverse effects can still occur with long-term use [39]. Most notably, children may have deceleration of growth velocity with the long-term use of corticosteroids [40]. In adults, long-term use of inhaled corticosteroids (ICS) may lead to accelerated loss of bone mass and possible ophthalmic side-effects (such as increased intraocular pressure and/or cataracts) [41]. The most commonly used inhaled steroids include beclomethasone, fluticasone, budesonide and mometasone. Nebulized delivery of respiratory solutions provides the best delivery of medications to the lower airways when compared with metered-dose inhalers or dry powder inhalers. Proper inhaler technique with or without the use of spacer devices may provide equivalent effects with powder/inhaled forms of steroids as compared to nebulizer administrations [42].

Topical formulations of steroids are available for use and have been utilized therapeutically for a wide variety of dermatologic conditions. Like inhaled forms, topical use of steroids provides local effects on the skin with some systemic absorption. Consequently, local effects of steroids are maximized, while systemic side-effects are minimized. However, use of a large amount of topical steroids, especially if continued over a long period of time, can result in significant systemic side-effects (as is the case with inhaled steroids) [43]. A number of vehicles are available for the topical delivery of steroids including ointments, creams, lotions, gels, foams and wet dressings. Topical steroids have been classified on the basis of their potency into 7 categories viz. least potent, low potency, lower-mid potency, medium potency, high potency, very high potency, and super-high potency. Using the correct vehicle and potency of topical steroids is of utmost importance as inadvertent use of a weak steroid preparation may lead to treatment failure, while use of a very potent topical preparation can lead to thinning and atrophy of the skin [44]. It is important to bear in mind that the potency of topical steroids is determined not only by the dermatologic diagnosis, but also by the area and extent of the skin that is affected. For instance, genital skin or intertriginous areas are exquisitely sensitive to topical steroids, which make them suitable candidates for lower potency topical steroids. On the other hand, skin of palms and soles have thick stratum corneum (the uppermost layer of epidermis), which necessitates the use of more potent topical steroids.

5. Therapeutic use in respiratory disorders

Steroids have been approved for the use of various respiratory diseases for both pediatric and adult populations. Both systemic and inhaled formulations of steroids have been utilized for the treatment of various respiratory disorders. In most disorders, steroids exert a therapeutic effect through their anti-inflammatory or immunosuppressive effects [21]. In many diseases, steroids can be given in the form of short intermittent courses; examples include hypersensitivity pneumonitis, eosinophilic pneumonitis, allergic bronchopulmonary aspergillosis (ABPA), etc. In some diseases, such as bronchial asthma or chronic obstructive pulmonary disease (COPD), inhaled steroids are continued on a long-term basis as a maintenance therapy. Systemic steroid therapy may also be required on a long-term basis in patients with systemic disorders or diseases refractory to other therapies, for instance sarcoidosis or collagen vascular diseases. In many diseases requiring long-term immunosuppression, steroid-sparing agents (such as azathioprine, mycophenolate, cyclosporine, tacrolimus, etc.) can be introduced to taper off steroids and mitigate their long-term side-effects [45].

In the following lines, we discuss the use of corticosteroids in the management of various respiratory disorders. A general overview of each of these diseases is provided and along with a holistic view of how steroid therapy works in conjunction with other components of management.

5.1. Asthma

Bronchial asthma is a chronic inflammatory disorder of bronchi and bronchioles that results in intermittent and reversible bronchospasm [46]. Clinical features of the disorder include recurrent episodes of chest tightness, wheezing and shortness of breath. Most patients have a diurnal variation in their symptoms with worsening shortness of breath and cough towards the end of the day. Over time, patients tend to develop bronchial smooth muscle hypertrophy, goblet cell hyperplasia with hypersecretion of mucus, recruitment of eosinophils and a state of chronic inflammation within the airways. Genetic predisposition to type I hypersensitivity has been demonstrated in most patients with asthma, although environmental factors also play a central role in triggering attacks of asthma [47]. Asthma has been classified into multiple subtypes depending on the type of triggers that precipitate attacks of asthma viz. atopic asthma, non-atopic asthma, drug-induced asthma, occupational asthma, and exercise-induced asthma. Atopic asthma is characterized by a personal or family history of atopy, allergic rhinitis, eczema and hypersensitivity to allergens, such as pollens or dust mites [48]. In non-atopic asthma, patients do not have hypersensitivity responses to allergens; instead, attacks of asthma are precipitated by factors such as viral infections, cold temperature, inhaled gases (e.g. sulfur dioxide), etc. Drug-induced asthma is precipitated by drugs such as NSAIDs or aspirin, which tip the balance towards increased synthesis of leukotrienes with consequent bronchospasm. Likewise, occupational asthma is reportedly precipitated by exposure to chemicals (e.g. anhydrides, isocyanates, acids) in various industries, such as paints, varnishes, adhesives and resins. Exercise-induced asthma is precipitated by exercise and diagnostic testing at rest may be normal in such cases [49]. Irrespective of the type of asthma, the core pathogenesis underlying all these types of asthma is similar.

The pathogenesis of asthma entails an inflammatory response affecting the bronchi and bronchioles, which is chiefly driven by a type 2 helper T (T_H2) lymphocytes. When an environmental allergen is inhaled, antigen-presenting cells (APCs) engulf the allergen and present it to T lymphocytes. As a consequence of this, a T_H2 cell-mediated inflammatory response is mounted. T_H2 cells produce an array of cytokines including interleukin (IL)-2, IL-4, IL-5 and IL-13. IL-2 acts upon other T lymphocytes to differentiate them into T_H2 cells and promote an amplified response [50]. IL-4 activates B lymphocytes and promotes immunoglobulin class switching to immunoglobulin E (IgE) production. IL-5 acts on bone marrow to increase differentiation and proliferation of eosinophils. Eotaxin is another cytokine produced by airway epithelial cells and serves to recruit eosinophils. IL-13 is believed to stimulate mucus production from mucus glands and goblet cells. Through these cytokines, T_H2 promote a humoral immune response that results in production of high circulating levels of allergen-specific IgE. IgE binds to mast cells and cross-linking of mast cell-bound IgE results in degranulation of mast cells with release of histamine, tryptase and heparin sulfate. Histamine is a potent bronchoconstrictor and is the chief mediator of bronchoconstrictor in atopic asthma. Repeated exposure to the same allergen results in stronger activation of T_H2 lymphocytes. A state of chronic inflammation persists within the bronchioles and results in *airway remodeling*, which is a histopathological hallmark of chronic asthma [51].

Numerous pharmacologic and non-pharmacologic modalities are used in the management of patients with asthma. Non-pharmacologic approaches include avoidance of allergens by removing carpets from houses, avoiding exposure to animal dander, using personal protective equipment while at work (in cases of occupational asthma), maintaining a clean environment (reducing exposure to dust mites), and so on. Pharmacologic treatment options include short-acting β_2-adrenoceptor agonists (SABA), short-acting muscarinic antagonists (SAMA), long-acting β_2-adrenoceptor agonists (LABA), ICS, phosphodiesterase (PDE) inhibitors (such as theophylline), anti-leukotrienes (such as montelukast), systemic corticosteroids, and immunotherapy (such as omalizumab and mepolizumab) [52]. SABA causes bronchodilation by stimulating β_2-adrenergic receptors on the smooth muscle layer of bronchioles. As β_2-adrenoceptors are G-protein coupled receptors (GPCRs), their stimulation (G_s) results in activation of adenylyl cyclase and increased levels of cyclic adenosine monophosphate (cAMP) inside smooth muscle cells. This in turn activates protein kinase A and results in phosphorylation of myosin light chain kinase, which essentially deactivates this enzyme. Consequently, dephosphorylation of myosin light chain occurs via the unregulated action of myosin light chain phosphatase, which causes smooth muscle relaxation and bronchodilation. PDE inhibitors (such as theophylline and aminophylline) act in a similar manner by inhibiting degradation of cAMP (caused by PDE), which results in increased level of cAMP in smooth muscle cells [53]. This results in bronchodilation in the same manner as SABA, except that the β_2-adrenoceptor and adenylyl cyclase are not involved in this pathway. SAMA causes bronchodilation by blocking muscarinic receptors and preventing vagal stimulation. Moreover, SAMA also blocks muscarinic

M_3 receptors present on smooth muscle cells of bronchioles and prevent bronchoconstriction in response to a variety of stimuli. Anti-leukotrienes effectively block bronchoconstriction in response to leukotrienes C_4, D_4 and E_4 by either blocking their target receptors (montelukast) or reducing their synthesis (zileuton). Omalizumab is a humanized monoclonal antibody directed against free circulating IgE and reduces levels of IgE, thereby reducing sensitivity to allergens [54]. Mepolizumab is an antibody that binds IL-5 and blocks the signaling pathways activated by IL-5 [55]. While mepolizumab reduces activation and recruitment of eosinophils, its exact mechanism of action in the treatment of asthma remains unclear.

Corticosteroids act through multiple pathways in controlling asthma and are useful in the treatment of acute exacerbations of asthma as well as long-term maintenance therapy [56]. Systemic and ICS act in a similar manner and their chief effect is reduction of airway inflammation by blocking the NFκB pathway. Corticosteroids reduce the expression of the enzyme phospholipase A_2, which results in decreased synthesis of arachidonic acid and its metabolites [21]. Reduced levels of leukotrienes promote bronchodilation and relieve airway obstruction. Anti-inflammatory activity of corticosteroid over a long period of time can retard airway remodeling, thereby reducing smooth muscle cell hypertrophy, thickening of the basement membrane, and goblet cell hyperplasia [56]. Corticosteroids also have immunosuppressive properties, which enable them to reduce levels of IgE and inhibit proliferation of T_H2 and B lymphocytes [31]. By reducing transcription of IL-4 and IL-5, corticosteroids also inhibit eosinophil recruitment and activation. Furthermore, by blocking the synthesis of IL-13, mucus secretion is reduced, which can further relieve airway obstruction.

Corticosteroids form a cornerstone of the management of asthma. Management of acute exacerbation of asthma requires accurate assessment of the severity of the exacerbation and appropriate triage [57]. Airway, breathing and circulation need to be secured as in any other emergency condition. Inhaled oxygen and SABA therapy are the first and foremost in the management of acute exacerbations. Intravenous terbutaline (β_2-agonist) may also be used. Systemic corticosteroids should also be administered to all patients with a moderate to severe acute exacerbation of asthma, although their onset of action is after several hours. If patients do not respond to acute SABA therapy, intravenous magnesium sulfate and/or aminophylline infusion may also be considered. Patients with signs of fatigue (such as mental status changes or normalization of arterial carbon dioxide levels) may require endotracheal intubation and mechanical ventilation. In patients with long-standing asthma, a stepwise approach to therapy has been proposed [58]. Again, accurate assessment of asthma control is essential to tailor therapy to individual patients. The first step of therapy consists of non-pharmacologic measures and rescue medication (inhaled SABA) as needed. The second step is to add a low-dose ICS (controlled medication) along with a rescue medication (inhaled SABA) as needed. The third step is to either add LABA along with ICS or to increase the dose of ICS to medium dose. The fourth step is to use LABA along with medium-dose ICS therapy, or to add another agent (such as an anti-leukotriene or a PDE inhibitor). The fifth step is to use high-dose ICS therapy along with LABA with or without other agents mentioned in step 4. The sixth step is the use of systemic corticosteroids and/or immunotherapy along with other therapies as mentioned in steps 1–4. Generally, refer to an asthma specialist should be considered for patients who persistently require step 4 or higher therapies [59].

5.2. Chronic obstructive pulmonary disease

COPD refers to a group of obstructive lung diseases which are characterized by progressive and irreversible limitation to airflow in the setting of a chronic inflammatory state of the airways and/or lung parenchyma. Generally, emphysema and chronic bronchitis are two entities included under the heading of COPD, although these entities are not mutually exclusive and may co-exist in a patient. Emphysema is characterized by destruction of the wall and interstitium of the lung parenchyma leading to irreversible dilatation and enlargement of acini, thereby leading to air trapping within the lungs [60]. Depending on the etiology of emphysema, it can affect either whole of the respiratory acinus (pan-acinar emphysema) or portions of it (centriacinar, distal acinar or irregular emphysema). Clinically, patients with emphysema have been referred to as 'pink puffers' as they tend to have a lean built, breath with pursed lips, are often tachypneic, and appear pink due to hypercapnia (carbon dioxide retention). In contrast, chronic bronchitis is characterized by the presence of a productive cough for ≥3 consecutive months over a period of at least 2 years [61]. Interestingly, chronic bronchitis has a 'clinical' definition as opposed to emphysema, which is defined on the basis of morphologic and histopathological features. Patients with chronic bronchitis often have pathology affecting the larger airways (i.e. bronchi) as opposed to the air-space (parenchymal) disease seen in patients with emphysema. 'Blue bloaters' is a term used to refer to patients with chronic bronchitis as they often have resting cyanosis due to hypoxemia and polycythemia, and fluid retention due to right-sided heart failure ('cor pulmonale'). All patients with COPD do have a number of features in common. All patients have a demonstrable obstructive defect on pulmonary function testing, which differentiates them from those with restrictive lung diseases. Moreover, patients with COPD generally have a progressive, irreversible obstructive process, which differentiates them from the intermittent, reversible obstruction seen in patients with asthma [62]. From a physiologic standpoint, all patients with COPD have a higher than normal lung compliance, which increases the tendency for alveoli to collapse, and makes expiration difficult. Air trapping results in elevated residual volume and increased total lung capacity, but a reduced forced vital capacity. Consequently, patients have an elevated functional residual capacity at rest. Moreover, as the disease process progresses, patients with emphysema develop a defect in diffusion of gases and impaired gas exchange. All these processes increase the work of breathing and impair oxygenation and ventilation [63].

Cigarette smoking has been implicated as the main etiologic factor in the pathogenesis of COPD [64]. Exposure to inhaled pollutants and toxins leads to production of free radicals and oxidant stress that can damage the airway epithelial lining. On-going exposure to such inhaled pollutants leads to accumulation of inflammatory cells (such as neutrophils, macrophages and lymphocytes) with release of proteolytic enzymes and a cascade of pro-inflammatory cytokines. This process of active chronic inflammation leads to destruction of elastin contained in the pulmonary interstitium, which leads to dilatation of acini — the hallmark feature of emphysema. Cigarette smoke in particular has been shown to inhibit α_1-antitrypsin — an enzyme that inhibits neutrophilic elastase and prevents destruction of elastin. Inhibition of α_1-antitrypsin by cigarette smoking leads to unregulated activity of neutrophilic elastase and consequent destruction of acini. Similarly, in patients with congenital deficiency of α_1-antitrypsin, pan-acinar emphysema sets in early in life, in the absence of any history of cigarette smoking [65]. In patients with chronic bronchitis, cigarette smoking leads to hyperplasia of mucus-secreting glands in the larger airways; this is an adaptive response of the body to the irritants contained in cigarette smoke. Accumulation of mucus plugs, co-existent emphysema and bronchiolitis results in airflow obstruction in patients with clinical features of chronic bronchitis [63]. In cases of both emphysema and chronic bronchitis, the core feature of pathogenesis is on-going exposure to inhaled toxins and a state of chronic inflammation within the smaller airways [60]. This explains why smoking cessation is the most important therapeutic intervention in patients with COPD and reduces overall mortality in such patients.

Corticosteroids have an important role in the overall management of patients with COPD. As is the case with asthma, corticosteroids provide a therapeutic effect in patients with COPD by inhibiting bronchoconstriction, promoting bronchodilation, suppressing the immune response, and having an overall anti-inflammatory effect [66]. In patients with acute exacerbation of COPD, SABA and SAMA are the first-line therapeutic agents. The use of non-invasive positive pressure ventilation (NIPPV) can reduce the need for endotracheal intubation and reduces overall mortality in such patients. Systemic corticosteroids and antibiotics also have an important role in the treatment of acute exacerbation of COPD, although the onset of their action is delayed. Nebulized corticosteroids (such as budesonide) may also be added along with other therapies. In patients with refractory respiratory failure or contraindications to NIPPV, endotracheal intubation and mechanical ventilation may become necessary. In the management of patients with stable COPD, ICS are a cornerstone of therapy. The optimal therapy for such patients is based on their degree of airflow limitation (quantified by the forced expiratory volume in first second of expiration [FEV_1]) and clinical symptoms (quantified by the COPD assessment test [CAT] and/or modified Medical Research Council [mMRC] scores) [67]. The Global Initiative for Chronic Obstructive Lung Disease (GOLD) classifies patients into one of four stages (I–IV) depending on their degree of airflow limitation ($FEV_1 \geq 80\%$, FEV_1 50–79%, FEV_1 30–49% and $FEV_1 < 30\%$ respectively). In patients with GOLD stage III–IV COPD, ICS should be used in conjunction with other therapies [68]. As in patients with asthma, SABA or SAMA are used as rescue medications as needed. LAMA alone or LABA combined with ICS may be combined with ICS depending on the degree of airflow limitation and clinical symptoms in individual patients. Roflumilast, a PDE inhibitor, may also be used in patients with COPD who have frequent exacerbations despite other treatment modalities [69]. In patients with advanced COPD, lung volume reduction surgery or lung transplant may be needed to improve quality of life [70]. In patients with advanced COPD who have a limited life expectancy and/or contraindications to lung transplant, hospice care may be the best strategy to improve patients' symptoms.

5.3. Pneumonia

Pneumonia is a term often used to indicate an infection affecting the pulmonary parenchyma. Pneumonitis is a term that specifically refers to any inflammatory process affecting the pulmonary parenchyma, whether infective in origin or otherwise. However, in different publications, the two terms are often used interchangeably. For the purpose of this chapter, we use the term 'pneumonia' to refer specifically to infections affecting the pulmonary parenchyma.

Pneumonia is an extremely common illness affecting approximately 450 million people a year and is also a leading cause of death among all parts of the world and across all age groups [71]. In the United States, pneumonia alone accounts for almost one-sixth of all deaths. These figures seem plausible as the epithelial lining of the lungs are continuously exposed to the atmosphere which contains a high burden of pollutants and microbes. Impairment in host immunity, mucociliary apparatus and/or cough reflex can predispose people to the development of pneumonia. Acute bacterial pneumonias tend to have an acute onset of a lobar pneumonia with exudation of fibropurulent material in the alveoli and hepatization (consolidation) of lungs. Intracellular microbes cause an *atypical pneumonia* with a subacute presentation and mononuclear interstitial infiltrates. Chronic pneumonia is usually secondary to fastidious mycobacteria or fungal infections, which lead to granulomatous inflammation and possible cavitation of lung parenchyma. A variety of microbial pathogens can cause pneumonia and the predisposition to infection with a particular organism is determined by several factors, such as age, co-morbidities, vaccination status, use of immunosuppressive drugs, exposure to animals, presence of microbial reservoirs, hospitalization status, presence of endotracheal or tracheostomy tube, alcoholism, smoking, malnutrition, and so on and so forth [72]. *Streptococcus pneumoniae, Haemophilus influenzae, Moraxella catarrhalis, Legionella pneumophila, Chlamydia pneumoniae, Mycoplasma pneumoniae, Staphylococcus aureus, Pseudomonas aeruginosa, Klebsiella pneumoniae, Mycobacterium tuberculosis* and *Pneumocystis jiroveci* are some of the well-known causative organisms of pneumonia. While the aforementioned list is by no means exhaustive, a causative organism cannot be isolated in most cases of community acquired pneumonia (CAP) [73]. A number of explanations have been proposed to explain this phenomenon with the most likely explanation being that a significant proportion of patients have pneumonia secondary to viruses, which cannot be isolated by routine microbiological methods.

Corticosteroids are not routinely used in all cases of pneumonia. From a theoretical perspective, the use of corticosteroids in patients with pneumonia would seem counterintuitive. Pneumonia is an infection of the pulmonary parenchyma and use of antimicrobials seems to be the prime management. Corticosteroids have been avoided in most cases of pneumonia due to concerns that their immunosuppressive effects may actually worsen the underlying infection. However, corticosteroids do have a role to play in selected patients with pneumonia. The most well-established use of corticosteroids is in patients with severe *Pneumocystis jiroveci* pneumonia as defined by a resting arterial partial pressure of oxygen (PaO_2) of less than 70 mm Hg or an alveolar–arterial (A–a) gradient of PaO_2 of 35 mm Hg or more (both on room air) [74]. In such patients, corticosteroids have been shown to provide a clear benefit in terms of overall mortality and reduction in respiratory failure. Apart from this, there have been several studies that have assessed the use of steroids in patients with severe pneumonia in general. A randomized placebo-controlled trial by Torres et al. demonstrated that the use of a short course of methylprednisolone among patients with severe CAP reduced treatment failure [75]. A meta-analysis of 12 randomized clinical trials published in 2015 concluded that the use of systemic corticosteroids in adults hospitalized with CAP may reduce overall mortality by 3%, decrease hospital stay by 1 day and cut need for mechanical ventilation by 5% [76]. Clinical guidelines generally recommend that steroids be considered for all patients with CAP requiring hospitalization, especially those requiring admission to the intensive care unit, although the benefits and harms should be weighed on a case-by-case basis.

5.4. Allergic bronchopulmonary aspergillosis

ABPA is a pulmonary disorder characterized by a hypersensitivity reaction to the allergens of the fungus *Aspergillus fumigatus,* which occurs in patients with a history of bronchial asthma or cystic fibrosis (CF). [77] ABPA has been reported to occur in 1–3% of patients with asthma, while in patients with CF, its prevalence may be as high as 10% [78]. *A. fumigatus* is a spore-forming mold that occurs ubiquitously in nature. This fungus is medically important because it has been implicated in a number of diseases viz. ABPA, aspergilloma, invasive pulmonary aspergillosis, allergic fungal rhinosinusitis and bronchial asthma. In patients with long-standing asthma or CF, *A. fumigatus* spores can grow within the lumen of airways and lead to the formation of hyphae (molds). These fungal hyphae can trigger an IgE-mediated hypersensitivity which results in bronchial inflammation and airway destruction. Clinically, ABPA manifests as a worsening of asthma or CF with patients complaining of wheezing and cough. Laboratory investigations may reveal eosinophilia and elevated levels of total IgE. Skin prick tests to *Aspergillus* and precipitins to *A. fumigatus* are positive. Radiologic studies may reveal fleeting pulmonary opacities in the acute stage and signs of central bronchiectasis in longstanding cases. Mucus plugging within the larger airways may be visible on roentgenograms and computed tomograms may lead to a characteristic "finger-in-glove" appearance [77]. A diagnosis of ABPA should be suspected in patients with a history of previously controlled asthma or CF, who develop unexplained worsening of their disease. Diagnostic criteria have been published in the literature in order to enable clinicians to vouchsafe a diagnosis of ABPA with certainty [79].

Management of ABPA entails the achievement of two separate goals: (a) attenuating the hypersensitivity response to *A. fumigatus;* and (b) decreasing the overall burden of *A. fumigatus* allergens. Systemic corticosteroid therapy is useful to achieve the former goal, while antifungal therapy (typically itraconazole) is required for the latter [77]. Prednisone in a dose of 0.5–2.0 mg/kg/day (or an equivalent) is often employed as first-line therapy. This dosage is maintained for a period of 1–2 weeks, beyond which the dosage can be modified to an alternate day regimen. Depending on the patient's response, dose of steroids can be reduced slowly and gradually weaned off over a period of 2–3 months. In patients who relapse when the dose of corticosteroids is reduced, itraconazole therapy can be especially useful [80]. As discussed previously for asthma and COPD, steroids afford a therapeutic effect in ABPA owing to their anti-inflammatory, immunosuppressive and bronchodilator effects. Recent studies have explored the role of omalizumab in the management of ABPA [81]. Small-scale studies suggest that omalizumab may be useful as a steroid-sparing agent in patients with either asthma or CF who develop chronic ABPA [82].

5.5. Sarcoidosis

Sarcoidosis is a multisystem disorder of unknown etiology characterized by the formation of non-caseating epithelioid cell granuloma. This disorder occurs 10 times more frequently among African Americans as compared to Caucasians and the incidence is higher among young and middle-aged women. Interestingly, this disease affects non-smokers more often than people who smoke. Most commonly, the disease may be discovered incidentally when a chest radiograph reveals bilateral hilar lymphadenopathy. Patients may also present with a variety of clinical features including uveitis, xerophthalmia, parotidomegaly, xerostomia, lupus pernio, skin nodules, erythema nodosum, hypercalcemia, cardiac conduction system abnormalities, hepatomegaly and pulmonary infiltration. Given the undetermined etiology of sarcoidosis, it is a histopathological diagnosis of exclusion [83]. Nevertheless, two clinical variants of sarcoidosis are well-recognized and may suggest a diagnosis of sarcoidosis in the absence of histopathological evidence. Heerfordt-Waldenström syndrome refers to a constellation of clinical findings viz. fever, uveitis, parotidomegaly and facial palsy. Uveoparotid fever is another term used to refer to this syndrome and, in the appropriate setting, may obviate the need for a biopsy [84]. Another variant of sarcoidosis, Löffgren's syndrome, has been classically described in the literature, although it may be somewhat less specific as compared to uveoparotid fever. Löffgren's syndrome refers to a triad of erythema nodosum, arthralgia (or arthritis) and bilateral hilar lymphadenopathy [85]. Generally, women who present with Löffgren's syndrome tend to have a better prognosis compared to others. The diagnosis of sarcoidosis requires histopathological evaluation and is one of exclusion since its etiology is unknown. The hallmark feature on biopsies is the presence of non-caseating granuloma in different organs and tissues of the body without an alternative explanation. Laboratory investigations may also reveal elevated levels of ACE, although this is a non-specific finding. The differential diagnosis includes all granulomatous diseases, such as tuberculosis, histoplasmosis, berylliosis, silicosis and cat-scratch disease [83].

Management of sarcoidosis is dependent upon the severity and extent of the disease at the time of diagnosis. Pulmonary sarcoidosis has been traditionally described to have four stages [86]. Stage I refers to the presence of hilar lymphadenopathy and/or mediastinal lymphadenopathy in the absence of any lung infiltration. Stage II refers to the presence of pulmonary reticular opacities (predominantly in upper lung zones) along with hilar and/or mediastinal lymphadenopathy. Stage III refers to the presence of pulmonary fibrosis and/or reticular infiltrates with resolution of hilar and/or mediastinal lymphadenopathy. Stage IV refers to an advanced stage of "burnt out" disease in which diffuse pulmonary fibrosis with volume loss and bronchiectasis is evident in the absence of any lymphadenopathy. Fortunately, a substantial proportion of patients with pulmonary sarcoidosis do not require treatment as most of them have asymptomatic, non-progressive disease. Treatment is necessary for patients who have severe disease at the time of presentation, those who report bothersome symptoms, or those who demonstrate evidence of progressive disease upon follow-up [87]. Likewise, in patients with extra-pulmonary disease, treatment is generally indicated to prevent end-organ damage. First-line treatment is to begin prednisone at a dose of approximately 40 mg/day (0.6 mg/kg) and continue for about 4–6 weeks. If there is no clinical and/or radiographic improvement, this dose of prednisone (or an equivalent steroid) can be continued for another 4 weeks. Once the patient shows evidence of clinical improvement, reduction in dosage of steroids can be started. There is no evidence available to support a particular steroid tapering schedule. Most clinicians would gradually reduce the dose of prednisone to 10–15 mg/day (approximately 0.2 mg/kg); this maintenance dose of prednisone (or an equivalent steroid) would then be continued for a period of approximately 6 months with frequent monitoring of pulmonary function tests (PFTs) and radiologic studies. The usual duration of treatment with prednisone (or equivalent steroid) is almost 1 year. In cases where patients have disease refractory to steroids, patients experience relapses when steroids are tapered, or patients develop serious adverse effects related to steroids, steroid-sparing immunosuppressive agents (methotrexate, azathioprine or biologic agents) can be tried [88]. For patients who are at risk of steroid-induced adverse effects and have stage I-II pulmonary disease (or evidence of slowly progressive disease), inhaled corticosteroid therapy may be a feasible alternative to systemic corticosteroids [89]. Budesonide 800–1600 mcg inhaled twice daily has been most studied in this context. Fluticasone propionate 500–1000 mcg inhaled twice daily is also a possible alternative option.

5.6. Collagen vascular diseases

Collagen vascular diseases comprise of a group of disorders characterized by auto-immunity to antigens contained within blood vessels and extracellular matrix of various organs. A large number of diseases affecting connective tissue of the body are included under this heading. A substantial proportion of rheumatologic diseases and auto-immune vasculitides are included in this category with the most notable ones being systemic sclerosis (SSc), polymyositis (PM), dermatomyositis (DM), systemic lupus erythematosus (SLE), rheumatoid arthritis (RA), granulomatosis with polyangiitis (GPA), eosinophilic granulomatosis with polyangiitis (EGPA), microscopic polyangiitis (MPA), Goodpasture syndrome (GPS) and relapsing polychondritis (RPC). Sometimes, vascular diseases are also included in this category irrespective of whether auto-immunity is implicated in pathogenesis or not.

Nearly all collagen vascular diseases can affect the lung in a variety of ways. This is not surprising since the lungs are rich in both connective tissue and blood vessels. Abundant pulmonary vasculature is necessary for gaseous exchange, while abundant collagen and elastin fibers in the interstitium are necessary to support the dynamic chest wall–lung breathing system [90]. In the following lines, we briefly discuss the spectrum of pulmonary pathologies seen in various collagen vascular diseases and the role of steroids in their management.

SSc is a disorder characterized by progressive fibrosis affecting multiple organs of the body including the skin, kidneys, lungs and other organs [91]. Within the pulmonary system, SSc can lead to the development of ground-glass opacities, which can slowly progress to fibrosis of the lung parenchyma. The most common pattern of pulmonary fibrosis seen in SSc is similar to that of usual interstitial pneumonitis (UIP) and may be histologically indistinguishable from rheumatoid lung or idiopathic pulmonary fibrosis (IPF). In some cases, SSc may involve the lung in a pattern similar to that of idiopathic non-specific interstitial pneumonitis (NSIP). Progressive pulmonary impairment in SSc is a sign of worse prognosis and mandates aggressive treatment [92]. The decision to start treatment with immunosuppressive agents is based on clear evidence of progressive pulmonary damage as demonstrated by radiologic worsening or decline in pulmonary function as measured by PFTs. Two pharmacologic agents have been studied for the treatment of SSc-related interstitial lung disease (ILD): mycophenolate and cyclophosphamide [93]. Mycophenolate is often prescribed as monotherapy and the usual duration of immunosuppressive therapy is approximately 2 years. Cyclophosphamide therapy can be given as intravenous injections or oral therapy and it is generally combined with corticosteroid therapy. Oral cyclophosphamide is given daily and necessitates a higher cumulative dosage of the drug; on the other hand, intravenous cyclophosphamide is given once monthly and allows a lower cumulative dosage with a lower incidence of adverse effects.

Cyclophosphamide therapy is continued for a few months and thereafter, it is transitioned to an alternative immunosuppressive agent (such as azathioprine or mycophenolate). Most clinicians prefer a daily oral dosage of low-dose prednisone (7.5–10 mg) along with cyclophosphamide as it is associated with a lower incidence of scleroderma renal crisis. However, some small studies have also reported the use of pulse-dose methylprednisolone along with cyclophosphamide [94]. Generally, pulse steroid therapy should be reserved for patients with SSc who have another organ-threatening manifestation necessitating their use.

PM and DM are auto-immune diseases that primarily affect muscles and skin, but in severe cases, involvement of other organ systems (including the respiratory system) can occur. The pathogenesis of PM entails a primary injury to skeletal muscles that is mediated by T lymphocytes, while in DM, immune complex deposition occurs in blood vessels and skin followed by complement activation that leads to injury and inflammation of the skin and muscles [95]. Pulmonary manifestations may be due to aspiration pneumonitis (a consequence of bulbar muscle weakness), respiratory failure (secondary to diaphragmatic involvement or chest wall muscle weakness) and/or acute alveolitis. ILD associated with PM or DM has been associated with the presence of antibodies against aminoacyl-transfer ribonucleic acid (tRNA)–synthetase and can occur as part of the antisynthetase syndrome [96]. The spectrum of ILD associated with PM/DM ranges from a chronic, slowly progressive UIP to an acute interstitial pneumonitis with diffuse alveolar damage (DAD); NSIP or bronchiolitis obliterans organizing pneumonitis (BOOP) can also occur [97]. Depending on the severity of the disease, glucocorticoid therapy alone or in association with other immunosuppressive agents may be required. Since most patients with PM/DM require systemic glucocorticoid therapy, such corticosteroid therapy may suffice for the pulmonary manifestations as well in many cases. In patients with severe disease at baseline or rapidly progressive ILD, pulse-dose methylprednisolone therapy followed by systemic glucocorticoid therapy (such as prednisone 1 mg/kg/day) along with cyclophosphamide (or other immunosuppressive agents) may be required. Intravenous immunoglobulin (IVIG) and/or rituximab have also been used in severe cases [98]. In most patients who receive glucocorticoid therapy, another immunosuppressive agent (usually azathioprine or mycophenolate) is also started at the same time and continued for a prolonged period of time (as glucocorticoids are tapered off).

SLE is a systemic auto-immune disease with protean manifestations that can affect nearly every organ-system of the body, but, occurs more frequently in women. Diagnosis is based on exclusion of alternative diagnoses and by applying the classification criteria proposed by the American College of Rheumatology (1997) or Systemic Lupus International Collaborating Clinics (2012) [99]. Pulmonary manifestations of SLE include pleuritis or pleural effusions, pulmonary hypertension, diffuse alveolar hemorrhage (DAH), acute interstitial pneumonitis, ILD and/or shrinking lung syndrome (SLS) [100]. ILD associated with SLE can take one of several histologic forms including NSIP, UIP, BOOP, lymphocytic interstitial pneumonitis (LIP), follicular bronchitis and/or nodular lymphoid hyperplasia. The general approach to the management of these pulmonary manifestations is similar to that for PM/DM associated ILD. Aggressive immunosuppressive therapy (i.e. pulse steroid therapy along with cyclophosphamide, rituximab or IVIG) is used for patients with acute interstitial pneumonitis or DAH. Plasmapheresis may also be employed for the management of patients with

DAH. NSAID therapy (if not contraindicated) is used for patients with pleuritis [101]. Long-term immunosuppressive therapy may be required for patients with ILD or SLS.

RA is an auto-immune disorder that results in chronic, symmetric, progressive, erosive polyarthritis which can affect any synovial joint of the body. Extra-articular manifestations of this disease are common and occur in 20–40% of affected patients. Pulmonary manifestations may include arthritis of the cricoarytenoid joints, vasculitis affecting the recurrent laryngeal nerve, bronchiolitis obliterans, pleuritis with pleural effusions, pulmonary nodules, pulmonary hypertension and/or UIP [102]. Management of RA is with disease modifying anti-rheumatoid drugs and/or biologic agents [103]. NSAIDs may be used for management of pain. Short courses of systemic corticosteroids are used to manage acute exacerbations of RA. Systemic corticosteroid therapy is also useful for patients who develop rheumatoid vasculitis or bronchiolitis obliterans. ILD associated with RA is treated in a similar fashion as that due to SLE or PM/DM [104].

GPA, EGPA and MPA are small-vessel vasculitides associated with the presence of antineutrophil cytoplasmic antibodies (ANCA). GPA is a necrotizing, granulomatous vasculitis that frequently affects the nose, paranasal sinuses, upper airways, lungs and kidneys [105]. EGPA is a granulomatous vasculitis that is often associated with a history of asthma and eosinophilia, but can involve multiple organ-systems of the body [106]. MPA is another ANCA-related small-vessel vasculitis that is non-granulomatous and can affect multiple organ-systems of the body, although it usually spares the paranasal sinuses and upper airways [107]. GPS is an auto-immune disorder characterized by the formation of auto-antibodies against type IV collagen present in basement membrane. This disease principally affects the alveolar and glomerular basement membranes resulting in DAH and rapidly progressive glomerulonephritis respectively [108]. DAH and/or DAD can also occur in GPA, EGPA or MPA. Treatment of these disorders entails aggressive immunosuppression; pulse steroid therapy is combined with either rituximab or cyclophosphamide therapy. IVIG and/or plasmapheresis are also used in conjunction with immunosuppression. Patients who receive cyclophosphamide therapy are usually switched over to an alternative immunosuppressive agent, such as azathioprine or methotrexate. Patients who received rituximab initially may be maintained on the same agent or switched over to azathioprine or methotrexate [109].

RPC is a rare auto-immune disease that leads to inflammation and destruction of cartilaginous structures of the body. Auricular chondritis (sparing the earlobe), nasal chondritis (may lead to saddle-nose deformity), scleritis (or episcleritis), orbital pseudotumor, non-erosive arthritis, laryngeal inflammation, tracheal stricture, bronchial obstruction with post-obstructive pneumonia, and/or mitral or aortic regurgitation are some of the prominent clinical features of this disease [110]. Approximately one-third of cases occur in association with other rheumatologic diseases or malignancy. Patients with auricular or nasal chondritis and/or arthritis in the absence of other organ involvement can be treated with NSAIDs alone. Systemic corticosteroid therapy is used in patients with life or organ-threatening disease [111]. Dapsone or other immunosuppressive agents may be used in combination with, or in place of, corticosteroids; evidence does not support the use of any particular immunosuppressive agent over others. Surgical treatment or airway stenting may be required in patients who develop laryngeal or tracheal disease [112].

5.7. Eosinophilic pneumonitis

Eosinophilic pneumonitis may present either as an acute eosinophilic pneumonia or a more indolent chronic eosinophilic pneumonia. Patients with acute idiopathic eosinophilic pneumonia generally present with an acute febrile illness and progressive respiratory failure [113]. Most patients have a history of new onset or resumption of cigarette smoking, although heavy inhalational exposure to fine sand and dust may also precipitate this illness. Peripheral eosinophilia is generally absent at presentation, although it may develop later in the disease. Computed tomography usually shows bilateral patchy ground-glass opacities or reticular infiltrates. Bronchoalveolar lavage (BAL) may reveal a preponderance of eosinophils. Lung biopsies usually show marked eosinophilic infiltration of the interstitium and alveolar spaces with DAD and absence of hemorrhage or granuloma [114]. Treatment is with systemic corticosteroid therapy (usually prednisone 1 mg/kg) continued for a period of 2 weeks followed by a gradual taper over the next 4 weeks. Most patients respond dramatically to steroids within 24–72 hours and respiratory failure resolves rapidly [115].

Chronic eosinophilic pneumonia is an idiopathic disorder that presents with cough, fever, dyspnea and wheezing that progress over a period of several weeks to months. Radiologic findings of this disorder have been classically described as the "photographic negative of pulmonary edema" i.e. bilateral peripheral pleural-based opacities [116]. BAL reveals a predominance of eosinophils with the eosinophil count often exceeding 25% of leukocyte count. BAL and/or lung biopsy are also useful in excluding alternative causes, such as drug-induced or infectious causes. Treatment of chronic eosinophilic pneumonia is similar to that for acute eosinophilic pneumonia, although systemic corticosteroid therapy is generally tapered slowly over a period of 6 months (or more) [117].

5.8. Lymphocytic interstitial pneumonitis

LIP is characterized by benign polyclonal proliferation of lymphocytes with infiltration of pulmonary interstitium and alveolar spaces with lymphocytes and plasma cells. This disorder often occurs in association with rheumatologic diseases or human immunodeficiency virus (HIV) infection [118]. Patients may be asymptomatic or they may present with cough, dyspnea and/or constitutional symptoms. Radiologic studies may reveal ground-glass opacities, centrilobular nodules (or masses), septal thickening and/or lung cysts. Thoracoscopic or open lung biopsies are necessary in most cases to confirm the diagnosis and exclude alternative diseases [119]. Treatment of patients with asymptomatic disease may be watchful waiting with frequent monitoring. For patients with symptomatic disease, systemic corticosteroid therapy (usually prednisone 0.5 mg/kg/day) is used and gradually tapered over a period of 6–12 months. For patients who do not respond to steroids or relapse during taper, other immunosuppressive agents (azathioprine, cyclosporine, cyclophosphamide or rituximab) may be used [120]. For patients with HIV infection, highly active antiretroviral therapy is used as first-line treatment (instead of corticosteroid therapy). However, corticosteroid therapy will be needed for patients with HIV infection who continue to experience worsening LIP despite antiretroviral therapy [121]. Infrequently, LIP may undergo malignant transformation and evolve into a pulmonary lymphoma.

5.9. Hypersensitivity pneumonitis

Hypersensitivity pneumonitis (also known as extrinsic allergic alveolitis) refers to a group of diseases that develop secondary to numerous agricultural dusts, microorganisms, bioaerosols and/or reactive chemical species. Prompt diagnosis of hypersensitivity pneumonitis is important as the disease is reversible in its early stages. Correct diagnosis is usually based on a compatible exposure history, clinical assessment, radiographic findings and response to avoidance of the suspected etiologic agent [122]. Acute hypersensitivity pneumonitis often occurs following heavy exposure to an inciting agent and is usually confused with CAP. Patients present with fever, chest pain, cough and dyspnea about 6 hours following exposure. In most cases, symptoms improve within a few days after cessation of exposure to inciting agent, although radiographic resolution requires several weeks. Skin testing to allergens is not useful and serum precipitins may have a high false negative rate. Bronchoscopy with BAL shows lymphocytosis exceeding 20% (often >50%) and the BAL CD4+/CD8+ ratio is usually decreased to less than 1.0 [123]. Characteristic radiographic findings on computed tomography include mid-to-upper zone predominance of centrilobular ground-glass or nodular opacities with signs of air-trapping. Histopathological findings may reveal poorly formed granulomas and/or a patchy mononuclear infiltration near the alveolar walls [124]. Subacute hypersensitivity pneumonitis presents with productive cough, dyspnea, fatigue, anorexia, and weight loss. Most patients have mixed obstructive and restrictive abnormalities on PFTs with a reduction in diffusion capacity. Radiographic findings may include diffuse micronodules, ground-glass opacities, or mild fibrotic changes predominantly involving the middle to upper lung zones. Bronchoscopy with BAL may reveal lymphocytosis and negative cultures. Lung biopsy may reveal poorly formed, noncaseating granulomas in the pulmonary interstitium with fibrosis and bronchiolitis [125]. Removal of the inciting agent results in complete resolution of findings over a longer period of time (weeks to months) and most patients require systemic glucocorticoid therapy. In the chronic progressive form of hypersensitivity pneumonitis, patients present with cough, dyspnea, fatigue, and weight loss. Physical examination may reveal digital clubbing and hypoxemia. Radiographic studies will show widespread pulmonary fibrosis; BAL may reveal lymphocytosis. Lung biopsy is necessary to demonstrate granulomatous pneumonitis, diffuse interstitial pneumonitis, bronchiolitis obliterans and distal destruction of alveoli (honey-combing) with densely fibrotic zones [126]. At this stage, removal of exposure to the inciting agent will only lead to partial improvement. Corticosteroid therapy (usually 0.5–1 mg/kg/day of prednisone) should be prescribed to all symptomatic patients with hypersensitivity pneumonitis. Gradual tapering of steroid dosage can be started after 2 weeks and tapered over the ensuing 2–4 weeks in most patients [127]. In patients with chronic hypersensitivity pneumonitis and extensive pulmonary fibrosis, lung transplantation may be a viable treatment option.

5.10. Idiopathic interstitial pneumonitis

IIP refer to a group of idiopathic ILDs that are characterized by infiltration of the pulmonary interstitium with inflammatory cells and consequently result in progressive fibrosis. IIP is a broad umbrella category that includes a number of different disease entities with distinct histologic patterns, natural course and prognosis [128]. The American Thoracic Society (ATS) and

European Respiratory Society (ERS) classification [129] has recognized 6 major IIPs: (i) idiopathic pulmonary fibrosis (IPF); (ii) idiopathic NSIP; (iii) cryptogenic organizing pneumonitis (COP); (iv) respiratory bronchiolitis (RB) associated ILD; (v) acute interstitial pneumonitis (AIP); and (vi) desquamative interstitial pneumonitis (DIP). Two other ILDs are also included in the ATS/ERS classification as rare IIP viz. idiopathic LIP and idiopathic pleuroparenchymal fibroelastosis (PPFE). A category of unclassifiable IIP is also included in the ATS/ERS classification which is reserved for those IIPs which do not fit the criteria for any specific category of IIP.

IPF and idiopathic NSIP are both ILDs that run a chronic course with most patients experiencing symptoms for many months prior to diagnosis. IPF usually presents in the sixth to seventh decades of life. Typical radiologic findings include bibasilar subpleural fibrosis with traction bronchiectasis and honeycombing in the later stages. IPF is characterized histologically by a UIP pattern with a temporal and geographical heterogeneity, patchy involvement of the lung parenchyma, presence of architectural distortion and fibroblast foci and absence of features suggesting an alternative pattern [130]. Two novel tyrosine kinase inhibitors—pirfenidone and nintedanib—have been approved for the treatment of IPF [131]. Despite this, the overall prognosis for IPF remains poor. Systemic corticosteroid therapy is often employed for patients who develop acute infective exacerbation of IPF, although high quality evidence in support of this practice is lacking [132]. Idiopathic NSIP is a distinct clinical entity and tends to have a subacute presentation and a better prognosis as compared to IPF. Histologically, NSIP is characterized by temporal and geographical homogeneity with uniform involvement of the lung parenchyma, mononuclear cell infiltration of the interstitium and relative preservation of lung architecture [133]. The term "non-specific" is used because the histologic appearance of NSIP lacks the characteristic features of UIP, DIP, RB-ILD or AIP. Radiologic findings include bibasilar subpleural reticular shadowing with traction bronchiectasis, ground-glass opacities and absence of honeycombing. Alternative causes of NSIP, such as collagen vascular diseases, drugs and infections, need to be excluded. Treatment of NSIP is with systemic corticosteroid therapy, usually prednisone 1 mg/kg, gradually tapered over 6–12 months [134]. Pulse-dose methylprednisolone therapy has also been used in those with severe disease on presentation. In patients who relapse or remain refractory despite systemic corticosteroid therapy, a second immunosuppressive agent is added to prednisone.

Cigarette smokers tend to have a number of subclinical pulmonary interstitial abnormalities identifiable on histopathology [135]. These subclinical abnormalities do not meet the criteria for any particular ILD or IIP. Smoking-related ILD include RB-ILD, DIP and Langerhans cell histiocytosis. Langerhans cell histiocytosis is a separate disease entity and is generally not included under the heading of IIP. Both DIP and RB-ILD occur in smokers, usually with a smoking history of over 30 pack-years, most often in the third to fourth decades of life; men are more commonly affected [136]. In DIP, radiologic studies reveal bilateral ground-glass opacities without the peripheral reticular shadowing typical of UIP. In RB-ILD, radiologic findings may include scattered ground-glass opacities along with bronchial wall thickening. Lung biopsy in DIP shows uniform histopathological findings and lacks the patchy nature typical of IPF. Honeycombing is characteristically absent and a striking feature is the presence of numerous "smokers' macrophages" within the distal airspaces [137]. DIP is actually a misnomer as these macrophages were originally believed to be desquamated pneumocytes. A *smoker macrophage* is a macrophage that contains fine brown pigment flecked with tiny blackish particles; these cytoplasmic particles stain well with Prussian blue (iron content) and periodic acid Schiff (polysaccharides) stains. RB-ILD has a histopathological appearance somewhat similar to DIP in that numerous smoker macrophages are noted; however, these pigmented macrophages are abundant within the lumen of respiratory bronchioles [138]. Moreover, the histopathological findings seen in RB-ILD have a *bronchiolocentric* distribution, whereas DIP tends to affect the lung in a rather uniform and diffuse manner. The management of DIP and RB-ILD is similar; smoking cessation is the first line of management [139]. For patients who continue to experience symptoms and have worsening PFTs, systemic corticosteroid therapy is used. Rarely, other immunosuppressive agents may be used if patients do not improve, although evidence in this regard is scarce. Given the considerable overlap between RB-ILD and DIP, some researchers have suggested that the two categories may be merged together into a single group [140].

COP is the term applied to the idiopathic form of BOOP. This clinical disorder is characterized by an inflammatory pneumonitis and a proliferative bronchiolitis that results in excessive proliferation of granulation tissue within the smaller airways [141]. COP often presents with an acute or subacute clinical picture and mimics CAP with a lack of response to antibiotics. Patients are most often in their fifth or sixth decades of life and both sexes are affected equally. In many cases, a flu-like illness may precede the onset of COP. As is the case with other IIP, secondary causes of organizing pneumonia (such as drugs, collagen vascular diseases and infections) need to be excluded. PFTs reveal a restrictive defect with impairment of gaseous exchange (diffusion capacity). Radiologic studies show multiple patchy ground-glass opacities or peripheral consolidations [142]. Bronchoscopy with BAL is often performed to exclude other diagnoses such as infections, drug-induced pneumonitis, hypersensitivity pneumonitis, chronic eosinophilic pneumonitis and malignancy. In COP itself, BAL typically reveals a "mixed pattern" of increased cellularity (i.e. smaller proportion of macrophages and higher proportions of lymphocytes, neutrophils and eosinophils). Although transbronchial lung biopsy may be performed at the time of bronchoscopy, most patients suspected of having COP or other ILD require a thoracoscopic or open lung biopsy (i.e. via thoracotomy) to yield adequate specimens for histopathological evaluation [143]. Systemic corticosteroid therapy is the mainstay of treatment. Prednisone 1 mg/kg/day is usually started, unless the patient has severe symptoms or frank respiratory failure in which cases, IV methylprednisolone 500–1000 mg/day for 5 days may be used initially. Patients usually respond clinically to corticosteroids within a few days to a few weeks. Corticosteroid therapy is generally tapered over a period of 6–12 months. Other immunosuppressive agents may be used in patients who have COP refractory to steroids, or those who relapse frequently despite moderate doses of corticosteroids [144].

AIP (also known as Hamman-Rich syndrome) has a much more aggressive and acute disease course as compared to other ILD and it is similar to acute respiratory distress syndrome (ARDS) in terms of its worse prognosis. In fact, AIP differs from ARDS only in that it has no identifiable triggering event (i.e. it is idiopathic); otherwise, the histological pattern of AIP is identical to that for ARDS (DAD) [145]. Clinically, it presents with acute onset of rapidly worsening respiratory failure with diffuse airspace shadowing on plain radiographs. Computed tomography reveals bilateral diffuse ground glass opacities and/or consolidations with lobular sparing. The histologic hallmark of AIP is DAD as characterized by diffuse airspace organization with or without the formation of hyaline membranes and alveolar septal thickening (due to diffuse organizing fibrosis) with a geographic and temporal homogeneity [146]. As for other IIP, cultures should be negative and granulomas, viral inclusions or eosinophils should be absent on histopathology. AIP requires aggressive treatment with high doses of glucocorticoids—typically methylprednisolone 1–2 g/day in divided doses for 3–5 days, followed by systemic glucocorticoid therapy for several weeks to months [147]. The mortality of AIP is almost 50%, and even in patients who survive the acute illness, recurrence of AIP or progression to a chronic ILD frequently occurs [148].

5.11. Laryngotracheitis (croup)

Laryngotracheitis (also known as croup) is a viral infection caused by parainfluenza viruses (most commonly, type 1) and often affects children in the first 3 years of life with a slight predisposition for boys. Clinical symptoms include low-grade fever, dyspnea, inspiratory stridor and a characteristic *barking* cough. In older children, hoarseness may also be noticeable. In some cases, inflammation may extend to the lower airways and result in laryngotracheobronchitis or even superimposed bacterial laryngotracheobronchopneumonitis [149]. While croup is typically caused by parainfluenza viruses, other viruses may also cause croup in certain cases; these include respiratory syncytial virus, influenza virus, rhinoviruses and human metapneumoviruses [150]. Plain chest radiographs may show narrowing of the subglottic area, frequently referred to as the *steeple* sign—owing to its resemblance to the steeple of a church). It should be noted here that croup is different from bacterial tracheitis, acute epiglottitis and viral bronchiolitis. Bacterial tracheitis is a bacterial infection of the trachea that results in a thick purulent exudate in the trachea, frequently with involvement of the lower airways (tracheobronchopneumonitis) [151]. Acute epiglottitis is an infection that was frequently caused by *Haemophilus influenzae* prior to the widespread use of the "Hib" vaccine. Most cases in vaccinated children and adults are caused by streptococcal or staphylococcal infections. Epiglottitis generally has a more rapid onset and aggressive course than croup and children tend to have high-grade fever and a toxic appearance [152]. Airway obstruction may be precipitated by physical examination or manipulative procedures, such as laryngoscopy. Viral bronchiolitis is an infection that usually occurs in infants and children below the age of 2 years. Most infections are caused by respiratory syncytial virus and present with fever, cough, dyspnea and wheezing [153]. Bronchiolitis is treated with supportive care only and corticosteroids have no role in management.

Treatment of croup involves supportive care with humidified oxygen therapy and anti-pyretics, adequate hydration, corticosteroids and nebulized epinephrine [154]. A strong body of evidence suggests that the use of *either* nebulized budesonide or single-dose dexamethasone provides benefits in terms of reducing length of hospital stay and decreasing visits to the emergency department [155]. The Westley croup score can be used to grade the severity of croup [156]. Patients with mild croup may be managed at home with a single dose of oral dexamethasone 0.6 mg/kg. Patients with moderate croup may be admitted to the hospital and administered an intramuscular or intravenous dose of dexamethasone along with repeated nebulizations of epinephrine [157]. In patients with severe croup and impending respiratory failure, admission to the intensive care unit may be necessary with a plan for endotracheal intubation in the presence of anesthesiologist and/or otorhinolaryngologist.

5.12. Exacerbation of cystic fibrosis

CF is an autosomal recessive disorder that results from genetic mutations in the cystic fibrosis transmembrane conductance regular (*CFTR*) chloride channel. CF is the most common lethal genetic disorder in the European population with an incidence of about 1 in 2500 live births [158]. The most common genetic mutation responsible for CF worldwide is the ΔF508 mutation which results in deletion of a phenylalanine residue at the 508′ position of the *CFTR* channel. This mutation has a prevalence of about 70% in patients with CF. Interestingly, of the 2000 mutations described in *CFTR*, only 4 of the remaining mutations have a prevalence of greater than 1% [159]. In some parts of the world, mutations other than the ΔF508 mutation are relatively common; for instance, the G551D mutation is common in the Middle East region [160–164]. Despite the development of novel targeted therapies for CF patients [165], the median survival for CF patients remains at 37 years—although it has been consistently improving over the past few decades [166]. In patients with CF, defective functioning of the CFTR gene results in protean manifestations, such as sinonasal polyposis, bronchiectasis, chronic pancreatitis with pancreatic insufficiency, CF-related diabetes mellitus, gut pathologies (meconium ileus, meconium ileus equivalent and intestinal atresia), osteoporosis, malnutrition, infertility and delayed puberty [159]. However, the most disabling of these manifestations is lung disease; defective mucociliary clearance leads to recurrent and persistent infections with virulent organisms, resulting in progressive and cumulative lung damage and development of bronchiectasis and end-stage lung disease [166].

Patients with CF frequently present with recurrent and disabling infective exacerbations of their lung disease. The microbiologic agents implicated in pneumonia and lower respiratory tract infections among patients with CF are distinct from that of the general population [167–170]. The management of pulmonary disease in patients with CF is best carried out in dedicated CF centers with a multidisciplinary team that is experienced in the care of such patients [171]. In patients presenting with acute infective exacerbations of CF, good evidence is available to substantiate the role of antibiotics, pulmonary toilet, bronchodilators, ventilatory support and mucolytics [172]. The use of corticosteroids in the management of patients with CF is controversial. Systematic reviews of randomized controlled trials suggest that the use of inhaled or systemic corticosteroid on a chronic basis in patients with CF without evidence of asthma or ABPA causes more harm than meaningful benefits [173, 174]. However, in patients with CF who present with an acute infective exacerbation, some data suggest that short-term corticosteroid therapy may be beneficial. In a randomized controlled trial, Tepper and colleagues demonstrated that use of a short course of intravenous hydrocortisone in patients with acute infective exacerbation of CF provided a greater and sustained improvement in pulmonary function [175]. However, guidelines from the CF Foundation conclude that larger studies would be needed to further evaluate the efficacy of corticosteroids in acute exacerbations of CF vis-à-vis their safety [176].

5.13. Acute respiratory distress syndrome

ARDS is the development of acute hypoxic respiratory failure in response to an identifiable inciting event, which is characterized pathologically by a diffuse inflammatory process involving the lung that leads to increased vascular permeability, generalized alveolar edema, loss of aerated tissue and markedly decreased lung compliance [177]. ARDS can occur in response to a wide range of etiologies including sepsis, acute pancreatitis, trauma, drowning, burns, aspiration, transfusion-related acute lung injury, and so on; however, all these clinical entities are grouped together under the heading of ARDS as their clinical management is similar [178]. Clinically, ARDS presents with worsening hypoxemia and respiratory failure that develops within 24–72 hours of an inciting event. Patients typically have severe tachypnea and hypoxemia with accessory muscle use and respiratory distress on examination; chest auscultation may reveal bilateral diffuse crackles. Plain radiographs reveal bilateral airspace shadowing, which may be patchy in the initial stages, and coalesce later to a more homogeneous pattern in later stages. Arterial blood gas analysis will typically show respiratory alkalosis with hypoxemia and an elevated A–a gradient. The degree of hypoxemia can be quantified by the ratio of PaO_2 to the fraction of inspired oxygen (FiO_2) [179]. Computed tomography reveals widespread airspace opacities that may coalesce and are more prominent in the dependent parts of the lung. Histopathologically, the hallmark feature of ARDS is DAD (similar to AIP) with or without the presence of focal alveolar hemorrhage and hyaline membranes [180]. As per the Berlin definition, ARDS can be diagnosed if a patient has impairment in oxygenation (as measured by a PaO_2/FiO_2 ratio of ≤300 mm Hg) with bilateral airspace opacities on chest radiographs (not fully explained by lung collapse, pulmonary nodules or pleural effusions) that started within a week of a known clinical insult and are not secondary to cardiac failure or fluid overload as assessed by an objective assessment method (such as echocardiography) [181]. The PaO_2/FiO_2 ratio can be used to quantify the oxygenation impairment and stratify the severity of ARDS into severe ($PaO_2/FiO_2 \leq 100$ mm Hg), moderate (PaO_2/FiO_2 101–200 mm Hg) or mild (PaO_2/FiO_2 201–300 mm Hg) [182].

Management of ARDS is centered on mechanically ventilating patients with lung protective strategies. Low tidal volume ventilation is the mainstay of management while tolerating permissive hypercapnia and using high PEEP to maximize alveolar recruitment and prevent atelectasis [183]. In patients with very severe ARDS, prone positioning techniques and extracorporeal membrane oxygenation may be necessary to support life [184]. The use of corticosteroids in patients with ARDS is controversial and remains contentious to date. There is good evidence to suggest that corticosteroids should <u>not</u> be used >14 days after onset of ARDS as there is no demonstrable benefit and clear evidence of harm [185]. Moreover, in patients who develop ARDS due to a *steroid-responsive* etiology, corticosteroids should be used early in the course of the disease [186]. In patients with severe ARDS secondary to a disease process that is not treated with corticosteroids, initiation of systemic corticosteroids early (<14 days) in the course of the disease may offer some benefit. Several meta-analyses have been published to evaluate the impact of steroids on mortality in ARDS and their results have been conflicting. Three meta-analyses suggest that there is no benefit of steroids in terms of overall mortality, but, they help to improve gas oxygenation, reduce duration of mechanical ventilation and decrease overall stay in the ICU [187–189]. Two other meta-analyses reported that use of systemic corticosteroids provided a reduction in overall mortality and reduced the duration of mechanical ventilation [190, 191]. In the light of such conflicting evidence, use of systemic corticosteroids in patients with severe ARDS remains at the discretion of the treating clinician. Critical care physicians should assess each case individually and decide whether to administer corticosteroids or not based on their perceived benefits and possible adverse effects.

5.14. Lung transplantation and transplant-related complications

Lung transplant is used as a treatment modality for a wide variety of disorders that lead to end-stage lung disease with the most common ones being COPD, IPF, CF, α_1-antitrypsin deficiency and idiopathic pulmonary arterial hypertension [192]. Both single-lung and double-lung transplantation procedures are increasingly being performed; however, the availability of donor lungs is the main limiting factor to the number of procedures that can be performed. The basic selection criteria for lung transplantation include: (a) the presence of severe lung disease for which medical therapy is unavailable or ineffective and mortality without transplantation is estimated to be >50% within 2 years; (b) satisfactory psychosocial support system; (c) likelihood to withstand lung transplant surgery is >80%; and (d) absence of other comorbidities that would limit life expectancy in the first 5 years post-transplantation [193]. Absolute contraindications to lung transplant include psychosocial problems or non-adherence to medical therapy, cigarette smoking, alcohol dependency, substance abuse, uncontrolled or untreatable infection, malignancy in the last 2 years, uncorrectable bleeding diathesis, significant coronary artery disease that is not amenable to revascularization, significant dysfunction of other vital organs, severe obesity (body mass index ≥35 kg/m^2), active infection with *Mycobacterium tuberculosis*, or significant deformity of the chest wall or spine that would be expected to cause a severe restrictive defect post-transplant [194]. Apart from these absolute contraindications, there are a number of other diseases or conditions that are considered relative contraindications to lung transplant. Interestingly, use of systemic corticosteroids perioperatively was prohibited in the past due to concerns of poor healing of the newly formed anastomosis [195]. However, most evidence has shown that use of prednisone in doses of up to 0.3 mg/kg pre-transplantation does not increase the risk of complications [196].

Corticosteroids are an important part of immunosuppressive therapy for patients undergoing lung transplantation. At the time of the surgical procedure, an initial dose of 500–1000 mg of methylprednisolone is administered intravenously as soon as the donor allograft's vasculature and bronchus are anastomosed to the recipient's respective structures, and allograft reperfusion is established. Corticosteroid therapy is then continued at a dose of 0.5–1 mg/kg/day of prednisone (or equivalent) and gradually tapered down to a goal of 5–10 mg/day of prednisone (or equivalent) over a period of 6 months [197]. Depending on the transplant center's protocols and characteristics of the recipient (age, primary lung disease, panel reactive antibodies, etc.), induction therapy may or may not be administered post-transplantation. For induction therapy, the most commonly used agents are basiliximab, alemtuzumab or anti-thymocyte globulin [198]. Pre-medication with acetaminophen, diphenhydramine and corticosteroids (methylprednisolone 125 mg IV once) is required prior to infusion of alemtuzumab or anti-thymocyte globulin. Maintenance immunosuppression is then employed with a combination regimen consisting of a glucocorticoid (usually prednisone), a calcineurin inhibitor (usually tacrolimus or cyclosporine) and an anti-metabolite (usually mycophenolate or azathioprine) [199]. Occasionally, an mTOR (mechanistic target of rapamycin) inhibitor, such as sirolimus or everolimus, may also be used be as part of the maintenance immunosuppressive regimen; however, mTOR inhibitors should not be used in the first 3 months post-lung transplant as they may lead to fatal bronchial dehiscence [200].

Transplant rejections represent a significant problem in the world of transplantology. Corticosteroid therapy forms an integral component of the management of both acute and chronic graft rejections. In general terms, a graft rejection is the immune response of the recipient to the donor's graft, which results in dysfunction and failure of the transplanted organ. From a pathological perspective, graft rejection can be cell-mediated or humoral graft rejection depending on whether cytotoxic T lymphocytes or antibodies are implicated in immunopathogenesis respectively. In chronologic terms, rejection is classified into hyperacute, acute or chronic rejection based on temporality [201].

Hyperacute rejection occurs within 24 hours of transplantation (usually in the first few minutes to hours) and results in severe hypoxemia and other signs of graft failure. Such a graft rejection occurs due to preformed circulating antibodies in the recipient that are directed against antigens of the donor. Treatment involves therapeutic plasma exchange (to remove preformed antibodies), IVIG (to bind circulating antibodies & prevent them from interacting with transplanted tissues) and rituximab (to deplete B lymphocytes and prevent further formation of antibodies) [202]. All patients who develop hyper-acute rejection are already on high-dose steroids as part of their usual post-transplant care. Additional therapies, such as bortezomib (proteasome inhibitor) or eculizumab (monoclonal antibody to C5 complement protein), are also employed in most cases. While the outcome of hyperacute rejection is dismal in most cases, HLA typing and "virtual cross-match" of donor and recipient have made it a rare occurrence [203].

Acute lung allograft rejection usually occurs within the first 6–12 months of transplantation and it is cell-mediated in most cases. In acute cellular lung graft rejection, treatment is with pulse-dose methylprednisolone along with intensification of the maintenance immunosuppressive regimen [204]. Patients with persistent graft rejection may be treated with repeated courses of pulse-dose methylprednisolone along with other therapies, such as anti-thymocyte globulin, alemtuzumab and/or mTOR inhibitors (sirolimus or everolimus). Cases of acute humoral lung graft rejection developing weeks to months after transplantation are less common. Such cases are managed with a combination of therapeutic modalities including pulse-dose methylprednisolone, therapeutic plasma exchange, IVIG, rituximab and/or intensification of maintenance immunosuppression [205]. Empiric antibiotics are often initiated in patients with acute lung graft rejection until results of microbiologic and histopathological studies are available.

Chronic lung transplant rejection remains a major source of late morbidity and mortality for lung transplant recipients [206]. Chronic lung allograft rejection may manifest as either bronchiolitis obliterans or a restrictive allograft syndrome. Bronchiolitis obliterans is the predominant subtype of chronic lung graft rejection and has a worse prognosis [207]. It is usually detected as an obstructive defect on PFTs. Histopathologically, fibrosis in the lower airways (bronchioles) with formation of dense scar tissue is typical [208]. In some patients, an unexplained obstructive defect on PFTs is noted in the absence of definitive histopathological evidence of bronchiolitis obliterans; such patients are termed to have bronchiolitis obliterans syndrome. In restrictive allograft syndrome, patients have a demonstrable restrictive defect on PFTs and evidence of fibrotic changes involving the upper lung lobes [209]. In most cases, chronic lung allograft rejection is irreversible and most patients eventually require retransplantation [210]. However, several therapeutic options may be tried in such patients (depending on the transplant center's preferences) including intensification of the immunosuppressive regimen, addition of azithromycin, use of montelukast, use of mTOR inhibitors, trial of anti-thymocyte globulin, total lymphoid irradiation or extracorporeal photophoresis [211].

6. Adverse effects

The adverse effects of corticosteroid therapy are significant and, in most circumstances, these effects are a compelling reason to limit the dose and/or duration of their use [18]. In many of the chronic diseases discussed in this chapter, toxicities of steroid therapy are a major source of morbidity. Additionally, most patients with such chronic diseases are often on immunosuppressive therapy or other toxic medications that may lead to cumulative toxicity. While systemic glucocorticoid therapy is associated with the most number of adverse effects, inhaled glucocorticoid therapy can also have some adverse effects, although they tend to be generally less severe [40–42]. Moreover, some of the adverse effects of corticosteroids do not manifest until complications develop. For instance, loss of bone mineral density may go on unchecked until a patient develops vertebral collapse [212]. Luckily, most of the adverse effects of steroids are potentially reversible with time once corticosteroids are discontinued.

Side effects of systemic corticosteroids pertain to almost all systems of the body. Long-term corticosteroid therapy can cause skin thinning, dermal atrophy and purpura, especially on the dorsum of hand and forearm [213]. Dermal atrophy is a consequence of reduced collagen synthesis due to inhibition of protein synthesis. Purpura is a combined consequence of dermal atrophy and increased fragility of vessels, which predisposes to bleed in response to minor stress. In a case–control study, Karagas and co-workers reported that the risk of non-melanoma skin cancer was increased among patients who used corticosteroids [214]. Cushingoid striae occur due to overstretching of the skin with rupture of vessels within the skin. Steroid-induced acne is also a well-known dermatologic adverse effect of steroids [215]. Ophthalmic adverse effects of corticosteroids include cataracts, increased intraocular pressure and development of glaucoma [216]. Cataracts most commonly occur in a posterior subcapsular location and are often bilateral [41]. Central serous chorioretinopathy is another rare ophthalmic side effect of corticosteroids [217]. Redistribution of body fat with truncal obesity, buffalo hump and moon facies (Cushingoid features) develop when corticosteroids are used over a long period of time in high doses [218]. Prolonged periods of hyperglycemia predispose patients to the development of diabetes mellitus and central adiposity, which in turn leads to increasing insulin resistance. Insulin resistance and hyperinsulinemia lead to increased synthesis of very low-density lipoproteins and increase triglyceride levels and adipose tissue in the body [219]. Moreover, since many pharmacologically used corticosteroids have weak mineralocorticoid properties, they can lead to fluid retention, hypertension, hypokalemia and mild metabolic alkalosis. All these effects can culminate in accelerated atherosclerosis and increased incidence of cerebrovascular events and coronary artery disease [220]. Moreover, fluid retention and hypertension can worsen cardiac failure. Fluid retention can also be problematic in patients with pre-existing renal disease. In the gastrointestinal system, corticosteroids can lead to a number of adverse effects including gastritis and gastrointestinal bleeding [221]. Corticosteroids may also impair healing of peptic ulcers and mask signs of gastrointestinal perforation; however, in patients taking glucocorticoids alone, routine use of proton pump inhibitors is not recommended [222]. Proton pump inhibitors should be given to patients who are taking corticosteroids along with either aspirin or other NSAIDs [223]. Fatty liver is another adverse consequence of prolonged corticosteroid use. In the musculoskeletal system, glucocorticoids lead to accelerated bone loss due to decreased osteogenesis and increased osteolysis [224]. Corticosteroid use can lead to osteoporotic fractures; interestingly, vertebral fractures have been reported in patients treated with glucocorticoids, even with a normal bone mineral density [225]. Avascular necrosis, especially of the head of femur, is a serious adverse effect of glucocorticoid therapy [226]. In children, prolonged use of corticosteroids can lead to slowed growth or even, permanent growth impairment [227]. Corticosteroids can also lead to myopathy, which manifests as proximal muscle weakness, although muscle enzymes (serum creatine kinase) are within normal limits [228]. With respect to the reproductive system, corticosteroid use may lead to menstrual irregularities and decreased fertility in both sexes [229]. Moreover, use of high doses of corticosteroids during the first trimester of pregnancy may elevate the risk of cleft palate slightly [230]. The risk of fetal intrauterine growth restriction is also elevated in women who take corticosteroids throughout pregnancy [231]. Corticosteroids have also been shown to have a number of adverse effects on the central nervous system, especially when used in high doses [232]. Neuropsychiatric effects may include feeling of euphoria, anxiety, depression, mania, delirium or even psychosis. In a study by Shin et al. [233], patients with RA who were treated with oral glucocorticoids had a higher risk of having cognitive impairment. In another study by Keenan and colleagues [234], use of corticosteroids was associated with an adverse outcome on explicit memory at a period of 1 year. Last, but not the least, the immune system is also adversely affected by glucocorticoid therapy and immunosuppression leads to an increased risk of infections, decreased response to vaccines, poor wound healing and lymphopenia [235, 236]. Neutrophilia seen with corticosteroid therapy is a mere consequence of demargination of the neutrophil pool.

Close monitoring of such patients for the development of adverse effects is essential [237]. Routine monitoring should include blood pressure charting, weight charting, regular physical examination, lipid profile and fasting plasma glucose. Determination of bone mineral density and monitoring of intraocular pressure should be considered for patients who are receiving high doses of corticosteroids for a prolonged duration [238]. Specifically, patients with pre-existing co-morbid conditions, such as diabetes mellitus, hypertension, dyslipidemia, heart failure, peptic ulcer disease and osteoporosis, are at a much higher risk of developing adverse effects and must be monitored vigilantly [239].

In summary, corticosteroid therapy is a double-edged sword in patients with chronic diseases who are dependent on steroids. Adverse effects pertaining to nearly every system of the body can occur with the use of corticosteroids, which mandates that patients be treated with the lowest possible dose of corticosteroids for the minimum duration possible. Inhaled corticosteroid therapy can provide a therapeutic effect in many airway disorders, while reducing the risk of many steroid-induced adverse effects at the same time. Thus inhaled therapy for airway disorders should be preferred over systemic corticosteroid therapy, whenever possible.

Conflict of interest

The authors have no conflict of interests to disclose. The authors have no conflict of interests to disclose.

Abbreviations

A–a	alveolar–arterial
ABPA	allergic bronchopulmonary aspergillosis
ACE	angiotensin converting enzyme
ACTH	adrenocorticotrophic hormone
AIP	acute interstitial pneumonitis
ALT	alanine aminotransferase
ANCA	antineutrophil cytoplasmic antibody
APC	antigen presenting cell
ARDS	acute respiratory distress syndrome
ATP	adenosine 1,4,5-triphosphate
ATS	American Thoracic Society
BAL	bronchoalveolar lavage
BOOP	bronchiolitis obliterans organizing pneumonitis
cAMP	cyclic adenosine monophosphate
CAP	community acquired pneumonia
CAT	COPD assessment test
CF	cystic fibrosis
CFTR	cystic fibrosis transmembrane conductance regulator
COP	cryptogenic organizing pneumonitis
COPD	chronic obstructive pulmonary disease
DAD	diffuse alveolar damage
DAH	diffuse alveolar hemorrhage
DIP	desquamative interstitial pneumonitis
DM	dermatomyositis
EGPA	eosinophilic granulomatosis with polyangiitis

ERS	European Respiratory Society
FEV_1	forced expiratory volume in first second of expiration
FiO_2	fraction of inspired oxygen
GOLD	Global Initiative for Chronic Obstructive Lung Disease
GPA	granulomatosis with polyangiitis
GPCR	G-protein coupled receptor
GPS	Goodpasture syndrome
GRE	glucocorticoid-response elements
HIV	human immunodeficiency virus
ICS	inhaled corticosteroids
IgE	immunoglobulin E
IL	interleukin
ILD	interstitial lung disease
IPF	idiopathic pulmonary fibrosis
IVIG	intravenous immunoglobulin
LABA	long-acting β_2-adrenoceptor agonist
LAMA	long-acting muscarinic antagonists
LIP	lymphocytic interstitial pneumonitis
mMRC	modified Medical Research Council scale
MPA	microscopic polyangiitis
mTOR	mechanistic target of rapamycin
NFκB	nuclear factor-κB
NIPPV	non-invasive positive pressure ventilation
NSAID	non-steroidal anti-inflammatory drug
NSIP	non-specific interstitial pneumonitis
OPG	osteoprotegerin
PAMPs	pathogen-associated molecular patterns
PDE	phosphodiesterase
PECAM-1	platelet–endothelial cell adhesion molecule-1
PFT	pulmonary function test
PM	polymyositis

PPFE	pleuroparenchymal fibroelastosis
PRR	pattern recognition receptor
PTH	parathyroid hormone
RA	rheumatoid arthritis
RAAS	renin–angiotensin–aldosterone system
RANK	receptor activator for nuclear factor-κB
RANKL	receptor activator for nuclear factor-κB ligand
RB	respiratory bronchiolitis
RPC	relapsing polychondritis
SABA	short-acting β_2-adrenoceptor agonist
SAMA	short-acting muscarinic antagonists
SGPT	serum glutamate-pyruvate transaminase
SLE	systemic lupus erythematosus
SLS	shrinking lung syndrome
SSc	systemic sclerosis
T_H1	type 1 helper T
T_H2	type 2 helper T
tRNA	transfer ribonucleic acid
UIP	usual interstitial pneumonitis

Author details

Ibrahim A. Janahi[1,2,3]*, Abdul Rehman[4] and Noor Ul-Ain Baloch[5]

*Address all correspondence to: ijanahi@hamad.qa

1 Clinical Pediatrics, Weill-Cornell Medical College, Ar-Rayyan, Qatar

2 Pediatric Pulmonology, Department of Pediatrics, Hamad General Hospital, Doha, Qatar

3 Medical Research Center, Hamad Medical Corporation, Doha, Qatar

4 Internal Medicine Section, Department of Medicine, Hamad Medical Corporation, Doha, Qatar

5 Department of Internal Medicine, Rutgers-New Jersey Medical School, University Hospital, Newark, United States

References

[1] Barwick TD, Malhotra A, Webb JA, Savage MO, Reznek RH. Embryology of the adrenal glands and its relevance to diagnostic imaging. Clinical Radiology. 2005;**60**(9):953-959

[2] De Diego AM, Gandia L, Garcia AG. A physiological view of the central and peripheral mechanisms that regulate the release of catecholamines at the adrenal medulla. Acta Physiologica. 2008;**192**(2):287-301

[3] Burchard K. A review of the adrenal cortex and severe inflammation: Quest of the "eucorticoid" state. Journal of Trauma and Acute Care Surgery. 2001;**51**(4):800-814

[4] Prigent H, Maxime V, Annane D. Science review: Mechanisms of impaired adrenal function in sepsis and molecular actions of glucocorticoids. Critical Care. 2004;**8**(4):243

[5] Jiang G, Zhang BB. Glucagon and regulation of glucose metabolism. American Journal of Physiology. Endocrinology and Metabolism. 2003;**284**(4):E671-E678

[6] Kajiura H, Takata H, Kuriki T, Kitamura S. Structure and solution properties of enzymatically synthesized glycogen. Carbohydrate Research. 2010;**345**(6):817-824

[7] Roach PJ, Depaoli-Roach AA, Hurley TD, Tagliabracci VS. Glycogen and its metabolism: Some new developments and old themes. Biochemical Journal. 2012;**441**(3):763-787

[8] McCowen KC, Malhotra A, Bistrian BR. Stress-induced hyperglycemia. Critical Care Clinics. 2001;**17**(1):107-124

[9] Tamaki T, Uchiyama S, Uchiyama Y, Akatsuka A, Roy RR, Edgerton VR. Anabolic steroids increase exercise tolerance. American Journal of Physiology. Endocrinology and Metabolism. 2001;**280**(6):E973-E981

[10] Kim W, Flamm SL, Di Bisceglie AM, Bodenheimer HC. Serum activity of alanine aminotransferase (ALT) as an indicator of health and disease. Hepatology. 2008;**47**(4):1363-1370

[11] Clarke B. Normal bone anatomy and physiology. Clinical Journal of the American Society of Nephrology. 2008;**3**(Suppl. 3):S131-S139

[12] Wada T, Nakashima T, Hiroshi N, Penninger JM. RANKL–RANK signaling in osteoclastogenesis and bone disease. Trends in Molecular Medicine. 2006;**12**(1):17-25

[13] Canalis E, Delany AM. Mechanisms of glucocorticoid action in bone. Annals of the New York Academy of Sciences. 2002;**966**(1):73-81

[14] Sapolsky RM, Romero LM, Munck AU. How do glucocorticoids influence stress responses? Integrating permissive, suppressive, stimulatory, and preparative actions. Endocrine Reviews. 2000;**21**(1):55-89

[15] Angus DC, Van Der Poll T. Severe sepsis and septic shock. New England Journal of Medicine. 2013;**369**(9):840-851

[16] Paul M, Mehr AP, Kreutz R. Physiology of local renin-angiotensin systems. Physiological Reviews. 2006;**86**(3):747-803

[17] Atlas SA. The renin-angiotensin aldosterone system: Pathophysiological role and pharmacologic inhibition. Journal of Managed Care Pharmacy. 2007;**13**(8 Supp B):9-20

[18] Schäcke H, Döcke WD, Asadullah K. Mechanisms involved in the side effects of glucocorticoids. Pharmacology & Therapeutics. 2002;**96**(1):23-43

[19] Newell-Price J, Bertagna X, Grossman AB, Nieman LK. Cushing's syndrome. The Lancet. 2006;**367**(9522):1605-1617

[20] Nieman LK, Turner ML. Addison's disease. Clinics in Dermatology. 2006;**24**(4):276-280

[21] Barnes PJ. How corticosteroids control inflammation: quintiles prize lecture 2005. British Journal of Pharmacology. 2006;**148**(3):245-254

[22] Hotamisligil GS. Inflammation and metabolic disorders. Nature. 2006;**444**(7121):860

[23] Mogensen TH. Pathogen recognition and inflammatory signaling in innate immune defenses. Clinical Microbiology Reviews. 2009;**22**(2):240-273

[24] Van der Ven BC, Yates RM, Russell DG. Intraphagosomal measurement of the magnitude and duration of the oxidative burst. Traffic. 2009;**10**(4):372-378

[25] Serhan CN, Chiang N, Van Dyke TE. Resolving inflammation: Dual anti-inflammatory and pro-resolution lipid mediators. Nature Reviews. Immunology. 2008;**8**(5):349

[26] Serhan CN, Chiang N. Endogenous pro-resolving and anti-inflammatory lipid mediators: A new pharmacologic genus. British Journal of Pharmacology. 2008;**153**(S1):S200-S215

[27] Sprague AH, Khalil RA. Inflammatory cytokines in vascular dysfunction and vascular disease. Biochemical Pharmacology. 2009;**78**(6):539-552

[28] Bogatcheva NV, Sergeeva MG, Dudek SM, Verin AD. Arachidonic acid cascade in endothelial pathobiology. Microvascular Research. 2005;**69**(3):107-127

[29] Meirer K, Steinhilber D, Proschak E. Inhibitors of the arachidonic acid cascade: Interfering with multiple pathways. Basic & Clinical Pharmacology & Toxicology. 2014;**114**(1):83-91

[30] Stahn C, Löwenberg M, Hommes DW, Buttgereit F. Molecular mechanisms of glucocorticoid action and selective glucocorticoid receptor agonists. Molecular and Cellular Endocrinology. 2007;**275**(1):71-78

[31] Yamamoto Y, Gaynor RB. Role of the NF-kB pathway in the pathogenesis of human disease states. Current Molecular Medicine. 2001;**1**(3):287-296

[32] Hermoso MA, Cidlowski JA. Putting the brake on inflammatory responses: The role of glucocorticoids. IUBMB Life. 2003;**55**(9):497-504

[33] Busillo JM, Cidlowski JA. The five Rs of glucocorticoid action during inflammation: Ready, reinforce, repress, resolve, and restore. Trends in Endocrinology and Metabolism. 2013;**24**(3):109-119

[34] Hoes JN, Jacobs JW, Boers M, Boumpas D, Buttgereit F, Caeyers N, Choy EH, Cutolo M, Da Silva JA, Esselens G, Guillevin L. EULAR evidence-based recommendations on the

management of systemic glucocorticoid therapy in rheumatic diseases. Annals of the Rheumatic Diseases. 2007;**66**(12):1560-1567

[35] Czock D, Keller F, Rasche FM, Häussler U. Pharmacokinetics and pharmacodynamics of systemically administered glucocorticoids. Clinical Pharmacokinetics. 2005;**44**(1):61-98

[36] Samtani MN, Jusko WJ. Comparison of dexamethasone pharmacokinetics in female rats after intravenous and intramuscular administration. Biopharmaceutics & Drug Disposition. 2005;**26**(3):85-91

[37] Badsha H, Edwards CJ. Intravenous pulses of methylprednisolone for systemic lupus erythematosus. Seminars in Arthritis and Rheumatism. 2003;**32**(6):370-377

[38] Buttgereit F, Wehling M, Burmester GR. A new hypothesis of modular glucocorticoid actions: Steroid treatment of rheumatic diseases revisited. Arthritis & Rheumatology. 1998;**41**(5):761-767

[39] Derendorf H, Nave R, Drollmann A, Cerasoli F, Wurst W. Relevance of pharmacokinetics and pharmacodynamics of inhaled corticosteroids to asthma. European Respiratory Journal. 2006;**28**(5):1042-1050

[40] Zhang L, Prietsch SO, Ducharme FM. Inhaled corticosteroids in children with persistent asthma: Effects on growth. Evidence-Based Child Health: A Cochrane Review Journal. 2014;**9**(4):829-930

[41] Wang JJ, Rochtchina E, Tan AG, Cumming RG, Leeder SR, Mitchell P. Use of inhaled and oral corticosteroids and the long-term risk of cataract. Ophthalmology. 2009; **116**(4):652-657

[42] Dubus JC, Marguet C, Deschildre A, Mely L, Le Roux P, Brouard J, Huiart L. Local side-effects of inhaled corticosteroids in asthmatic children: Influence of drug, dose, age, and device. Allergy. 2001;**56**(10):944-948

[43] Hengge UR, Ruzicka T, Schwartz RA, Cork MJ. Adverse effects of topical glucocorticosteroids. Journal of the American Academy of Dermatology. 2006;**54**(1):1-5

[44] Ference JD, Last AR. Choosing topical corticosteroids. American Family Physician. 2009;**79**(2):135-140

[45] Del Rosso J, Friedlander SF. Corticosteroids: Options in the era of steroid-sparing therapy. Journal of the American Academy of Dermatology. 2005;**53**(1):S50-S58

[46] Janahi IA, Bener A, Bush A. Prevalence of asthma among Qatari schoolchildren: International study of asthma and allergies in childhood, Qatar. Pediatric Pulmonology. 2006;**41**(1):80-86

[47] Bener A, Janahi IA, Sabbah A. Genetics and environmental risk factors associated with asthma in schoolchildren. European Annals of Allergy and Clinical Immunology. 2005; **37**(5):163-168

[48] Agache I, Akdis C, Jutel M, Virchow JC. Untangling asthma phenotypes and endotypes. Allergy. 2012;**67**(7):835-846

[49] Rajan JP, Wineinger NE, Stevenson DD, White AA. Prevalence of aspirin-exacerbated respiratory disease among asthmatic patients: A meta-analysis of the literature. Journal of Allergy and Clinical Immunology. 2015;**135**(3):676-681

[50] Holgate ST. Innate and adaptive immune responses in asthma. Nature Medicine. 2012; **18**(5):673-683

[51] Holgate ST. The sentinel role of the airway epithelium in asthma pathogenesis. Immunological Reviews. 2011;**242**(1):205-219

[52] Fanta CH. Asthma. New England Journal of Medicine. 2009;**360**(10):1002-1014

[53] Dror RO, Pan AC, Arlow DH, Borhani DW, Maragakis P, Shan Y, Xu H, Shaw DE. Pathway and mechanism of drug binding to G-protein-coupled receptors. Proceedings of the National Academy of Sciences. 2011;**108**(32):13118-13123

[54] Olin JT, Wechsler ME. Asthma: Pathogenesis and novel drugs for treatment. BMJ. 2014; **349**:g5517

[55] Ortega HG, Liu MC, Pavord ID, Brusselle GG, FitzGerald JM, Chetta A, Humbert M, Katz LE, Keene ON, Yancey SW, Chanez P. Mepolizumab treatment in patients with severe eosinophilic asthma. New England Journal of Medicine. 2014;**371**(13):1198-1207

[56] Durrani SR, Viswanathan RK, Busse WW. What effect does asthma treatment have on airway remodeling? Current perspectives. Journal of Allergy and Clinical Immunology. 2011;**128**(3):439-448

[57] Lazarus SC. Clinical practice. Emergency treatment of asthma. New England Journal of Medicine. 2010;**363**(8):755-764

[58] Bateman ED, Hurd SS, Barnes PJ, Bousquet J, Drazen JM, FitzGerald M, Gibson P, Ohta K, O'byrne P, Pedersen SE, Pizzichini E. Global strategy for asthma management and prevention: GINA executive summary. European Respiratory Journal. 2008;**31**(1):143-178

[59] Bush A, Fleming L. Diagnosis and management of asthma in children. BMJ. 2015;**350**:h996

[60] MacNee W. ABC of chronic obstructive pulmonary disease: Pathology, pathogenesis, and pathophysiology. BMJ. 2006;**332**(7551):1202

[61] de Oca MM, Halbert RJ, Lopez MV, Perez-Padilla R, Tálamo C, Moreno D, Muiño A, Jardim JR, Valdivia G, Pertuzé J, Menezes AM. Chronic bronchitis phenotype in subjects with and without COPD: The PLATINO study. European Respiratory Journal. 2012; **40**(1):28-36

[62] Kim V, Pechulis RM, Abuel-Haija M, Solomides CC, Gaughan JP, Criner GJ. Small airway pathology and bronchoreversibility in advanced emphysema. COPD: Journal of Chronic Obstructive Pulmonary Disease. 2010;**7**(2):93-101

[63] O'donnell DE, Banzett RB, Carrieri-Kohlman V, Casaburi R, Davenport PW, Gandevia SC, Gelb AF, Mahler DA, Webb KA. Pathophysiology of dyspnea in chronic obstructive pulmonary disease: A roundtable. Proceedings of the American Thoracic Society. 2007;**4**(2):145-168

[64] Yoshida T, Tuder RM. Pathobiology of cigarette smoke-induced chronic obstructive pulmonary disease. Physiological Reviews. 2007;**87**(3):1047-1082

[65] Yang P, Sun Z, Krowka MJ, Aubry MC, Bamlet WR, Wampfler JA, Thibodeau SN, Katzmann JA, Allen MS, Midthun DE, Marks RS. Alpha1-antitrypsin deficiency carriers, tobacco smoke, chronic obstructive pulmonary disease, and lung cancer risk. Archives of Internal Medicine. 2008;**168**(10):1097-1103

[66] Alsaeedi A, Sin DD, McAlister FA. The effects of inhaled corticosteroids in chronic obstructive pulmonary disease: A systematic review of randomized placebo-controlled trials. American Journal of Medicine. 2002;**113**(1):59-65

[67] Rodriguez-Roisin R. COPD exacerbations·5: Management. Thorax. 2006;**61**(6):535-544

[68] Rabe KF, Hurd S, Anzueto A, Barnes PJ, Buist SA, Calverley P, Fukuchi Y, Jenkins C, Rodriguez-Roisin R, Van Weel C, Zielinski J. Global strategy for the diagnosis, management, and prevention of chronic obstructive pulmonary disease: GOLD executive summary. American Journal of Respiratory and Critical Care Medicine. 2007;**176**(6):532-555

[69] Wedzicha JA, Calverley PM, Rabe KF. Roflumilast: A review of its use in the treatment of COPD. International Journal of Chronic Obstructive Pulmonary Disease. 2016;**11**:81-90

[70] Meyers BF, Patterson GA. Chronic obstructive pulmonary disease• 10: Bullectomy, lung volume reduction surgery, and transplantation for patients with chronic obstructive pulmonary disease. Thorax. 2003;**58**(7):634-638

[71] Höffken G, Lorenz J, Kern W, Welte T, Bauer T, Dalhoff K, Dietrich E, Ewig S, Gastmeier P, Grabein B, Halle E. Epidemiology, diagnosis, antimicrobial therapy and management of community-acquired pneumonia and lower respiratory tract infections in adults. Guidelines of the Paul-Ehrlich-Society for Chemotherapy, the German respiratory society, the German Society for Infectiology and the competence network CAPNETZ Germany. Pneumologie (Stuttgart, Germany). 2009;**63**(10):e1

[72] Marrie TJ. Community-acquired pneumonia: Epidemiology, etiology, treatment. Infectious Disease Clinics of North America. 1998;**12**(3):723-740

[73] Jain S, Self WH, Wunderink RG, Fakhran S, Balk R, Bramley AM, Reed C, Grijalva CG, Anderson EJ, Courtney DM, Chappell JD. Community-acquired pneumonia requiring hospitalization among US adults. New England Journal of Medicine. 2015;**373**(5):415-427

[74] Ewald H, Raatz H, Boscacci R, Furrer H, Bucher HC, Briel M. Adjunctive corticosteroids for pneumocystis jiroveci pneumonia in patients with HIV infection. Cochrane Database of Systematic Reviews. 2015;**4**:CD006150

[75] Torres A, Sibila O, Ferrer M, Polverino E, Menendez R, Mensa J, Gabarrús A, Sellarés J, Restrepo MI, Anzueto A, Niederman MS. Effect of corticosteroids on treatment failure among hospitalized patients with severe community-acquired pneumonia and high inflammatory response: A randomized clinical trial. JAMA. 2015;**313**(7):677-686

[76] Siemieniuk RA, Meade MO, Alonso-Coello P, Briel M, Evaniew N, Prasad M, Alexander PE, Fei Y, Vandvik PO, Loeb M, Guyatt GH. Corticosteroid therapy for patients hospitalized

with community-acquired pneumonia: A systematic review and meta-analysis. Annals of Internal Medicine. 2015;**163**(7):519-528

[77] Janahi IA, Rehman A, Al-Naimi AR. Allergic bronchopulmonary aspergillosis in patients with cystic fibrosis. Annals of Thoracic Medicine. 2017;**12**(2):74

[78] Maturu VN, Agarwal R. Prevalence of Aspergillus sensitization and allergic bronchopulmonary aspergillosis in cystic fibrosis: Systematic review and meta-analysis. Clinical & Experimental Allergy. 2015;**45**(12):1765-1778

[79] Agarwal R, Chakrabarti A, Shah A, Gupta D, Meis JF, Guleria R, Moss R, Denning DW. Allergic bronchopulmonary aspergillosis: Review of literature and proposal of new diagnostic and classification criteria. Clinical & Experimental Allergy. 2013;**43**(8):850-873

[80] Reddy A, Greenberger PA. Allergic bronchopulmonary aspergillosis. The Journal of Allergy and Clinical Immunology. In Practice. 2017;**5**(3):866-867

[81] Tanou K, Zintzaras E, Kaditis AG. Omalizumab therapy for allergic bronchopulmonary aspergillosis in children with cystic fibrosis: A synthesis of published evidence. Pediatric Pulmonology. 2014;**49**(5):503-507

[82] Wong R, Wong M, Robinson PD, Fitzgerald DA. Omalizumab in the management of steroid dependent allergic bronchopulmonary aspergillosis (ABPA) complicating cystic fibrosis. Paediatric Respiratory Reviews. 2013;**14**(1):22-24

[83] Baughman RP, Culver DA, Judson MA. A concise review of pulmonary sarcoidosis. American Journal of Respiratory and Critical Care Medicine. 2011;**183**(5):573-581

[84] Dua A, Manadan A. Heerfordt's syndrome, or uveoparotid fever. New England Journal of Medicine. 2013;**369**(5):458

[85] Grunewald J, Eklund A. Sex-specific manifestations of Lofgren's syndrome. American Journal of Respiratory and Critical Care Medicine. 2007;**175**(1):40-44

[86] Mihailovic-Vucinic V, Jovanovic D. Pulmonary sarcoidosis. Clinics in Chest Medicine. 2008;**29**(3):459-473

[87] Schutt AC, Bullington WM, Judson MA. Pharmacotherapy for pulmonary sarcoidosis: A Delphi consensus study. Respiratory Medicine. 2010;**104**(5):717-723

[88] Korsten P, Strohmayer K, Baughman RP, Sweiss NJ. Refractory pulmonary sarcoidosis-proposal of a definition and recommendations for the diagnostic and therapeutic approach. Clinical Pulmonary Medicine. 2016;**23**(2):67-75

[89] Paramothayan S, Jones PW. Corticosteroid therapy in pulmonary sarcoidosis: A systematic review. JAMA. 2002;**287**(10):1301-1307

[90] Kim EA, Lee KS, Johkoh T, Kim TS, Suh GY, Kwon OJ, Han J. Interstitial lung diseases associated with collagen vascular diseases: Radiologic and histopathologic findings. Radiographics. 2002;**22**(Suppl 1):S151-S165

[91] Ferri C, Valentini G, Cozzi F, Sebastiani M, Michelassi C, La Montagna G, Bullo A, Cazzato M, Tirri E, Storino F, Giuggioli D. Systemic sclerosis: Demographic, clinical, and serologic features and survival in 1,012 Italian patients. Medicine. 2002;**81**(2):139-153

[92] Bouros D, Wells AU, Nicholson AG, Colby TV, Polychronopoulos V, Pantelidis P, Haslam PL, Vassilakis DA, Black CM, Du Bois RM. Histopathologic subsets of fibrosing alveolitis in patients with systemic sclerosis and their relationship to outcome. American Journal of Respiratory and Critical Care Medicine. 2002;**165**(12):1581-1586

[93] Kowal-Bielecka O, Landewé R, Avouac J, Chwiesko S, Miniati I, Czirjak L, Clements P, Denton C, Farge D, Fligelstone K, Földvari I. EULAR recommendations for the treatment of systemic sclerosis: A report from the EULAR scleroderma trials and research group (EUSTAR). Annals of the Rheumatic Diseases. 2009;**68**(5):620-628

[94] Khanna D, Denton CP. Evidence-based management of rapidly progressing systemic sclerosis. Best Practice & Research. Clinical Rheumatology. 2010;**24**(3):387-400

[95] Dalakas MC, Hohlfeld R. Polymyositis and dermatomyositis. The Lancet. 2003;**362**(9388): 971-982

[96] Katzap E, Barilla-LaBarca ML, Marder G. Antisynthetase syndrome. Current Rheumatology Reports. 2011;**13**(3):175

[97] Fathi M, Lundberg IE, Tornling G. Pulmonary complications of polymyositis and dermatomyositis. Seminars in Respiratory and Critical Care Medicine. 2007;**28**(4):451-458

[98] Schnabel A, Reuter M, Biederer J, Richter C, Gross WL. Interstitial lung disease in polymyositis and dermatomyositis: Clinical course and response to treatment. Seminars in Arthritis and Rheumatism. 2003;**32**(5):273-284

[99] Yu C, Gershwin ME, Chang C. Diagnostic criteria for systemic lupus erythematosus: A critical review. Journal of Autoimmunity. 2014;**48**:10-13

[100] Keane MP, Lynch JP. Pleuropulmonary manifestations of systemic lupus erythematosus. Thorax. 2000;**55**(2):159-166

[101] Feng PH. Systemic lupus erythematosus. Annals of the New York Academy of Sciences. 2007;**1108**(1):114-120

[102] Firestein GS. Evolving concepts of rheumatoid arthritis. Nature. 2003;**423**(6937):356-361

[103] Smolen JS, Landewé R, Breedveld FC, Dougados M, Emery P, Gaujoux-Viala C, Gorter S, Knevel R, Nam J, Schoels M, Aletaha D. EULAR recommendations for the management of rheumatoid arthritis with synthetic and biological disease-modifying antirheumatic drugs. Annals of the Rheumatic Diseases. 2010;**69**(6):964-975

[104] Tanaka N, Kim JS, Newell JD, Brown KK, Cool CD, Meehan R, Emoto T, Matsumoto T, Lynch DA. Rheumatoid arthritis–related lung diseases: CT findings. Radiology. 2004;**232**(1):81-91

[105] Jennette JC, Falk RJ, Gasim AH. Pathogenesis of ANCA vasculitis. Current Opinion in Nephrology and Hypertension. 2011;**20**(3):263

[106] Vaglio A, Buzio C, Zwerina J. Eosinophilic granulomatosis with polyangiitis (Churg–Strauss): State of the art. Allergy. 2013;**68**(3):261-273

[107] Jennette JC, Thomas DB, Falk RJ. Microscopic polyangiitis (microscopic polyarteritis). Seminars in Diagnostic Pathology. 2001;**18**(1):3-13

[108] Salama AD, Levy JB, Lightstone L, Pusey CD. Goodpasture's disease. The Lancet. 2001;**358**(9285):917-920

[109] Collard HR, Schwarz MI. Diffuse alveolar hemorrhage. Clinics in Chest Medicine. 2004; **25**(3):583-592

[110] Hazra N, Dregan A, Charlton J, Gulliford MC, D'Cruz DP. Incidence and mortality of relapsing polychondritis in the UK: A population-based cohort study. Rheumatology. 2015;**54**(12):2181-2187

[111] Yoo JH, Chodosh J, Dana R. Relapsing polychondritis: Systemic and ocular manifestations, differential diagnosis, management, and prognosis. Seminars in Ophthalmology. 2011;**26**(4-5):261-269

[112] Rafeq S, Trentham D, Ernst A. Pulmonary manifestations of relapsing polychondritis. Clinics in Chest Medicine. 2010;**31**(3):513-518

[113] Philit F, Etienne-Mastroïanni B, Parrot A, Guérin C, Robert D, Cordier JF. Idiopathic acute eosinophilic pneumonia: A study of 22 patients. American Journal of Respiratory and Critical Care Medicine. 2002;**166**(9):1235-1239

[114] Shorr AF, Scoville SL, Cersovsky SB, Shanks GD, Ockenhouse CF, Smoak BL, Carr WW, Petruccelli BP. Acute eosinophilic pneumonia among US military personnel deployed in or near Iraq. JAMA. 2004;**292**(24):2997-3005

[115] Allen J. Acute eosinophilic pneumonia. Seminars in Respiratory and Critical Care Medicine. 2006;**27**(2):142-147

[116] Vivero F, Ciocchini C, Gandini MJ, Wehbe L. Chronic eosinophilic pneumonia. Revista de la Facultad de Ciencias Medicas (Cordoba, Argentina). 2012;**69**(1):42-46

[117] Rhee CK, Min KH, Yim NY, Lee JE, Lee NR, Chung MP, Jeon K. Clinical characteristics and corticosteroid treatment of acute eosinophilic pneumonia. European Respiratory Journal. 2013;**41**(2):402-409

[118] Panchabhai TS, Farver C, Highland KB. Lymphocytic interstitial pneumonia. Clinics in Chest Medicine. 2016;**37**(3):463-474

[119] Becciolini V, Gudinchet F, Cheseaux JJ, Schnyder P. Lymphocytic interstitial pneumonia in children with AIDS: High-resolution CT findings. European Radiology. 2001; **11**(6):1015-1020

[120] Fishback N, Koss M. Update on lymphoid interstitial pneumonitis. Current Opinion in Pulmonary Medicine. 1996;**2**(5):B97

[121] Dufour V, Wislez M, Bergot E, Mayaud C, Cadranel J. Improvement of symptomatic human immunodeficiency virus-related lymphoid interstitial pneumonia in patients receiving highly active antiretroviral therapy. Clinical Infectious Diseases. 2003;**36**(10): e127-e130

[122] Ismail T, Mcsharry C, Boyd G. Extrinsic allergic alveolitis. Respirology. 2006;**11**(3):262-268

[123] Mohr LC. Hypersensitivity pneumonitis. Current Opinion in Pulmonary Medicine. 2004;**10**(5):401-411

[124] Bourke SJ, Dalphin JC, Boyd G, McSharry C, Baldwin CI, Calvert JE. Hypersensitivity pneumonitis: Current concepts. European Respiratory Journal. 2001;**18**(32 suppl):81s-92s

[125] Selman M, Pardo A, King Jr TE. Hypersensitivity pneumonitis: Insights in diagnosis and pathobiology. American Journal of Respiratory and Critical Care Medicine. 2012;**186**(4):314-324

[126] Zacharisen MC, Schlueter DP, Kurup VP, Fink JN. The long-term outcome in acute, subacute, and chronic forms of pigeon breeder's disease hypersensitivity pneumonitis. Annals of Allergy, Asthma & Immunology. 2002;**88**(2):175-182

[127] Matar LD, McAdams HP, Sporn TA. Hypersensitivity pneumonitis. American Journal of Roentgenology. 2000;**174**(4):1061-1066

[128] Flaherty KR, Toews GB, Travis WD, Colby TV, Kazerooni EA, Gross BH, Jain A, Strawderman RL, Paine R, Flint A, Lynch JP. Clinical significance of histological classification of idiopathic interstitial pneumonia. European Respiratory Journal. 2002; **19**(2):275-283

[129] Travis WD, King TE, Bateman ED, Lynch DA, Capron F, Center D, Colby TV, Cordier JF, DuBois RM, Galvin J, Grenier P. American Thoracic Society/European Respiratory Society international multidisciplinary consensus classification of the idiopathic interstitial pneumonias. American Journal of Respiratory and Critical Care Medicine. 2002;**165**(2):277-304

[130] Gross TJ, Hunninghake GW. Idiopathic pulmonary fibrosis. New England Journal of Medicine. 2001;**345**(7):517-525

[131] Raghu G, Rochwerg B, Zhang Y, Garcia CA, Azuma A, Behr J, Brozek JL, Collard HR, Cunningham W, Homma S, Johkoh T. An official ATS/ERS/JRS/ALAT clinical practice guideline: Treatment of idiopathic pulmonary fibrosis. An update of the 2011 clinical practice guideline. American Journal of Respiratory and Critical Care Medicine. 2015;**192**(2):e3-19

[132] Ryerson CJ, Cottin V, Brown KK, Collard HR. Acute exacerbation of idiopathic pulmonary fibrosis: Shifting the paradigm. European Respiratory Journal. 2015;**46**(2):512-520

[133] Tabaj GC, Fernandez CF, Sabbagh E, Leslie KO. Histopathology of the idiopathic interstitial pneumonias (IIP): A review. Respirology. 2015;**20**(6):873-883

[134] Flaherty KR, Martinez FJ. Nonspecific interstitial pneumonia. Seminars in Respiratory and Critical Care Medicine. 2006;**27**(6):652-658

[135] Jin GY, Lynch D, Chawla A, Garg K, Tammemagi MC, Sahin H, Misumi S, Kwon KS. Interstitial lung abnormalities in a CT lung cancer screening population: Prevalence and progression rate. Radiology. 2013;**268**(2):563-571

[136] Vassallo R, Ryu JH. Smoking-related interstitial lung diseases. Clinics in Chest Medicine. 2012;**33**(1):165-178

[137] Craig PJ, Wells AU, Doffman S, Rassl D, Colby TV, Hansell DM, Du Bois RM, Nicholson AG. Desquamative interstitial pneumonia, respiratory bronchiolitis and their relationship to smoking. Histopathology. 2004;**45**(3):275-282

[138] Fraig M, Shreesha U, Savici D, Katzenstein AL. Respiratory bronchiolitis: A clinicopathologic study in current smokers, ex-smokers, and never-smokers. American Journal of Surgical Pathology. 2002;**26**(5):647-653

[139] Park JS, Brown KK, Tuder RM, Hale VA, King TE Jr, Lynch DA. Respiratory bronchiolitis-associated interstitial lung disease: Radiologic features with clinical and pathologic correlation. Journal of Computer Assisted Tomography. 2002;**26**(1):13-20

[140] Wells AU, Nicholson AG, Hansell DM, du Bois RM. Respiratory bronchiolitis-associated interstitial lung disease. Seminars in Respiratory and Critical Care Medicine. 2003;**24**(5):585-594

[141] Wells AU. Cryptogenic organizing pneumonia. Seminars in Respiratory and Critical Care Medicine. 2001;**22**(4):449-460

[142] Vasu TS, Cavallazzi R, Hirani A, Sharma D, Weibel SB, Kane GC. Clinical and radiologic distinctions between secondary bronchiolitis obliterans organizing pneumonia and cryptogenic organizing pneumonia. Respiratory Care. 2009;**54**(8):1028-1032

[143] Kim SJ, Lee KS, Ryu YH, Yoon YC, Choe KO, Kim TS, Sung KJ. Reversed halo sign on high-resolution CT of cryptogenic organizing pneumonia: Diagnostic implications. American Journal of Roentgenology. 2003;**180**(5):1251-1254

[144] Lazor R, Cordier JF. Cryptogenic organizing pneumonia. Clinical Pulmonary Medicine. 2005;**12**(3):153-161

[145] Bouros D, Nicholson AC, Polychronopoulos V, Du Bois RM. Acute interstitial pneumonia. European Respiratory Journal. 2000;**15**(2):412-418

[146] Mukhopadhyay S, Parambil JG. Acute interstitial pneumonia (AIP): Relationship to Hamman-rich syndrome, diffuse alveolar damage (DAD), and acute respiratory distress syndrome (ARDS). Seminars in Respiratory and Critical Care Medicine. 2012; **33**(5):476-485

[147] Bonaccorsi A, Cancellieri A, Chilosi M, Trisolini R, Boaron M, Crimi N, Poletti V. Acute interstitial pneumonia: Report of a series. European Respiratory Journal. 2003;**21**(1): 187-191

[148] Vourlekis JS, Brown KK, Cool CD, Young DA, Cherniack RM, King Jr TE, Schwarz MI. Acute interstitial pneumonitis: Case series and review of the literature. Medicine. 2000; **79**(6):369-378

[149] Cherry JD. Clinical practice. Croup. New England Journal of Medicine. 2008;**358**(4): 384-391

[150] Roe M, O'Donnell DR, Tasker RC. Acute laryngotracheobronchitis. Paediatric Respiratory Reviews. 2003;**4**(3):267-269

[151] Al-Mutairi B, Kirk V. Bacterial tracheitis in children: Approach to diagnosis and treatment. Paediatrics & Child Health. 2004;**9**(1):25-30

[152] Shah RK, Roberson DW, Jones DT. Epiglottitis in the Hemophilus influenzae type B vaccine era: Changing trends. Laryngoscope. 2004;**114**(3):557-560

[153] Fernandes RM, Bialy LM, Vandermeer B, Tjosvold L, Plint AC, Patel H, Johnson DW, Klassen TP, Hartling L. Glucocorticoids for acute viral bronchiolitis in infants and young children. Cochrane Database of Systematic Reviews. 2013;**6**:CD004878

[154] Brown JC. The management of croup. British Medical Bulletin. 2002;**61**(1):189-202

[155] Russell KF, Liang Y, O'Gorman K, Johnson DW, Klassen TP. Glucocorticoids for croup. Cochrane Database of Systematic Reviews. 2011;**1**:CD001955

[156] Rajapaksa S, Starr M. Croup: Assessment and management. Australian Family Physician. 2010;**39**(5):280

[157] Petrocheilou A, Tanou K, Kalampouka E, Malakasioti G, Giannios C, Kaditis AG. Viral croup: Diagnosis and a treatment algorithm. Pediatric Pulmonology. 2014;**49**(5):421-429

[158] Farrell PM. The prevalence of cystic fibrosis in the European Union. Journal of Cystic Fibrosis. 2008;**7**(5):450-453

[159] Janahi IA, Rehman A. Clinical manifestations of cystic fibrosis and their management. In: Robertson L, editor. Cystic and Idiopathic Pulmonary Fibrosis: Risk Factors, Management and Long-Term Health Outcomes. Hauppauge, NY: Nova Publishers, Inc; 2016. pp. 1-56

[160] Wahab AA, Janahi IA, Hebi S, Al-Hamed M, Kambouris M. Cystic fibrosis in a child from Syria. Annals of Tropical Paediatrics. 2002;**22**(1):53-55

[161] Molinski SV, Gonska T, Huan LJ, Baskin B, Janahi IA, Ray PN, Bear CE. Genetic, cell biological, and clinical interrogation of the CFTR mutation c. 3700 a> G (p. Ile1234Val) informs strategies for future medical intervention. Genetics in Medicine. 2014;**16**(8): 625-632

[162] Abdul-Wahab A, Janahi IA, Abdel-Rahman MO. Sweat chloride concentration in cystic fibrosis patients with cystic fibrosis trans-membrane conductance regulator I1234V mutation. Saudi Medical Journal. 2009;**30**(8):1101-1102

[163] Zahraldin K, Janahi IA, Ben-Omran T, Alsulaiman R, Hamad B, Imam A. Two Qatari siblings with cystic fibrosis and apparent mineralocorticoid excess. Annals of Thoracic Medicine. 2015;**10**(1):69

[164] Wahab AA, Janahi IA, Marafia MM. Pseudo-Bartter's syndrome in an Egyptian infant with cystic fibrosis mutation N1303K. Journal of Tropical Pediatrics. 2004;**50**(4):242-244

[165] Rehman A, Baloch NU, Janahi IA. Lumacaftor-ivacaftor in patients with cystic fibrosis homozygous for Phe508del CFTR. New England Journal of Medicine. 2015;**373**(18):1783

[166] Dodge JA, Lewis PA, Stanton M, Wilsher J. Cystic fibrosis mortality and survival in the UK: 1947-2003. European Respiratory Journal. 2007;**29**(3):522-526

[167] Janahi IA, Abdulwahab A, Sittana SE, Bush A. Rapidly progressive lung disease in a patient with cystic fibrosis on long-term azithromycin: Possible role of mycoplasma infection. Journal of Cystic Fibrosis. 2005;**4**(1):71-73

[168] Janahi IA, Rehman A. The cystic fibrosis airway microbiome and pathogens. In: Sriramulu D, editor. Progress in Understanding Cystic Fibrosis. Rijeka, Croatia: InTech Publishers, Inc; 2017. pp. 45-71

[169] Wahab AA, Janahi IA, Marafia MM, El-Shafie S. Microbiological identification in cystic fibrosis patients with CFTR I1234V mutation. Journal of Tropical Pediatrics. 2004;**50**(4):229-233

[170] Abdul WA, Janahi IA, El-Shafie SS. Achromobacter xylosoxidans isolated from the sputum of a patient with cystic fibrosis mutation I1234V with Pseudomonas Aeruginosa. Saudi Medical Journal. 2004;**25**(6):810

[171] Borowitz D, Robinson KA, Rosenfeld M, Davis SD, Sabadosa KA, Spear SL, Michel SH, Parad RB, White TB, Farrell PM, Marshall BC. Cystic Fibrosis Foundation evidence-based guidelines for management of infants with cystic fibrosis. Journal of Pediatrics. 2009;**155**(6):S73-S93

[172] Flume PA, Mogayzel PJ Jr, Robinson KA, Goss CH, Rosenblatt RL, Kuhn RJ, Marshall BC, Clinical Practice Guidelines for Pulmonary Therapies Committee. Cystic fibrosis pulmonary guidelines: Treatment of pulmonary exacerbations. American Journal of Respiratory and Critical Care Medicine. 2009;**180**(9):802-808

[173] Döring G, Flume P, Heijerman H, Elborn JS, Consensus Study Group. Treatment of lung infection in patients with cystic fibrosis: Current and future strategies. Journal of Cystic Fibrosis. 2012;**11**(6):461-479

[174] Balfour-Lynn IM, Welch K. Inhaled corticosteroids for cystic fibrosis. Cochrane Database of Systematic Reviews. 2016;**8**:CD001915

[175] Tepper RS, Eigen H, Stevens J, Angelicchio C, Kisling J, Ambrosius W, Heilman D. Lower respiratory illness in infants and young children with cystic fibrosis. Pediatric Pulmonology. 1997;**24**(1):48-51

[176] Flume PA, O'sullivan BP, Robinson KA, Goss CH, Mogayzel PJ Jr, Willey-Courand DB, Bujan J, Finder J, Lester M, Quittell L, Rosenblatt R. Cystic fibrosis pulmonary guidelines: Chronic medications for maintenance of lung health. American Journal of Respiratory and Critical Care Medicine. 2007;**176**(10):957-969

[177] Force AD. Acute respiratory distress syndrome. JAMA. 2012;**307**(23):2526-2533

[178] Ferguson ND, Davis AM, Slutsky AS, Stewart TE. Development of a clinical definition for acute respiratory distress syndrome using the Delphi technique. Journal of Critical Care. 2005;**20**(2):147-154

[179] Ware LB, Matthay MA. The acute respiratory distress syndrome. New England Journal of Medicine. 2000;**342**(18):1334-1349

[180] Thille AW, Esteban A, Fernández-Segoviano P, Rodriguez JM, Aramburu JA, Peñuelas O, Cortés-Puch I, Cardinal-Fernández P, Lorente JA, Frutos-Vivar F. Comparison of the berlin definition for acute respiratory distress syndrome with autopsy. American Journal of Respiratory and Critical Care Medicine. 2013;**187**(7):761-767

[181] Ferguson ND, Fan E, Camporota L, Antonelli M, Anzueto A, Beale R, Brochard L, Brower R, Esteban A, Gattinoni L, Rhodes A. The berlin definition of ARDS: An expanded rationale, justification, and supplementary material. Intensive Care Medicine. 2012;**38**(10):1573-1582

[182] Kangelaris KN, Calfee CS, May AK, Zhuo H, Matthay MA, Ware LB. Is there still a role for the lung injury score in the era of the berlin definition ARDS? Annals of Intensive Care. 2014;**4**(1):4

[183] Meade MO, Cook DJ, Guyatt GH, Slutsky AS, Arabi YM, Cooper DJ, Davies AR, Hand LE, Zhou Q, Thabane L, Austin P. Ventilation strategy using low tidal volumes, recruitment maneuvers, and high positive end-expiratory pressure for acute lung injury and acute respiratory distress syndrome: A randomized controlled trial. JAMA. 2008;**299**(6):637-645

[184] Brodie D, Bacchetta M. Extracorporeal membrane oxygenation for ARDS in adults. New England Journal of Medicine. 2011;**365**(20):1905-1914

[185] Steinberg KP, Hudson LD, Goodman RB, Hough CL, Lanken PN, Hyzy R, Thompson BT, Ancukiewicz M. Efficacy and safety of corticosteroids for persistent acute respiratory distress syndrome. New England Journal of Medicine. 2006;**354**(16):1671-1684

[186] Davis WB, Wilson HE, Wall RL. Eosinophilic alveolitis in acute respiratory failure: A clinical marker for a non-infectious etiology. Chest Journal. 1986;**90**(1):7-10

[187] Meduri GU, Marik PE, Chrousos GP, Pastores SM, Arlt W, Beishuizen A, Bokhari F, Zaloga G, Annane D. Steroid treatment in ARDS: A critical appraisal of the ARDS network trial and the recent literature. Intensive Care Medicine. 2008;**34**(1):61-69

[188] Peter JV, John P, Graham PL, Moran JL, George IA, Bersten A. Corticosteroids in the prevention and treatment of acute respiratory distress syndrome (ARDS) in adults: Meta-analysis. BMJ. 2008;**336**(7651):1006-1009

[189] Agarwal R, Nath A, Aggarwal AN, Gupta D. Do glucocorticoids decrease mortality in acute respiratory distress syndrome? A meta-analysis. Respirology. 2007;**12**(4):585-590

[190] Tang BM, Craig JC, Eslick GD, Seppelt I, McLean AS. Use of corticosteroids in acute lung injury and acute respiratory distress syndrome: A systematic review and meta-analysis. Critical Care Medicine. 2009;**37**(5):1594-1603

[191] Meduri GU, Bridges L, Shih MC, Marik PE, Siemieniuk RA, Kocak M. Prolonged glucocorticoid treatment is associated with improved ARDS outcomes: Analysis of individual patients' data from four randomized trials and trial-level meta-analysis of the updated literature. Intensive Care Medicine. 2016;**42**(5):829-840

[192] Burton CM, Milman N, Carlsen J, Arendrup H, Eliasen K, Andersen CB, Iversen M. The Copenhagen National Lung Transplant Group: Survival after single lung, double lung, and heart-lung transplantation. Journal of Heart and Lung Transplantation. 2005;**24**(11):1834-1843

[193] Weill D, Benden C, Corris PA, Dark JH, Davis RD, Keshavjee S, Lederer DJ, Mulligan MJ, Patterson GA, Singer LG, Snell GI. A consensus document for the selection of lung transplant candidates: 2014—An update from the pulmonary transplantation Council of the International Society for heart and lung transplantation. Journal of Heart and Lung Transplantation. 2015;**34**:1-15

[194] Nathan SD. Lung transplantation: Disease-specific considerations for referral. Chest Journal. 2005;**127**(3):1006-1016

[195] McAnally KJ, Valentine VG, LaPlace SG, McFadden PM, Seoane L, Taylor DE. Effect of pre-transplantation prednisone on survival after lung transplantation. Journal of Heart and Lung Transplantation. 2006;**25**(1):67-74

[196] Park SJ, Nguyen DQ, Savik K, Hertz MI, Bolman RM. Pre-transplant corticosteroid use and outcome in lung transplantation. Journal of Heart and Lung Transplantation. 2001;**20**(3):304-309

[197] Yusen RD, Edwards LB, Kucheryavaya AY, Benden C, Dipchand AI, Goldfarb SB, Levvey BJ, Lund LH, Meiser B, Rossano JW, Stehlik J. The registry of the International Society for Heart and Lung Transplantation: Thirty-second official adult lung and heart-lung transplantation report—2015; focus theme: Early graft failure. Journal of Heart and Lung Transplantation. 2015;**34**(10):1264-1277

[198] Swarup R, Allenspach LL, Nemeh HW, Stagner LD, Betensley AD. Timing of basiliximab induction and development of acute rejection in lung transplant patients. Journal of Heart and Lung Transplantation. 2011;**30**(11):1228-1235

[199] Lake KD. Immunosuppressive drugs and novel strategies to prevent acute and chronic allograft rejection. Seminars in Respiratory and Critical Care Medicine. 2001;**22**(5):559-580

[200] Groetzner J, Kur F, Spelsberg F, Behr J, Frey L, Bittmann I, Vogeser M, Ueberfuhr P, Meiser B, Hatz R, Reichart B. Airway anastomosis complications in de novo lung transplantation with sirolimus-based immunosuppression. Journal of Heart and Lung Transplantation. 2004;**23**(5):632-638

[201] Game DS, Warrens AN, Lechler RI. Rejection mechanisms in transplantation. Wiener Klinische Wochenschrift. 2001;**113**(20-21):832-838

[202] Masson E, Stern M, Chabod J, Thévenin C, Gonin F, Rebibou JM, Tiberghien P. Hyperacute rejection after lung transplantation caused by undetected low-titer anti-HLA antibodies. Journal of Heart and Lung Transplantation. 2007;**26**(6):642-645

[203] Bittner HB, Dunitz J, Hertz M, Bolman IIIMR, Park SJ. Hyperacute rejection in single lung transplantation—Case report of successful management by means of plasmapheresis and antithymocyte globulin treatment. Transplantation. 2001;**71**(5):649-651

[204] Chakinala MM, Trulock EP. Acute allograft rejection after lung transplantation: Diagnosis and therapy. Chest Surgery Clinics. 2003;**13**(3):525-542

[205] Otani S, Davis AK, Cantwell L, Ivulich S, Pham A, Paraskeva MA, Snell GI, Westall GP. Evolving experience of treating antibody-mediated rejection following lung transplantation. Transplant Immunology. 2014;**31**(2):75-80

[206] Shuhaiber JH, Kim JB, Hur K, Gibbons RD. Survival of primary and repeat lung transplantation in the United States. Annals of Thoracic Surgery. 2009;**87**(1):261-266

[207] Weber DJ, Wilkes DS. The role of autoimmunity in obliterative bronchiolitis after lung transplantation. American Journal of Physiology. Lung Cellular and Molecular Physiology. 2013;**304**(5):L307-L311

[208] Boehler A, Estenne M. Post-transplant bronchiolitis obliterans. European Respiratory Journal. 2003;**22**(6):1007-1018

[209] Sato M, Waddell TK, Wagnetz U, Roberts HC, Hwang DM, Haroon A, Wagnetz D, Chaparro C, Singer LG, Hutcheon MA, Keshavjee S. Restrictive allograft syndrome (RAS): A novel form of chronic lung allograft dysfunction. Journal of Heart and Lung Transplantation. 2011;**30**(7):735-742

[210] Strueber M, Fischer S, Gottlieb J, Simon AR, Goerler H, Gohrbandt B, Welte T, Haverich A. Long-term outcome after pulmonary retransplantation. Journal of Thoracic and Cardiovascular Surgery. 2006;**132**(2):407-412

[211] Benden C, Speich R, Hofbauer GF, Irani S, Eich-Wanger C, Russi EW, Weder W, Boehler A. Extracorporeal photopheresis after lung transplantation: A 10-year single-center experience. Transplantation. 2008;**86**(11):1625-1627

[212] Lane NE. An update on glucocorticoid-induced osteoporosis. Rheumatic Disease Clinics of North America. 2001;**27**(1):235-253

[213] Schoepe S, Schäcke H, May E, Asadullah K. Glucocorticoid therapy-induced skin atrophy. Experimental Dermatology. 2006;**15**(6):406-420

[214] Karagas MR, Cushing Jr GL, Greenberg ER, Mott LA, Spencer SK, Nierenberg DW. Non-melanoma skin cancers and glucocorticoid therapy. British Journal of Cancer. 2001;**85**(5):683-686

[215] Melnik B, Jansen T, Grabbe S. Abuse of anabolic-androgenic steroids and bodybuilding acne: An underestimated health problem. Journal der Deutschen Dermatologischen Gesellschaft. 2007;**5**(2):110-117

[216] Carnahan MC, Goldstein DA. Ocular complications of topical, peri-ocular, and systemic corticosteroids. Current Opinion in Ophthalmology. 2000;**11**(6):478-483

[217] Carvalho-Recchia CA, Yannuzzi LA, Negrão S, Spaide RF, Freund KB, Rodriguez-Coleman H, Lenharo M, Iida T. Corticosteroids and central serous chorioretinopathy. Ophthalmology. 2002;**109**(10):1834-1837

[218] Arnaldi G, Angeli A, Atkinson AB, Bertagna X, Cavagnini F, Chrousos GP, Fava GA, Findling JW, Gaillard RC, Grossman AB, Kola B. Diagnosis and complications of Cushing's syndrome: A consensus statement. The Journal of Clinical Endocrinology and Metabolism. 2003;**88**(12):5593-5602

[219] Garrapa GG, Pantanetti P, Arnaldi G, Mantero F, Faloia E. Body composition and metabolic features in women with adrenal incidentaloma or Cushing's syndrome. The Journal of Clinical Endocrinology and Metabolism. 2001;**86**(11):5301-5306

[220] Souverein PC, Berard A, Van Staa TP, Cooper C, Egberts AC, Leufkens HG, Walker BR. Use of oral glucocorticoids and risk of cardiovascular and cerebrovascular disease in a population based case–control study. Heart. 2004;**90**(8):859-865

[221] Rodríguez LA, Hernández-Díaz S. The risk of upper gastrointestinal complications associated with nonsteroidal anti-inflammatory drugs, glucocorticoids, acetaminophen, and combinations of these agents. Arthritis Research & Therapy. 2000;**3**(2):98-101

[222] Christensen S, Riis A, Nørgaard M, Thomsen RW, Tønnesen EM, Larsson A, Sørensen HT. Perforated peptic ulcer: Use of pre-admission oral glucocorticoids and 30-day mortality. Alimentary Pharmacology & Therapeutics. 2006;**23**(1):45-52

[223] Targownik LE, Thomson PA. Gastroprotective strategies among NSAID users: Guidelines for appropriate use in chronic illness. Canadian Family Physician. 2006; **52**(9):1100-1105

[224] Weinstein RS. Glucocorticoid-induced osteoporosis. Reviews in Endocrine & Metabolic Disorders. 2001;**2**(1):65-73

[225] Weinstein RS. Glucocorticoid-induced osteonecrosis. Endocrine. 2012;**41**(2):183-190

[226] Van Staa TP, Laan RF, Barton IP, Cohen S, Reid DM, Cooper C. Bone density threshold and other predictors of vertebral fracture in patients receiving oral glucocorticoid therapy. Arthritis & Rheumatology. 2003;**48**(11):3224-3229

[227] Lai HC, FitzSimmons SC, Allen DB, Kosorok MR, Rosenstein BJ, Campbell PW, Farrell PM. Risk of persistent growth impairment after alternate-day prednisone treatment in children with cystic fibrosis. New England Journal of Medicine. 2000;**342**(12):851-859

[228] Schakman O, Gilson H, Thissen JP. Mechanisms of glucocorticoid-induced myopathy. Journal of Endocrinology. 2008;**197**(1):1-10

[229] Whirledge S, Cidlowski JA. Glucocorticoids, stress, and fertility. Minerva Endocrinologica. 2010;**35**(2):109-125

[230] Hviid A, Mølgaard-Nielsen D. Corticosteroid use during pregnancy and risk of orofacial clefts. Canadian Medical Association Journal. 2011;**183**(7):796-804

[231] Sugden MC, Langdown ML, Munns MJ, Holness MJ. Maternal glucocorticoid treatment modulates placental leptin and leptin receptor expression and materno-fetal leptin physiology during late pregnancy, and elicits hypertension associated with hyperleptinaemia in the early-growth-retarded adult offspring. European Journal of Endocrinology. 2001;**145**(4):529-539

[232] Fardet L, Petersen I, Nazareth I. Suicidal behavior and severe neuropsychiatric disorders following glucocorticoid therapy in primary care. American Journal of Psychiatry. 2012;**169**(5):491-497

[233] Shin SY, Katz P, Wallhagen M, Julian L. Cognitive impairment in persons with rheumatoid arthritis. Arthritis Care & Research. 2012;**64**(8):1144-1150

[234] Keenan PA, Jacobson MW, Soleymani RM, Mayes MD, Yaldoo DT. The effect on memory of chronic prednisone treatment in patients with systemic disease. Neurology. 1996;**47**(6):1396-1402

[235] Cutolo M, Seriolo B, Pizzorni C, Secchi ME, Soldano S, Paolino S, Montagna P, Sulli A. Use of glucocorticoids and risk of infections. Autoimmunity Reviews. 2008;**8**(2):153-155

[236] Auphan N, DiDonato JA, Rosette C, Helmberg A, Karin M. Immunosuppression by glucocorticoids: Inhibition of NF-kappaB activity through induction of IkappaB synthesis. Science. 1995;**270**(5234):286-290

[237] Van der Goes MC, Jacobs JW, Boers M, Andrews T, Blom-Bakkers MA, Buttgereit F, Caeyers N, Cutolo M, Da Silva JA, Guillevin L, Kirwan JR. Monitoring adverse events of low-dose glucocorticoid therapy: EULAR recommendations for clinical trials and daily practice. Annals of the Rheumatic Diseases. 2010;**69**(11):1913-1919

[238] Sholter DE, Armstrong PW. Adverse effects of corticosteroids on the cardiovascular system. Canadian Journal of Cardiology. 2000;**16**(4):505-511

[239] Duru N, van der Goes MC, Jacobs JW, Andrews T, Boers M, Buttgereit F, Caeyers N, Cutolo M, Halliday S, Da Silva JA, Kirwan JR. EULAR evidence-based and consensus-based recommendations on the management of medium to high-dose glucocorticoid therapy in rheumatic diseases. Annals of the Rheumatic Diseases. 2013;**72**(12):1905-1913

Permissions

All chapters in this book were first published in CORTICOSTEROIDS, by InTech Open; hereby published with permission under the Creative Commons Attribution License or equivalent. Every chapter published in this book has been scrutinized by our experts. Their significance has been extensively debated. The topics covered herein carry significant findings which will fuel the growth of the discipline. They may even be implemented as practical applications or may be referred to as a beginning point for another development.

The contributors of this book come from diverse backgrounds, making this book a truly international effort. This book will bring forth new frontiers with its revolutionizing research information and detailed analysis of the nascent developments around the world.

We would like to thank all the contributing authors for lending their expertise to make the book truly unique. They have played a crucial role in the development of this book. Without their invaluable contributions this book wouldn't have been possible. They have made vital efforts to compile up to date information on the varied aspects of this subject to make this book a valuable addition to the collection of many professionals and students.

This book was conceptualized with the vision of imparting up-to-date information and advanced data in this field. To ensure the same, a matchless editorial board was set up. Every individual on the board went through rigorous rounds of assessment to prove their worth. After which they invested a large part of their time researching and compiling the most relevant data for our readers.

The editorial board has been involved in producing this book since its inception. They have spent rigorous hours researching and exploring the diverse topics which have resulted in the successful publishing of this book. They have passed on their knowledge of decades through this book. To expedite this challenging task, the publisher supported the team at every step. A small team of assistant editors was also appointed to further simplify the editing procedure and attain best results for the readers.

Apart from the editorial board, the designing team has also invested a significant amount of their time in understanding the subject and creating the most relevant covers. They scrutinized every image to scout for the most suitable representation of the subject and create an appropriate cover for the book.

The publishing team has been an ardent support to the editorial, designing and production team. Their endless efforts to recruit the best for this project, has resulted in the accomplishment of this book. They are a veteran in the field of academics and their pool of knowledge is as vast as their experience in printing. Their expertise and guidance has proved useful at every step. Their uncompromising quality standards have made this book an exceptional effort. Their encouragement from time to time has been an inspiration for everyone.

The publisher and the editorial board hope that this book will prove to be a valuable piece of knowledge for researchers, students, practitioners and scholars across the globe.

List of Contributors

Danka Svecova
Faculty of Medicine, Comenius University in Bratislava, Bratislava, Slovakia

Katiuska Satué Ambrojo and María Marcilla Corzano
Department of Animal Medicine and Surgery, School of Veterinary Medicine, University CEU-Cardenal Herrera, Valencia, Spain

Juan Carlos Gardon Poggi
Department of Animal Medicine and Surgery, Faculty of Veterinary and Experimental Sciences, Catholic University of Valencia "San Vicente Mártir", Valencia, Spain

Sanela Domuz Vujnović
School of Applied Medical Sciences, Prijedor, Republic of Srpska, Bosnia and Herzegovina

Adrijana Domuz
Primary Health Center, Srbac, Republic of Srpska, Bosnia and Herzegovina

Hanna Kalamarz-Kubiak
Genetic and Marine Biotechnology Department, Institute of Oceanology Polish Academy of Sciences, Sopot, Poland

Silvia Graciela Ruginsk
Department of Physiology, Biomedical Sciences Institute, Federal University of Alfenas, Minas Gerais, Brazil

Ernane Torres Uchoa
Department of Physiological Sciences, State University of Londrina, Parana, Brazil

Cristiane Mota Leite
University of North of Parana, Parana, Brazil

Clarissa Silva Martins
Federal University of Mato Grosso do Sul, Mato Grosso do Sul, Brazil
Department of Internal Medicine, Ribeirao Preto Medical School, University of Sao Paulo, Sao Paulo, Brazil

Leonardo Domingues de Araujo, Lucila Leico Kagohara Elias and José Antunes Rodrigues
Department of Physiology, Ribeirao Preto Medical School, University of Sao Paulo, Sao Paulo, Brazil

Margaret de Castro
Department of Internal Medicine, Ribeirao Preto Medical School, University of Sao Paulo, Sao Paulo, Brazil

Cheng Wang, Roel Oldenkamp, Ronald J.W. Oellers and Colin Logie
Radboud University Faculty of Science, Mathematics and Informatics, RIMLS, Nijmegen, The Netherlands

Wei Cheong Ngeow, Daniel Lim and Nurhalim Ahmad
Faculty of Dentistry, University of Malaya, Kuala Lumpur, Malaysia

Ibrahim A. Janahi
Clinical Pediatrics, Weill-Cornell Medical College, Ar-Rayyan, Qatar
Pediatric Pulmonology, Department of Pediatrics, Hamad General Hospital, Doha, Qatar
Medical Research Center, Hamad Medical Corporation, Doha, Qatar

Abdul Rehman
Internal Medicine Section, Department of Medicine, Hamad Medical Corporation, Doha, Qatar

Noor Ul-Ain Baloch
Department of Internal Medicine, Rutgers-New Jersey Medical School, University Hospital, Newark, United States

Index

www.ingramcontent.com/pod-product-compliance
Lightning Source LLC
LaVergne TN
LVHW061510220926
848485LV00017B/784
* 9 7 8 1 6 3 9 8 9 2 5 7 0 *